JUST PILLS

JUST PILLS

THE EXTRAORDINARY
STORY OF A REVOLUTION
IN ABORTION CARE

REBECCA KELLIHER

BEACON PRESS, BOSTON

BEACON PRESS
24 Farnsworth Street
Boston, Massachusetts
www.beacon.org

Beacon Press books
are published under the auspices of
the Unitarian Universalist Association of Congregations.

28 27 26 25 8 7 6 5 4 3 2 1

This book is printed on acid-free paper that meets the uncoated paper
ANSI/NISO specifications for permanence as revised in 1992.

Text design and composition by Kim Arney

This book is intended to be educational and informative. The author is not
a physician, and readers should not use this book as a substitute for medical
advice and/or treatment. The author and publisher disclaim all responsibility
for any liability, loss, or risk that may be associated with the application of
any of the contents of this book. Although the author and publisher have
made every effort to ensure that the information in this book was correct at
press time, the author and publisher assume no responsibility for any errors,
inaccuracies, omissions, or other inconsistencies within this book
and disclaim any liability to any party for any loss, damage,
or harm resulting from such errors or omissions.

*Library of Congress Cataloging-in-Publication
Data is available for this title.*
ISBN: 978-0-8070-1270-3; e-book: 978-0-8070-1273-4;
audiobook: 978-0-8070-1817-0

The authorized representative in the EU for product safety and
compliance is Easy Access System Europe 16879218, Mustamäe tee 50,
10621 Tallinn, Estonia: http://beacon.org/eu-contact.

To Maureen,
who teaches me to listen.

CONTENTS

CHAPTER I

THE PILL THAT MAKES YOUR PERIOD COME BACK

A round 1990 in São Paulo, Brazil, feminist psychology professor Margareth Arilha noticed something astounding: fewer dead women. More than 1,500 miles away in Fortaleza, a city in Brazil's northeastern state of Ceará, Assis Chateaubriand Maternity Hospital records indicated that, from 1988 to 1990, women admitted for "abortion-related complications" were surviving.[1] This reversed what had been a devastating trend until then.

In Brazil, as in most countries banning abortion in the 1980s, women who came to a hospital for care after self-inducing their abortions typically died within hours, even minutes.[2] Arilha wanted to know why these women at this small hospital were not. The women themselves told the hospital workers plainly why: they took pills called Cytotec, a brand name for the medication misoprostol.

Pharmacies across Brazil stocked Cytotec pills in packets of 28 tablets, with each tablet containing 200 mcg of misoprostol.[3] Researchers in Brazil would later find that, if one needed just four or so misoprostol pills for an abortion, then those pills cost about $6 at the time, much cheaper than the roughly $140 needed for a clandestine abortion procedure in a clinic.[4] That $140 was about how much the women known to be using misoprostol for their abortions earned in one month.[5] How did women find out these pills could help them? Because they were smart. On each Cytotec box was a black-and-white stick figure of a visibly pregnant person in a dress, a red line diagonally cutting across her body to say: if pregnant, do not take these pills.[6] Okay, but what if someone did not want to be pregnant?

1

In 1973, G. D. Searle & Company, an American pharmaceutical firm, had invented misoprostol, a synthetic prostaglandin, in a lab outside Chicago.[7] Prostaglandins were hormone-like substances found in the body, with synthetic versions (like misoprostol) mimicking them.[8] By the 1970s, scientists around the world were furiously researching prostaglandins, including their use for abortions.[9]

But Searle marketed Cytotec as a stomach ulcer treatment, not an abortion pill, calling this medication's ability to trigger contractions in pregnant people a side effect.[10] In 1986, Brazil's government authorized Cytotec to be sold over the counter as an ulcer treatment, ignoring those side effects on its warning label, while, north of the equator, the US Food and Drug Administration (FDA) looked likely to approve that same medication, also only for stomach ulcers.[11] Searle representatives, eager to sell their new miracle drug in Brazil, flew to São Paulo weeks after Cytotec's approval in the country, ready to market Cytotec to doctors at the World Congress of Gastroenterology in the city.[12] The company even supposedly placed a giant diorama of a stomach inside a conference hall to explain how these pills worked.[13] Abortion was not mentioned.

Brazil criminalized abortion in an 1890 penal code that was a painful remnant of colonization.[14] For centuries in much of the world, ending a pregnancy—or helping someone else do so—had not been a crime. One of the earliest recorded abortions hailed from around 1550 BCE in ancient Egypt.[15] But abortion criminalization began in many countries in the mid- to late-nineteenth century, largely when most of the imperial forces of Europe, like Portugal and Spain, thrust abortion bans on their colonies.[16]

Brazil updated its 1890 penal code in 1940 to at least allow a legal abortion for women and girls who could prove that they had been raped or suffered incest—or for a pregnant person whose life was deemed at risk.[17] Those who provided an illegal abortion faced up to four years in prison, and those who had an illegal abortion risked up to three years in prison.[18] Despite this, abortion in Brazil was common well before Cytotec. About 1.5 million women in Brazil had abortions each year, roughly the same as in the US at the time, even though abortion had been legal in the US since 1973 with *Roe v. Wade*.[19] Still, that 1.5 million estimate of the number of abortions in Brazil was considered an undercount given just how difficult it was to track a criminalized and, in a majority-Catholic country, highly stigmatized procedure.

Like most Brazilians, Arilha knew that if a woman had money, she could pay for an abortion, no matter what the law said. These abortion procedures were usually either a dilation and curettage (D&C), where a provider used surgical instruments to empty the person's uterus, or vacuum aspiration, still an invasive method but typically safer.[20] Poor women were left on their own, resorting to other means, like throwing themselves down stairs, punching their stomachs, exercising until collapse, or placing sharp objects inside their uteruses, risking perforation and infection that, if untreated, spelled almost-certain death. Yet not with Cytotec. Arilha saw it in those hospital numbers.

In 1988 at Assis Chateaubriand Maternity Hospital, about 12 percent of women hospitalized for abortion complications said they had taken Cytotec to end their pregnancies.[21] That shot up to 50 percent the next year, then 72 percent the year after that.[22] Women's use of misoprostol for abortions was not unique to that hospital, even to Fortaleza.[23] A 1993 study found a similar trend at seven public hospitals in Rio de Janeiro.[24] That research and others would soon confirm what many Brazilian women knew: misoprostol was an abortion pill.

When Arilha was eight, her grandmother told her the story about her unwanted pregnancy. Her grandmother had a safe abortion procedure in Austria years before moving to Brazil.[25] Once in Brazil, she underwent a second abortion beyond the law "in terrible conditions," Arilha recalled being told. Her grandmother was rushed to a hospital while she bled, only that hospital was a Catholic-affiliated facility strongly opposed to abortion.[26] Arilha's grandmother was pressured to name who provided her abortion. She refused, saying, "I'll die if necessary, but I won't tell—because the decision for the abortion was mine, and I'm not going to denounce the people that tried to help me."[27] Arilha remembered her grandmother like this: unashamed. "I had grown up in a home where [abortion] was discussed without a lot of fuss," she said in a 2018 interview in Portuguese translated to English. "And I couldn't conceive of it as a crime."[28]

When Arilha was a college student in the 1970s, the political tumult in Brazil molded her, as she joined protests against the country's dictatorship, meeting feminists with bold ideas like universal women's health care, including abortion care. "I remember perfectly well," she recalled. "They were organizing for non-violence, the right to abortion, the right to daycare."[29]

In the early 1980s, the dictatorship breathing its last gasp, Arilha and allies started strategizing to decriminalize abortion. They focused first on how to ensure at least the existing abortion law worked: that women who qualified for slim exceptions for legal abortions (rape, incest, or to save the pregnant person's life) would get that care. A year before Cytotec came to Brazil, the country's military rule toppled after more than two decades in power. Redemocratization began. Arilha, thrilled, believed that women having control over their bodies was inseparable from any true democracy.

It was around 1988 when she heard whispers of this pill, Cytotec, that women took to start their abortions at home, bleeding and cramping in what felt physically like a miscarriage. Some women went to hospitals afterwards for legal and mostly free miscarriage treatment, where a doctor safely emptied their uterus with a procedure to complete their abortions. There was even an adage that the pill was a "passport to the hospital."[30] But no Cytotec-as-abortifacient studies existed yet, and there were no package inserts or websites explaining how to use the pills to end pregnancies. Women needed to figure this out by themselves. Arilha thought this medication had enormous potential for women, but she worried that, with anti-abortion voices in Brazil, an anti-Cytotec campaign might foment in these information gaps about the pills. Media coverage from the US on that same pill did not exactly help.

On October 29, 1988, misoprostol hit the front page of the *New York Times* under the headline, "U.S. May Allow Anti-Ulcer Drug Tied to Abortion," and the subheading, "Opponents Threatening Boycott of Company."[31] The Brazilian press printed the article in Portuguese, the story reporting that the FDA was close to approving Cytotec as a stomach-ulcer medication.[32] But the article also mentioned that, in 1985, an FDA advisory committee discussed whether misoprostol should be approved, and an American anti-abortion group, the National Right to Life Committee (NRLC), called misoprostol a "death drug."[33]

In the early 1980s, Searle had indeed tested misoprostol on a small group of abortion-seekers in Germany, finding that the pill caused "uterine expulsion and bleeding."[34] But according to a Searle spokesperson in that New York Times article, this trial was "too small to indicate the likelihood that the drug would cause an abortion."[35] The FDA determined a label on the medication warning pregnant women not to use the pills should suffice. Dr. John C. Willke, then president of the NRLC, scathingly told The Times the pills "will be on the street literally days after it is made available on prescription," believing such a warning label would make it more likely that people seeking abortions would turn to this "death drug."[36]

These predictions put a spotlight on the medication in Brazil. The Catholic Church since the late nineteenth century had been arguing that abortion was murder, ignoring the life of the pregnant person.[37] And while the Church did not publicly take a stand against misoprostol's use for abortions in Brazil at this time, its influence in the country would be hard to overstate.[38] It was no coincidence that a 98-foot-tall sculpture of Jesus Christ overlooked Rio de Janeiro. Arilha needed to act fast if she sought to protect Cytotec.

But an anti-Cytotec campaign in Brazil would not only be driven by anti-abortion actors. A pharmacology professor, Dr. Helena Lutéscia Luna Coelho, who supported family planning, had an entirely different reaction from Arilha to those Fortaleza hospital records.[39] She thought misoprostol could be dangerous to women, and pushed Brazil's Ministry of Health to restrict Cytotec.[40] To make her case, Coelho and her students ran a study-of-sorts in Fortaleza, where they went to more than 100 pharmacies to ask pharmacists "for a solution to their (women) or their girlfriends' (men) unwanted pregnancies," as Coelho and her colleagues later wrote.[41] Almost all pharmacists recommended misoprostol, a fact that Coelho reported in a 1991 letter to the editor in *The Lancet*. Above her letter in that same issue of the prestigious, peer-reviewed medical journal was another letter to the editor on Cytotec: this time from Searle.

A company spokesperson wrote scoldingly of the reported "misuse of misoprostol as an abortifacient in Brazil" while responding to claims that this pill caused congenital disorders.[42] Those very claims added to Coelho's anxieties. Three women had by then reported to have taken misoprostol while pregnant to induce abortions, but the pills did not work (again, there was no information on how to use these pills effectively).[43] The women were then forced to carry their pregnancies to term, giving birth to babies that had slightly misshapen skulls.[44] This Searle spokesperson in his letter stated the company found no teratogenic effects in their trials and that reports from only three "mothers" were not enough to conclude such side effects were real.[45]

Yet these cases brought up many unanswered questions over the pills at the time. As Arilha worried, an information void fanned flames against misoprostol, word spreading among even her fellow feminists that this medication may be harmful.[46] Their criticisms touched on deeper fears.

About a year before Cytotec entered Brazil, yet another American reproductive health product stirred controversy. Brazil's Ministry of Health in 1984 authorized trials of a long-acting, reversible contraceptive implant known by its commercial name Norplant. Scientists at the Population Council, an international research nonprofit in New York, invented Norplant in the 1970s.[47] Norplant consisted of six, matchstick-like rods that, with a minor surgery, would be implanted under the skin of a woman's arm. For up to five years, rods continuously released a small amount of the hormone progestin into the woman's body to prevent pregnancy. The rods could be removed with another surgery.

But some Brazilian women in these trials reported that they had Norplant inserted into their arms without their informed consent, and several experienced painful side effects.[48] When some women asked their trial coordinators for their implant to be removed, they

reportedly were refused (the US in the 1990s would face a Norplant fiasco of its own, bringing attention to anti-Black racism in the
histories of certain reproductive health technologies).[49] Norplant's
rollout in Brazil looked to many feminists like another example of
male-dominated governments and Global North–based researchers
pushing aside women's bodily autonomy in the name of population
control.

Those supportive of population-control policies argued curbing
birth rates may reduce poverty, preserve environmental resources, even
prevent communist takeovers (a popular idea in the Cold War).[50] But
these policies were grounded in thinly veiled racist anxieties fixated on
the booming populations of developing countries, and largely white
men in the Global North were advocating for these measures.[51] During
the 1970s and 1980s in parts of the Global South, reports emerged of
low-income women of color being sometimes forcibly or coercively
sterilized in government-funded population-control programs.[52] The
1960s and 1970s US witnessed as well how some low-income women
of color, including Indigenous communities, were being forcibly sterilized under population-control auspices.[53] This all meant that, when
word of ethical concerns in those Norplant trials in Brazil got out,
feminists organized to shut the trials down, successfully doing so in
1986, just before misoprostol lit up on the national stage.[54]

And so, it was no surprise that many of these same feminists
viewed misoprostol warily. One longtime Brazilian feminist and bio-
ethics researcher, Sonia Corrêa, who played a prominent role in the
movement against population control at this time, later acknowl-
edged that, in hindsight, she got misoprostol wrong—with disastrous
consequences.[55] Because with even the feminist movement hesitating
to advocate for at least better understanding this pill before taking
drastic action, the state of Ceará, home to that hospital in Fortaleza,
banned all misoprostol sales on July 4, 1991, a year after Arilha noticed more women surviving self-induced abortions.[56]

The Ministry of Health about a week later clamped down on the
medication by ordering that all pharmacies in Brazil only sell misoprostol to people with a prescription.[57] The ministry struck a deal with
Biolab Laboratories, the company that began to make misoprostol in

Brazil after Searle, in which the production of misoprostol pills would dramatically slow down.[58] State officials in Rio de Janeiro restricted misoprostol sales to hospitals under tight controls.[59] An illegal market for Cytotec soon expanded in this backlash. With barriers to this pill suddenly falling into place, the voices of the women in those hospital records, and the many more unseen, those who took Cytotec to end their own pregnancies, were missing. What did *they* think and feel about this medication? Arilha set out to see.

In 1992, Arilha and her colleague, Regina Maria Barbosa, asked women they knew if *they* knew any women who used Cytotec. It was not hard to find people. They interviewed 14 women of varied socioeconomic classes, aged 18 to 40, all of whom had an abortion using misoprostol pills about six to 18 months prior to speaking with Arilha and her colleague.[60] Their accounts, which included no identifying details given abortion criminalization and stigma, remain one of the only first-person records of Brazilian women who used misoprostol to end their pregnancies at that time.

Most said they learned of Cytotec through friends. There were big differences in how each took pills (orally, vaginally, or orally and vaginally) and how many pills they used. Most took pills in roughly the first 13 weeks of pregnancy.[61] One woman took 64 tablets over four months until she ended her pregnancy at about 16 weeks at home.[62] All said they took Cytotec because it was their cheapest option. Some also thought the pills would be "less traumatic" than a procedure.[63] A few worried that, if they had a procedure, their gynecologist might find out about their abortion when examining them at a later appointment and mistreat them because of it.[64] All low-income women said they used these pills because "at least Cytotec doesn't kill," as 34-year-old Sandra Lucia stated.[65] Several thought of taking these pills not as inducing an abortion but as bringing their periods back. "The sensation you have is that your period is late and so you take medicine for it to come," said 27-year-old Fatima.[66] There was nuance.

Yet of the 14 women, only three described positive experiences with Cytotec. Those three took pills earlier in pregnancy (around seven to

10 weeks), knew what to expect from stories they heard about others who took the pills, and, critically, were not alone during their abortion process.[67] They experienced cramping and nausea, which they found tolerable.[68] One of the three took pills with her feminist gynecologist present.[69] Another was a nurse, as was her husband, who supported her throughout her abortion.[70] The third said that her boyfriend and friend were with her.[71] None of the three went to a hospital after they took pills.[72] Their stories would hold clues as to what, a decade later, abortion care with acompañantes would look like in much of Latin America. Acompañantes, or trained volunteer counselors, would learn to support people through their abortions with pills, whether with misoprostol alone or misoprostol and another abortion pill, mifepristone, as described in later chapters.

But in early 1990s Brazil, the 11 women who had negative experiences with these pills found "an almost total lack of information" terrifying.[73] Most took Cytotec secretly at home, alone in the night so as not to be discovered.[74] Several had intense cramping and did not know if or when to get help.[75] None thought that they would need to go to a hospital; they had used Cytotec to avoid hospitals and doctors. But eight, frightened by the abdominal pain and bleeding after taking pills, did go to a hospital while three chose not to.[76] Sandra Lucia, who said "at least Cytotec doesn't kill," had a stressful experience with pills and went to a hospital after taking them, only to be met with disdain: "I saw the doctor . . . and he was angry with me and said: 'Look, mother, you are pregnant, and we are here to take care of mothers who want children, not those who don't.' So, what could I do? I left and went home and just bled all night."[77]

The majority (10) of the women told Arilha and Barbosa that, if they had a choice, they would not take Cytotec again. The three women who had positive abortion experiences said the opposite. The only person in the group who had a distressing experience and nonetheless said that she would use Cytotec again was Sandra Lucia.

Arilha and her colleague wanted to know what doctors thought about this medication too. In 1992, they led two focus groups with 14 gynecologists in the São Paulo public health system.[78] All confirmed women had been using Cytotec for abortions, and all called it a "valuable therapeutic resource" for completing miscarriages, inducing labor, and treating postpartum hemorrhage, noting misoprostol's metamorphic and lifesaving uses.[79] With misoprostol's new restrictions, however, it became much harder for these doctors to get Cytotec for these other gynecological uses.[80] All voiced worries that the pill for abortions may lead to health problems that they may not know about yet. Nonetheless, the doctors recognized the public health benefits of an abortion pill.[81] "We used to have two hysterectomies a week," said one doctor. "Now we have one every six months." Like most abortion-seekers, these doctors did not know how to use the misoprostol pills for abortions. Some patients would come to them with intense bleeding after taking Cytotec, others with very little bleeding.[82] The doctors did not understand why.

It remains unknown today just how many doctors in Brazil told women about Cytotec in these early years before the pills became restricted—as it is unknown just how many women told each other about these pills and used them for an abortion, or bringing back a period. Aside from the documented Cytotec sales in the country, hospital admissions records, like those in Fortaleza, became the only reliable data on how many women were using misoprostol for abortions at that time.[83] What about the women who took Cytotec and never went to a hospital afterward? Who could not reach a hospital or did not want or need to go to one? And who maybe, just maybe, had abortions safely at home with the support they wanted around them, perhaps without, as Arilha might say, "a lot of fuss"?

Arilha and Barbosa ended their paper with another abortion pill, mifepristone, known as RU-486 at that time: "Given the apparent willingness of more Brazilian gynecologists to be involved with abortions induced by a non-invasive method, the ideal situation would be for RU486 to be introduced in Brazil for use with Cytotec, as it is being used in France."[84] Later chapters detail this pill's winding saga. But mifepristone could not reliably complete an abortion on its own. That pill worked better when paired with a prostaglandin, another medication. And misoprostol happened to be a prostaglandin—exactly what was needed.

Before Cytotec, researchers in Europe used a medication abortion regimen that injected prostaglandins into a woman's muscle a day or two days after she swallowed mifepristone. Side effects could be intense. Misoprostol pills replacing those injections would soon make abortions simpler and safer. Brazilian women started using misoprostol before researchers began giving women that pill with mifepristone, all under tight controls. Combining mifepristone with misoprostol would soon be considered the gold standard for a medication abortion, as will be detailed next. After years of research partnerships with grassroots feminist activists caring for people using both these pills in countries under near-total abortion bans, but especially using misoprostol, the World Health Organization (WHO) in 2022 said that people did not need a doctor or any licensed clinician to have a safe medication abortion early in pregnancy.[85] With the right information and medications, they could safely take mifepristone and misoprostol pills, or just misoprostol, at home by themselves.[86] This today is still revolutionary, with no country in the world as of 2024 having both mifepristone and misoprostol over the counter as abortion pills.

For a misoprostol-only abortion among people fewer than 12 weeks pregnant, the WHO as of this writing advised taking 800 mcg of misoprostol buccally (in the cheek), sublingually (under the tongue), or vaginally, with repeat doses as needed.[87] And for a misoprostol-only abortion among people at or past 12 weeks pregnant, the agency suggested repeat doses of 400 mcg of misoprostol taken buccally, sublingually, or vaginally every three hours.[88] The WHO stated that using mifepristone and misoprostol together generally worked better and was less painful.[89] While this information exists now, with the stamp of approval of a United Nations agency and ample studies demonstrating the safety of these methods, women in Brazil today have less access to misoprostol than they did three decades ago—and the post-*Dobbs* US should pay close attention.

By 1998, Brazil created an FDA equivalent, the National Health Surveillance Agency (Agência Nacional de Vigilância Sanitária in

Portuguese, or ANVISA), that put misoprostol on a list of the most restricted drugs.[90] That classification, which continues as I write in 2024, mandated misoprostol be sold to specially registered hospitals. Supplying or selling misoprostol beyond these rules was a crime punishable by 10 to 15 years in prison and a fine, a more severe penalty than for drug trafficking.[91] Then in the early 2000s, with internet use spreading, some people in Brazil began ordering misoprostol online under the country's still-existent abortion ban. ANVISA swiftly made it illegal in 2006 to share information online about misoprostol, an offense punishable again with prison time. "I say that in Brazil, misoprostol has been in jail since 1998," said feminist Sonia Corrêa in a 2021 interview in Portuguese translated to English.[92] She called this jailing a "jabuticaba," slang for an absurdity that could only happen in Brazil (a jabuticaba tree is indigenous to Brazil).

Indeed, even in countries and some US states post-*Dobbs* that almost entirely ban abortion, people still can, at least as I write, legally share information about how to correctly use misoprostol pills for abortions. That protection has been foundational for activists around the globe to organize sophisticated abortion-pills support networks. Brazil, considered the birthplace of people using misoprostol for abortions on their own, is today home to what many experts consider the worst restrictions in the world on that pill.[93] "Brazilian women actually found a solution with the use of misoprostol," said Arilha in a 2018 interview in Portuguese translated to English. "Today, misoprostol is in the hands of drug dealers. . . . Brazilian women can still not have abortions. They have to go underground and run completely unnecessary risks, legal and health risks, ultimately risking their own lives."[94]

What Arilha did not mention, perhaps did not know, was that some feminist activists in Brazil have for years taken serious legal risks to bring misoprostol to abortion-seekers, operating quietly by word of mouth, with no website or public presence. I spoke to several of them about the growth and diversity of such networks across Latin America and their reflections on the US post-*Dobbs*, mindful of what a rising far right without borders may mean for us all. As Arilha said, "abortion is a 'global saga.'"

This book traces the rich history of misoprostol as well as mifepristone, including the creative ways feminist activists have used these pills beyond the US for many years, though this book cannot possibly capture the nuances of these medications and the activism around them in every country. My hope is this history can help us better understand our tumultuous present to continue to demand equality and dignity, with these pills as one revolutionary tool already reshaping abortion and maternal health care around the globe. But to do that, we must rewind to what may be the first abortion medication, one that was not a pill at all.

CHAPTER 2

A PARENTHETICAL

In New York City around 1930, 27-year-old Sarah Ratner peered through her microscope at, of all things, human semen. She worked at Sloane Hospital for Women as a lab assistant while studying for a biochemistry doctorate at Columbia University. It was the Great Depression. At this fertility clinic, Ratner helped those struggling to become pregnant. Infertility was not well understood in the early 1930s, but artificial insemination held promise. Ratner stood out as one of the few scientists who had a uterus herself. An outsider self-described as "innately very shy," she could see what others could not.[1]

Ratner grew up in New York as the only daughter of Russian Jewish immigrants who fled poverty and persecution for the US. She landed a scholarship to Cornell University and gravitated to science. But her quiet temperament and status as the sole woman in most classes made it difficult for her to be heard. Ratner spoke deliberately throughout her life, so much so a colleague told her, "Sarah, I always know when you are calling because the phone rings more slowly."[2] American academia, however, held a dark side in the 1920s and 1930s. Some fertility research aligned with eugenics, a global movement of white elites to reproduce "good" races ("Nordic" white, not Jewish, not disabled, not queer) and decrease "inferior" races (just about anyone else).[3] Nazi Germany thrust eugenics to disastrous ends. Yet there were also eugenic US laws in the 1920s, such as one enacted in the US Supreme Court in 1927, the year *Buck v. Bell* allowed state-funded, forced sterilization of those mentally "unfit" to parent.[4]

The young Ratner approached fertility research differently from others in this era. And, in doing so, she noticed a pattern her senior (white male) scientists had not. Some women in the clinic where she worked were having contractions while being artificially inseminated, but others experienced no such contractions. Why? Instead of assuming the uterus to be the problem, Ratner turned her gaze to the semen, finding under her microscope a compound in semen that had never been identified before, one that triggered uterine contractions. She did not name this compound, but her discovery would be a silent breakthrough she would not receive full credit for. The scientists running that lab, Raphael Kurzrok and Charles C. Lieb, published a paper in 1930 announcing this compound, listing themselves as the authors. In parentheses and smaller type next to their names was "with the assistance of Sarah Ratner."[5]

"My career as a biochemist," Ratner would later say, "has been a more difficult one because of my sex." She struggled to find a job after her doctorate, though her male peers were quickly hired. Once, a male mentor praised Ratner by saying she "thinks like a man," to which she let out "a somewhat disdainful hrumph."[6] Ratner's biochemistry contributions eventually led to her election to the National Academy of Sciences at 71 years old. She still recalled that 1930 finding, saying it "constituted the first recorded description of the uterine contracting properties of a prostaglandin."[7]

Because a man would later name that compound a "prostaglandin," what Ratner recorded would form the foundation of the first known safe, effective abortion medication. One of today's abortion pills, misoprostol, is a synthetic (lab-made) prostaglandin. The compound's name did not hail from uteruses or people with them. In 1935 in Sweden, physiologist and pharmacologist Dr. Ulf von Euler (who later won a Nobel Prize for other work) coined the term "prostaglandin" after noticing these compounds in the prostate glands of monkeys, sheep, and goats, the prostate producing some fluid in semen.[8] Von Euler observed these compounds could also lower blood pressure and stimulate certain muscles. What that may mean for women was lost on him. And so, "prostaglandin" came from "prostate" and "gland," its masculinity holding delicious irony today.

Ratner sensed back in 1930 that this compound could transform women's reproductive lives one day. She just did not know how. It took three more decades before another young researcher pushed that idea forward. These next few chapters follow mostly white male scientists in the Global North at one start of medication abortion's journey, a history told from powerful halls of science and politics, halls that few who had or sought abortions could enter as equals, if at all. To draw from American Black queer feminist Audre Lorde, these spaces are the "master's house."[9] But abortion pills themselves are not necessarily the "master's tools." These stories unravel how these medications came to be and be controlled, as well as how grassroots feminist activists in mainly the Global South later took risks to reclaim pills and abortion, person by person, year by year, creating a bolder vision of care that continues today.

Almost four thousand miles away from New York City and thirty years after Ratner's first observation of a mysterious compound, 29-year-old gynecologist Dr. Marc Bygdeman received a rare sample. It was a prostaglandin.

This was 1963 in Stockholm, Sweden, at the Karolinska Institute, a research university. Bygdeman had just finished his residency and started his doctoral thesis. He did not know it yet, but his career would soon zero in on prostaglandins as abortion medications. Scientists at this point knew there were many types of prostaglandins, but not what each type did (or how many types existed). The compounds remained perplexing despite decades passing since Ratner and von Euler's work. World War II paused their 1930s research.[10] Shortly after the war, one of Bygdeman's mentors, Dr. Sune Bergström, studied prostaglandins to pick up where they left off.

Except the compounds' supply for lab research was comically strained. Bergström found himself importing tons of Icelandic sheep glands to extract the prostaglandins from these disembodied organs. Marine biologists, recognizing this demand, later plucked corals from the Gulf of Mexico after finding out they also contained prostaglandins. Not until the 1970s would researchers switch to synthetic compounds (sparing sheep and corals). With two other scientists, Bergström later won the 1982 Nobel Prize for his prostaglandin research; his speech did credit Ratner as a pioneer.[11]

In the early 1960s, a race to find better birth control pills also drove this prostaglandin demand among researchers. The first birth control pill hit the US market around 1960, upending staid attitudes of sexuality and challenging gender roles.[12] Although abortion was still mostly illegal in Sweden, booming contraceptive research in the 1960s led to another curiosity in the labs of Stockholm: the search for an abortion pill. A radical potential for such a pill may reside in prostaglandins, which Bygdeman would try to uncover using that rare sample.

Around 1963, Bygdeman's advisor, von Euler (the same von Euler who coined "prostaglandin"), gave him a prostaglandin that Bergström had prepared for in vitro studies. An abortion medication struck Bygdeman as undoubtedly critical. As a gynecologist working under Sweden's near-total abortion ban, he had witnessed the humiliation that women endured in asking for permission from a (male) doctor and the state to have a legal abortion procedure.[13] An at-home abortion method could potentially transform this, empowering and entrusting women.

Before Sweden decriminalized abortion, a woman who wanted to end her pregnancy under the ban's narrow exceptions needed to plead her case before the Royal Board of Health, a typically all-male, all-white committee.[14] Those exceptions included if a woman had been raped or her pregnancy threatened her life. A woman was expected to argue why she was "deserving" of this care while the board investigated her case, her unwanted pregnancy progressing all the while.[15] Similar to the government in the US, the Swedish government until around 1975 also funded ableist, sexist, and racist forced sterilization programs.[16] Forcing someone to give birth and forcing someone to never give birth sought the same end: control.

As a medical resident at Karolinska Hospital in the late 1950s, Bygdeman worked with a young midwife, Karin Birgitta Berg, who joined him in caring for countless women who had been denied an abortion under Sweden's ban. They shared this conviction that women should one day have the option of safe, legal at-home abortions. The two formed a friendship, then a courtship, then a marriage. "We thought in the same way," Bygdeman at age 89 told me of Berg in 2023. He sat in a wheelchair while we spoke, his wife of more than five decades in the next room, and when I asked who molded his views on abortion the most, he said Berg, a midwife there at his ear, urging change.

By 1969 in Stockholm, after testing prostaglandins on strips of uterine tissue in labs, Bygdeman narrowed down two prostaglandin types that stimulated contractions. Perhaps these could be the backbone of an abortion medication. He and a colleague decided to test prostaglandins in a few pregnant women who sought an abortion. These women, whose names we do not know today, gave informed consent, having been told the potential risks, including that they would likely experience painful contractions. Bygdeman convinced the Swedish government to allow this research to happen under Sweden's ban.

In May 1969 over a few days, 11 women who were 13 to 18 weeks pregnant came to the Karolinska Institute for a prostaglandin injection (there was no pill yet).[17] All had contractions for hours. Only three women fully expelled their uterine contents, as if miscarrying, becoming some of the first women known to safely have abortions with medications. For the other eight women, the prostaglandin started but did not finish a miscarriage; they then had an abortion procedure. All the women experienced vaginal bleeding and cramping for hours; most had diarrhea and nausea. While the women voiced relief to at least no longer be pregnant, this had been physically difficult. Bygdeman knew it was not enough that these prostaglandins seemed safe. Women should not have to suffer. It was discouraging. But changing the prostaglandin type, dose, and interval for women at different weeks in their pregnancies may yet unravel a less painful, more effective, and safe abortion medication.

In January 1970, Bygdeman and his colleagues published this small study in *The Lancet*, stressing it was "an exploratory investigation, and should not be taken as an indication of the final clinical effectiveness of the method."[18] That same *Lancet* issue included a piece by Dr. Sultan Karim about prostaglandins for "therapeutic abortions," the researcher having also recently used that compound to safely induce labor in pregnant people.[19] Prostaglandin research soon skyrocketed. About 500 laboratories around the world were studying the compounds by 1971, with scientific papers on prostaglandins published at a rate of roughly two a day that year.[20] "Prostaglandins have such new qualities and importance that they might mean as much in controlling the reproductive process as the introduction of penicillin meant in fighting infection," Dr. Reimert T. Ravenhold, then director of the Office of Population at the US Agency for International Development (USAID), told the *New York Times* in 1971.

The American pharmaceutical industry also had prostaglandin fervor. But not to find an abortion pill or even a new birth control pill, which the male-dominated industry by the 1970s worried could invite liability more than profit. Scientists as far back as the 1930s with von Euler's research noted that prostaglandins may lower blood pressure and offer similar nongynecological uses. Those possibilities, beyond women and their pesky uteruses, intrigued drug companies. In 1973, after studies suggested prostaglandins may treat stomach ulcers, G. D. Searle & Company of Skokie, Illinois, created its own synthetic prostaglandin in pill form: misoprostol.

We know that story.

Beyond the pharmaceutical industry, another player closely watched early 1970s prostaglandin research. The WHO declared in 1967 for the first time that unsafe abortion posed a public health crisis.[21] It estimated thousands of women, mostly poor women in the Global South, died each year of unsafe, self-induced abortions.[22] Yet given drug companies' apparent cool disinterest in possible solutions to that crisis, the WHO launched in 1972 its Special Program on Research, Development, and Research Training in Human Reproduction (HRP) with (mostly male) scientists focusing on finding reproductive health medications especially to help communities in the Global South, including searching for an abortion pill. WHO centers in India, Hungary, China, and Sweden (at the Karolinska Institute) did much of this early hunting for such a pill.

One of the HRP's inaugural task forces looked at prostaglandins for the "interruption of pregnancies," a euphemism for abortion.[23] Bygdeman's mentor, Bergström, chaired that task force (Bygdeman would hold the post years later). A WHO report in 1978 detailed one of the task force's goals was to find "a nonsurgical method of abortion, nontoxic to the woman and nonteratogenic in an effective dosage, reliably producing complete expulsion of the products of conception, suitable for application in a nonclinical setting, and economically accessible to women in all countries."[24]

But to slightly distance itself from erratic global politics, the HRP had an unusual funding structure. Governments with the most money could influence the WHO's priorities based on what they did or did not fund. And most countries still banned or severely restricted abortion at the HRP's 1972 launch (not until the following year did the US legalize abortion). So, to avoid diplomatic mishaps, the WHO's overall budget did not support the HRP's research.[25] Private donors and a few small, sympathetic governments did instead.[26] The HRP's biggest, private anonymous donor for years would be a Nebraskan: Susan Thompson Buffett, the first wife of American billionaire Warren Buffett and longtime advocate for abortion rights, wielding her wealth in philanthropy accordingly (after her 2004 death, the Susan Thompson Buffett Foundation continued supporting the HRP.).[27]

One night in 1975 in India, Bygdeman and two WHO center colleagues in the HRP stayed up late looking over their prostaglandin trial results. They realized in astonishment that there was "a success rate of practically 100% complete abortions" in women up to about seven weeks pregnant.[28] But there was still no abortion pill; a provider usually injected prostaglandin into women's bodies. And the side effects were still too painful. A lower dose of prostaglandin meant less intense side effects, only then the contractions might not be strong enough to complete a person's abortion. Bygdeman believed women deserved better.

Around 1981, he tried something different at Karolinska Hospital. There, 40 women who were up to seven weeks pregnant, who sought an abortion, who were otherwise healthy, and who had at least one prior pregnancy in their lives joined a study on at-home abortion.[29] Bygdeman's team gave each woman two suppositories, or dissolvable capsules, that contained a prostaglandin and that the women would use by themselves at home. Women were instructed to place the first suppository in their vaginas for about six hours, then the second suppository in their vaginas for six more hours. They were told what side effects to expect, and they received a prescription painkiller as well as anti-nausea medication. Nurses were on call nearby. If anything concerning happened, women could ring for help or return to the hospital.

Acting like fellow scientists, these 40 women recorded their side effects during their at-home abortions, taking their temperature and noting the start, duration, and amount of bleeding they experienced. All had two follow-up visits: the first appointment a week after using the prostaglandins, and the second the week after that. Since this method could take several hours or days, providers would determine by the second visit if a woman completed her abortion. If she had not, she would, with her consent, receive a procedure. All but one of the 40 women completed their abortions in what may have been the first study of at-home, safe medication abortions.[30] Though 24 women reported gastrointestinal side effects, only one considered these "disturbingly high."[31] Yet this was a small group of patients who had a prior pregnancy and so understood how contractions felt in their bodies based on their past, factors that may have shaped their tolerance. "The results of the present study indicate that termination of early pregnancy by self-treatment at home starts to be a reality at least in selected patients," co-wrote Bygdeman in a 1981 paper. "Almost all patients had a positive attitude to the treatment. The most common reasons were the anonymity of the therapy, the possibility of the husband to participate, and the more 'natural' procedure as compared to vacuum aspiration."[32]

This was a big deal. Bygdeman and the WHO's HRP had been hoping for this progress for more than a decade. Except the pain had not gone away. Sure, this group tolerated contractions. But would that be the same for hundreds, thousands, millions of people around the world? What about women without hospital access? What would they do if anything went wrong? There was something else, of course. These women used suppositories just fine. Except wouldn't a pill be simpler and, since that method would be noninvasive, safer?

In 1981, misoprostol was not yet in Brazilian women's hands or Bygdeman's purview. Prostaglandin research for at-home abortions was stuck, the potential of that compound that Ratner found in 1930 unrealized. Then the world—and Bygdeman—learned of mifepristone.

CHAPTER 3

THE DAWN OF RU-486

In 1980 in a laboratory in a Parisian suburb, Dr. Georges Teutsch, chief chemist at the $1.7 billion French pharmaceutical company Roussel-Uclaf, stumbled on an unassuming molecule.[1] As with all molecules they synthesized, Roussel-Uclaf named this one "RU" for "Roussel-Uclaf," then gave it a number based on how many molecules the company invented that far, resulting in "RU-486" ("486" was shorthand for the 38,486th molecule synthesized).[2] Its generic name was, and is, mifepristone.

Roussel-Uclaf was not at all hunting for an abortion pill. What the company sought was a controversy-free, money-making molecule. Mifepristone was, and is, an anti-progestin; it blocked the hormone progesterone in the uterus. Earlier research suggested an anti-progestin may reduce cortisol, another hormone. And a drug regulating cortisol could dominate a lucrative market for, say, treating Cushing's, a rare illness where people had too much cortisol.[3] But for people with uteruses, anti-progestins can do something else, something at least one person at Roussel-Uclaf, a part-time consultant, knew immediately.[4]

This scientist, Dr. Étienne-Émile Baulieu, had studied progesterone for years, while searching for a better birth control pill. The press would later fawningly call him the "father" of the abortion pill. Yet Teutsch disputed that title slightly to *Science* in 1989: "Étienne Baulieu is the father of the pill, but he is not the father of the compound."[5] Meanwhile, women in Brazil would not be hailed as "mothers" of the other abortion pill misoprostol, only criticized for "misusing" that pill, with RU-486 seizing far more press attention for decades.

By the time Baulieu heard in 1980 about RU-486, the 54-year-old French biochemist and endocrinologist had lived many lives. He joined the French Resistance as a Jewish teen growing up in France during World War II, changing his last name from Blum to Baulieu to hide his Jewish ancestry for survival.[6] He went back to school after the war to become a doctor, then a scientist. At 30, he became a tenured professor at the Faculté de Médecine in Paris and focused on hormones.[7] Yet it was while visiting New York City's Columbia University from 1961 to 1962 that he landed on a path to mifepristone. There, Baulieu met Dr. Gregory Pincus, one of the inventors of the birth control pill, a groundbreaking product which Searle had just released in the US as Enovid.[8]

Almost 30 years later, Searle introduced Cytotec, or misoprostol. But back when Pincus co-developed the birth control pill, contraceptives were still illegal in much of the US, so Searle strategically first received FDA approval for Enovid as a treatment for "menstrual irregularities," then attained FDA approval in 1960 to market that same medication as birth control.[9] The first version of the pill contained progestin and estrogen, with "progestin" as a synthetic progesterone.[10] The postwar baby boom in the US soon ended as use of the pill rapidly spread. By 1965, more than 6.5 million women in the US had tried birth control pills.[11] For the first time, women reliably, privately controlled if and when they got pregnant. A counterculture amid second-wave feminism swept through the decade. Women's paid labor force participation rate in the US skyrocketed, partially due to the birth control pill.[12] And the pill made money in a market where otherwise healthy people with uteruses took a medication once a day for years, potentially decades. In 1964, Searle earned $24 million in net profits from Enovid (about $235 million today).[13] It was a blockbuster drug.

So, when Baulieu met Pincus in 1961 at Columbia, he was starstruck. Pincus invited him to see birth control pill trials still underway in Puerto Rico. Baulieu, though flattered, later wrote, "It troubled me slightly that Hispanic women from a poor outlying territory were chosen for clinical trials."[14] But he went, and the data blew him away, convincing him that contraceptive research was the future. However, that queasiness Baulieu felt reflected a grim history.

The birth control pill trials in Puerto Rico began in 1956 with more than 1,500 women of color, most of whom were poor and not told the pill had potentially serious side effects, only that it would prevent pregnancy.[15] The women received the same 10 mg dose as in the first version of Enovid later sold in the US, a dose about four to 10 times higher than in today's typical birth control pill products.[16] Pincus and his colleagues chose that very high dose to be as certain as possible that the pill would work, which it did indeed.[17] But in Pincus's determination to get the pill approved in the US, he dismissed side effects Puerto Rican women reported. About a quarter of the study participants dropped out in the first year, some due to dizziness and nausea. Three women died in the trials, with no autopsies conducted to see what role the pills may have played.[18] It remains unclear if their deaths were tied to the pill.[19]

Once the pill made it to the US, some women did suffer concerning side effects, leading several feminist activists to successfully pressure Searle to cut Enovid's dosage in half to make the pill safer.[20] The company soon discontinued that product. Today's range of safe birth control pills is a far cry from Enovid's controversial start, which has since been criticized for following legacies of colonialism and eugenics.[21] By the mid-1980s when trials with RU-486 began, more guardrails around consent were in place than three decades prior. It would be paramount to Baulieu for this potential "abortion pill" not to repeat the birth control pill's early mistakes.

Back in 1970 after his inspiring (if somewhat jarring) meetings with Pincus, Baulieu's search for a new, better birth control pill turned to progesterone. His team in Paris found progesterone's receptor cells in the uterus.[22] Baulieu and other scientists argued a pregnancy started after a fertilized egg implanted on the uterine wall, and progesterone helped make this implantation happen, then kept the embryo in place on the uterine wall.[23] Baulieu believed blocking progesterone might stop a pregnancy from continuing or even starting. He wanted to find a fake key, or anti-progestin, an imposter to trick progesterone's receptors in the uterus into binding to that fake key and thus blocking the real progesterone. In the 1970s, no known anti-progestin existed.

Baulieu soon became head of a research unit at the French National Institute of Health and Medical Research (INSERM), France's equivalent of the US National Institutes of Health (NIH), and worked as a consultant at Roussel-Uclaf. He used the company's lab for anti-progestin research while his presence brought them clout. So, in 1980, when Baulieu learned that Roussel-Uclaf synthesized RU-486, he was thrilled that an anti-progestin had been discovered at last.[24] Baulieu later claimed that he suggested to some Roussel-Uclaf scientists a way to make that very molecule.[25] Teutsch challenged that claim but made clear that, once Roussel-Uclaf knew what RU-486 could do, the company would have thrown the molecule out: "If [Baulieu] had not been there, Roussel-Uclaf would not have developed the compound for this indication."[26]

That indication was abortion. But Baulieu did not think of the molecule as an abortion pill at first. He preferred the term "contragestive."[27] This was his hypothesis: If a woman took RU-486 for four days each month, starting two days before her period, a fertilized egg would not implant on the uterine wall. A woman would simply bring back her period each month. And as Baulieu and others argued a pregnancy did not start until implantation, this process would be menstrual regulation, not abortion. RU-486 would wear off a day or so later in the woman's body with no impact on future fertility. Baulieu thought RU-486 could similarly end a pregnancy up to about seven weeks (or three weeks after a missed period). By blocking progesterone, the uterine wall would no longer hold an embryo, which would detach in an early miscarriage—or, yes, an abortion. In 1980, these nuanced hypotheses had yet to be proven in people. But Baulieu did not want Roussel-Uclaf to abandon RU-486 before such studies even started.[28]

A self-identified feminist, Baulieu believed a woman should control her own body. Like Bygdeman, he abhorred doctors abusing women who sought abortions. As a resident in a 1950s French hospital when abortion was banned in the country, Baulieu flinched at male surgeons denying women anesthesia during abortion procedures, once hearing a doctor say, "Teach her a lesson she will remember."[29] But Baulieu did hold stigmatizing views about abortion that were consistent with his era and gender, quoting reproductive specialist Dr. Roger Short in Baulieu's 1991 co-authored book *The "Abortion Pill,"* "Abortion is like poverty: no one likes it, but it will always be with us."[30]

Globally, grassroots feminist activists in decades to come, many of whom had abortions themselves, challenged this negative assumption. Abortion stories would lift up a range of emotions people may feel about their abortions, from gratitude to guilt, distress to relief, shame to joy. Such activists would say all emotions, including all those felt at once, are valid. This conversation, however, was hardly present at Baulieu's time.

Just five years before mifepristone's synthesis, France legalized abortion for women up to 10 weeks pregnant in the 1975 Veil Act.[31] Prior, women faced prison time for illegal abortions, and even briefly, during World War II, the death penalty.[32] Women who could afford to travel to where abortion was legal did—or paid for a secret abortion procedure in France. Those without money were forced to give birth or self-induce an abortion invasively. The 1975 Veil Act was a major victory, but some feminists in France wanted more, calling for the full decriminalization of abortion in a 1971 manifesto.[33]

The Veil Act, aside from its 10-week ban, also mandated women wait seven days between asking for an abortion and accessing one. It required that procedures take place inside of hospitals with specially authorized "family planning" centers staffed by abortion-supportive providers.[34] This was partially due to a "conscience clause" that legally allowed doctors in France to refuse to perform an abortion as long as they gave the patient a referral.[35] The law thus implied that a doctor refusing to provide an abortion—rather than providing one—was an act of conscience.

But even supportive doctors in France were wary of performing abortions after the Veil Act. Their experiences with abortion under a ban had mostly been when women needed urgent care after an abortion gone wrong, leading pro-choice doctors to fear women hemorrhaging or going septic, and so they overburdened abortion procedures.[36] Post–Veil Act and pre-medication abortion, a woman having an abortion in France went under general anesthesia with a 48-hour hospital stay—for an otherwise safe, quick, simple procedure when done early in pregnancy.[37] This all meant that a doctor-less pill in France could be transformative—if Baulieu's hypotheses in 1980 were right.

Roussel-Uclaf's CEO, Dr. Edouard Sakiz, was an old friend of Baulieu's; they liked each other. But unlike Baulieu, Sakiz was a businessman before a scientist. He regretted that Roussel-Uclaf in the 1960s missed out on the contraceptive market, deciding not to research birth control pills supposedly because the company's leadership feared the Catholic Church's rebuke in majority-Catholic France.[38] Except Roussel-Uclaf wildly miscalculated public acceptance of "the pill" in France. What if RU-486 turned out similarly as a "contragestive," perhaps as an abortion pill?

This was one of the arguments Baulieu made to Sakiz to not throw out RU-486. At least temporarily convinced, Sakiz allowed the company's scientists to test mifepristone in animals in 1980 and 1981, finding it safe enough to test in controlled doses in women who were early in their pregnancies.[39] An elated Baulieu enlisted Dr. Walter Herrmann in Switzerland to lead the first mifepristone-only abortion trial in people.[40] Switzerland had one of the world's strictest ethics committees for medical research at the time, which was precisely why Baulieu tapped Herrmann. This inaugural RU-486 study, one that would surely be scrutinized, needed to be more ethical than those early birth control pill trials. In 1981, Herrmann gave 200 mg of mifepristone each day for four days to 11 women six to eight weeks pregnant.[41] Nine women finished their abortions after about four days. But the drug did not work for two women, who then needed procedures. One of those two took mifepristone and, thinking her abortion done, felt well enough to ski shortly after. While on the slopes, she bled heavily and panicked. A helicopter apparently airlifted her from the Alps to a clinic for an emergency procedure and blood transfusion.[42] This was not some miracle pill.

But Baulieu thought more tests could find the best dosage, raising that success rate. And he was eager to show off this molecule to the hyper competitive scientific community.

On April 19, 1982, in Paris's baroque French Academy of Sciences, he "breathed deeply of the dust of three centuries" and clicked through a clunky slideshow in that "stuffy" space with "terrible" acoustics.[43] This hall was not built for slideshows—or women. In 1666, King Louis XIV founded the academy while the French empire and slave trade brought his absolute monarchy ludicrous wealth.[44] For three centuries, women could not be academy members.[45] Yvonne Choquet-Bruhat would be the first woman invited to become a full member—in 1979, merely three years before Baulieu's presentation.[46]

It was mifepristone's debut, the moment to share the Swiss study. Except on that clunky slideshow, Baulieu could only display a sliver of RU-486's structure.[47] Roussel-Uclaf's patent forbade making the full structure public for another few months. Before his talk, Baulieu handed the academy a sealed envelope with the complete mifepristone structure inside, to be unsealed when Roussel-Uclaf's restriction expired. "My audience," he later wrote, "was not visibly impressed."[48] One professor snorted at Baulieu moments into his presentation, "After all, this is abortion. Nothing more!"[49]

The press had an altogether different reaction. The next day, a French paper wrote excitedly of RU-486 as a possible abortifacient as well as contraceptive, and the *New York Times* ran the story, "Birth Control: 4-Day Pill Is Promising in Early Test."[50] Anti-abortion groups in learning the news quickly argued RU-486 would trivialize abortion. Women would make bad decisions. They would have more sex (gasp!). They would have more abortions (gasp!). They would sell and buy mifepristone on a black market (a complicated reality later). A buzz around the little pill began.

Several Roussel-Uclaf executives, however, were frustrated at Baulieu speaking publicly about RU-486 as a "contragestive." Blurring lines between contraception and abortion seemed foolish if RU-486 were to have a shot in the world. The Catholic Church argued human life started at conception (not a scientific term), and some anti-abortion extremists already called birth control pills abortifacients, claiming these pills removed a fertilized egg from a person's uterus and that a fertilized egg was a human being (even though birth control pills worked by preventing fertilization). This messy contragestive space, the moments in a woman's body after fertilization and before implantation, held nuance that risked making mifepristone even more of a target.[51] Soon, Baulieu's "contragestive" concept fell out of favor.[52] RU-486 would become *the* abortion pill to much of the world's press. Only Baulieu made another misstep in his 1982 talk by suggesting that RU-486 could end a person's pregnancy on its own, no other medication needed. That stood on shaky ground.

In 1982, the WHO's HRP took keen notice when Baulieu reported the Swiss study. The results were imperfect but promising. If Roussel-Uclaf was serious about this pill, the company needed to run many more trials with hundreds of women around the world, which would be expensive and take time. The stakes were high. The WHO estimated in 1986 that maternal mortality in "developing countries" totaled 500,000 women each year, 15 to 20 percent from "illegal abortion attempts."[53] Medication abortion may be one lifesaving measure. Yet there was nothing stopping Roussel-Uclaf from abandoning RU-486 despite Baulieu's advocacy. After years of searching for a safe, at-home medication abortion method, the HRP now wanted to make sure the company did not turn its back on a medication it had stumbled upon.

Baulieu was friends with then director and co-founder of the WHO's HRP, Dr. Alexander Kessler, and liaised between Roussel-Uclaf and the WHO to conduct mifepristone trials on a bigger scale. In 1982, the WHO signed a deal with the company: the HRP would pay for and run RU-486 trials for "various uses" among its global centers, and Roussel-Uclaf would supply the mifepristone pills.[54] The company promised to sell mifepristone at a low cost to poorer WHO member nations that approved and requested the medication.[55] A clause in that contract proved prescient. If Roussel-Uclaf stopped selling mifepristone, it needed to supply the pill to the WHO or release its patent to another company of the WHO's choosing.[56]

This worked for both parties. The WHO researched abortifacients, but the agency was not a pharmaceutical company. To help bring into the world drugs with major public health benefits yet possibly low profit margins, the WHO did a delicate dance with the pharmaceutical industry. Roussel-Uclaf struck a similar agreement in 1982 with the Population Council, the nonprofit research institute in New York, allowing its scientists to use RU-486 for studies in the US and elsewhere.[57] The council would later play a critical role in mifepristone's path to America.

In Sweden around 1983, only two years after his small study on at-home abortions with prostaglandins, Bygdeman laid his hands on another rare sample: mifepristone. The Karolinska Institute was a WHO center under the HRP, so Bygdeman now had an RU-486 supply. He had been chasing after an abortion pill for years. Might this be it? He knew the 1981 Swiss study was a breakthrough. But a roughly 80 percent success rate among a few women was just nowhere near good enough to him. Mifepristone-only abortions needed to be at least as safe and effective as aspiration procedures, which had a nearly 98 percent success rate.[58]

The RU-486-only trials disappointed Bygdeman, their success rate hovering at 70 to 80 percent, sometimes lower.[59] But compared to side effects with prostaglandins, the side effects with RU-486 only were minimal. Researchers knew mifepristone halted a pregnancy's development. It also softened the cervix and started contractions, though it did not seem to fully empty the uterus. Bygdeman, then nearly 50, noticed that progesterone quieted the uterine muscle during a person's pregnancy, which made contractions less likely to happen. By blocking progesterone, mifepristone stopped that calming effect, and so the uterine muscle become more sensitive. He believed that another medication, taken a day or two after mifepristone, might then strengthen these contractions in the abortion seeker's body. The two medications could be synergistic.[60]

For almost two decades, Bygdeman had been studying compounds that did precisely that: triggered contractions. The idea "came very naturally to us," he told me in 2023. What about giving women a small dose of a prostaglandin a day or so after they swallowed RU-486? At the Karolinska Institute, 16 women up to about eight weeks pregnant who wanted an abortion took mifepristone. A day or two later, they received some prostaglandin, an amount five times smaller than in Bygdeman's earlier prostaglandin trials. Of the 16 women, 15 completed their abortions at a success rate of 95 percent, almost on par with aspirations.[61] All reported fewer and much less intense side effects than in prostaglandin-only trials—and no complications.[62] These abortions hurt a lot less. The one woman who did not complete her abortion had an aspiration.

Bygdeman was thrilled, closer to his and Berg's vision of at-home abortions. More trials may find the right dosage and push that success percentage up and side effects down, making medication abortion hopefully less painful and better. All that work on prostaglandins found a companion in RU-486. Bygdeman could not fathom Roussel-Uclaf not wanting to test this new pairing. Imagine the impact. Think of the women.

But Bygdeman's news did not go over well at Roussel-Uclaf.

CHAPTER 4

THE MORAL PROPERTY OF WOMEN

In October 1984 by Italy's glamorous Lake Como, Dr. Marc Bygdeman and Dr. Étienne-Émile Baulieu stepped into the thirteenth-century Villa Serbelloni. A princess had donated the villa to the Rockefeller Foundation for hosting scientific and literary luminaries.[1] That October at the villa about 15 scientists, almost entirely white men, would debate RU-486 and uteruses. For all the wonder of mifepristone in the press, if the medication's trial results continued to be as low as those in the 1981 Swiss study, then there would be no "abortion pill."

At the villa, Roussel-Uclaf's Sakiz listened anxiously to researchers sharing the same deflating results over and over until Bygdeman spoke. The Swedish scientist proudly announced a 95 percent success rate among a small group of women when pairing mifepristone with a prostaglandin.[2] A young gynecologist who recently joined the WHO's HRP, Dr. Paul Van Look, chimed in, arguing that Roussel-Uclaf and the WHO should clearly pursue trials with this new combined method. Why ever not? "I remember very well," Van Look told me almost four decades later. "Sakiz became extremely angry with me."

The CEO had an outburst. Sakiz furiously declared he wanted no studies with prostaglandins, only RU-486. "It was not appreciated *at all*," Bygdeman told me. Van Look did not understand why, but he had a theory: Roussel-Uclaf, unlike one of its biggest rivals, sold no prostaglandin product. Combining RU-486 with a competitor's drug therefore risked diluting Roussel-Uclaf's profits from this pill, Van Look speculated to me. He and Bygdeman were horrified. A few WHO centers ignored Sakiz and carried on testing this combined method regardless. And a year later, Bygdeman's phone rang in Stockholm. It was Sakiz cordially inviting him to Paris for dinner at an expensive restaurant. "And this time we were *highly* appreciated," Bygdeman told me. "Because they wanted to introduce the combined method on the market in France."

Roussel-Uclaf kept landing on that roughly 80 percent success rate for abortions with mifepristone alone when Bygdeman's 95 percent suddenly appealed to Sakiz.[3] By 1987, the WHO found nearly a 100 percent success rate in hundreds of women who took mifepristone, then, a day or two later, a suppository (not a pill) of a prostaglandin called gemeprost.[4] More WHO research among thousands of women around the globe confirmed this combined method worked and was safe in women up to nine weeks pregnant, barring a few rare contraindications.[5] On eventually being wined and dined in the city of lights with a smooth-talking Sakiz, Bygdeman scoffed to me, "It was a treatment quite different from the initial one. *That* was the start of the combined method."

In 1983, Dr. Elisabeth Aubény, a 51-year-old feminist gynecologist and abortion provider at Broussais Hospital in Paris, attended a meeting of France's family planning centers, the only places in the country that performed legal abortion procedures. Her jaw dropped when a fellow provider mentioned a Swiss trial for an abortion pill, RU-486. "We did not dare believe it," she told me at age 91 in 2023 through an interpreter. "It seemed miraculous to us and corresponded so much to the desires of women, who for so long have been asking for a drug to bring back their periods."

Aubény and French feminists had been fighting for abortion rights for years while critical of (male) doctor–(female) patient power imbalances. She became a gynecologist to change those dynamics. Around 1957, Aubény witnessed a woman die in a French hospital of a self-induced abortion. "It was awful," she told me. "She was dying, and she knew she was dying. And her husband was there next to her, and he was crying, saying, 'It is my fault, my fault.' And she had three children. Three little children." Aubény worked in the hospital's maternity ward and understood the "disaster" 1950s women suffered if they bore a child outside marriage, only to be denied jobs and ostracized, a cruelty that led many to self-induce and hurt themselves. "The abortion pill would make it possible to free oneself," Aubény told me. "To prevail of another choice without surgery and without anesthesia, one to be practiced by women themselves at home." She and fellow French feminist abortion providers immediately contacted Baulieu and Roussel-Uclaf's medical director, Dr. André Ulmann, who ran mifepristone's clinical trials at the company, telling the two men, "We are French. This pill is French. We have to make these trials. This is our chance."

Roussel-Uclaf hired the 36-year-old Ulmann in 1984 to focus on cardiovascular products when, that year, Sakiz asked him to oversee mifepristone instead. The company had already hired a male gynecologist for the job, but that person quit abruptly, refusing to work on an abortifacient. Ulmann, surprised at Sakiz's sudden request, told the CEO that he knew nothing about abortion. "And [Sakiz] said, 'That is no problem. You will learn,'" Ulmann recalled to me. But Ulmann did research steroid receptors, and mifepristone blocked one such receptor. He also suspected that Baulieu, who knew Ulmann, nudged Sakiz into picking him, somehow aware of Ulmann's views on abortion and correctly guessing that he would not abandon the pill. Ulmann thought RU-486 a prized invention. Yet Roussel-Uclaf dedicated no more than five employees to work on this mifepristone project full-time at once, with those five staff members (including Ulmann) managing clinical trials in France.[6] The company would invest little in the pill.

From 1984 to 1988, Aubény's Broussais Hospital team became the main center for these trials of mifepristone with a prostaglandin.[7] Roussel-Uclaf included their work in its application to the French Ministry of Health for mifepristone's approval. Like Baulieu, Aubény wanted mifepristone to travel around the world. But if a major problem happened at this stage, "I knew that the trials would be completely stopped, and all the hopes we had put in the revolutionary pill would disappear," she told me. "It was an enormous responsibility. And so, it seemed very urgent to be very, very careful in our tests to avoid any accidents as much as possible."

Those were four years of anxiety for Aubény. Roussel-Uclaf's protocols were strict. A woman with an early pregnancy and who wanted a medication abortion through these trials needed to visit a hospital's family planning center at least four times. French law required that a person's abortion take place in one of those centers like Aubény's, the law not imagining an at-home abortion. At the first visit, the woman needed to ask for a medication abortion, then French law required her to wait a week. She came back and took RU-486 pills in front of a doctor. At the third visit, she received an injection or vaginal suppository of a small amount of a prostaglandin, then stayed at the hospital for hours, bleeding and having what could be painful contractions until fully expelling her uterine contents in a toilet at the facility, finishing her abortion there before going home. During her fourth and final visit, a doctor confirmed with an exam that the person's abortion was complete.

These dizzying protocols stood in contrast to women in Brazil using over-the-counter misoprostol around the same time. "Doctors worried about what I call the 'cousin effect,'" wrote Baulieu in 1991 of early rigidity around RU-486 in France, revealing some of his own paternalism in the process. "A woman might receive the compound under controlled circumstances but, if she were allowed to take it home for whatever reason, she might change her mind, not take the compound, and leave it in her medicine cabinet. Some time later, her cousin, pregnant for months, asks her advice, and she remembers the magic pill."[8] Except what was so threatening about women helping each other?

Aubény believed that was the power of these medications all along. She was shocked at a post-*Dobbs* US when we spoke in April 2023. That month in France, where she still lived, there was a brief misoprostol shortage after some American state officials panic-ordered those pills to possibly pivot to a misoprostol-only regimen for medication abortions when mifepristone faced an existential threat in court.[9] An American anti-abortion group falsely claimed mifepristone was dangerous and sought to ban it more than 20 years after FDA approval, ignoring its global safety record.[10] "I am really sad for you, really, really sad," Aubény told me. The "you" was the US.

Aubény shook her head as she spoke with me, distressed when recalling her travels to New York in the early 1970s with fellow French doctors who supported abortion. New York was a vanguard to them; the state in 1970 legalized abortion up to 24 weeks in pregnancy, three years before *Roe*. Aubény came to the city to see a new abortion-clinic model. "We learned at this time from the US that we can do abortions outside of the hospital," she told me. "And now it is us who are on the other side. To see this go back, it is hard. I cannot understand [what is happening], but I think women in the US will have enough strength to stop this process, to stop what is going on." Then, as if impatient with the delay when speaking through an interpreter, Aubény asked me in English directly: "Do *you* think it will stop?"

In the late 1980s, while the French clinical trials wrapped up, RU-486 loomed large to American anti-abortion groups successfully growing their political power. The year that Roussel-Uclaf synthesized mifepristone, a so-called Moral Majority of white Evangelical Christians formed a critical voting bloc that helped elect Republican Ronald Reagan US president.[11] Reagan's anti-abortion stance, likely in addition to his thinly veiled racism, energized many previously politically disengaged Evangelicals to vote for him. Yet Reagan had not always been against abortion. He signed one of the country's most liberal abortion laws while governor of California before his presidential campaign.[12] Once Reagan entered the White House, however, abortion became increasingly partisan in US national politics during the 1980s, the anti-abortion movement aligning itself more with Republicans.[13] But RU-486 threatened this movement's winning streak.

Graphic, often medically inaccurate images of fetuses (the pregnant person absent) had been visceral, effective anti-abortion tools in the US to argue that abortion killed a human being. But mifepristone promised to end people's early pregnancies, so early that there was no fetus. "We're really a very simplistic, visually-oriented people," said

Dr. John Willke, president of the NRLC, one of the country's biggest anti-abortion groups, when asked about RU-486. "And if what [abortions] destroy in there doesn't look human, then it will make our job more difficult."[14]

Willke and his wife, Barbara Willke, had been credited with galvanizing a grassroots anti-abortion movement in the 1970s US thanks to their 1971 *Handbook on Abortion* replete with propaganda.[15] They spoke at American churches, schools, and town halls, sharing their book with photos of fetuses and abhorrent scientific inaccuracies (including that a woman could not get pregnant from rape).[16] Terrified of the RU-486 trials succeeding and securing the French government's approval, Willke later wrote furiously to the French prime minister that mifepristone contained "fetotoxicity."[17] He received no response.

The anti-abortion movement in France, however, was much smaller, quieter, and less funded than in the US. But even supporters of abortion in France worried about the "ethics" of an abortion pill that, some feared, might one day be sold in supermarkets (even though supermarkets in France sold cigarettes and bleach, far more dangerous to ingest than mifepristone).[18] Aubény was correct that any misstep in the trials could shut down such a highly scrutinized pill.

In 1987, Roussel-Uclaf applied at last to the French Ministry of Health for approval to sell RU-486 for inducing abortions in people up to seven weeks pregnant. Roussel-Uclaf's application stressed that mifepristone be used with a prostaglandin that combined method WHO trials continued to show safe and effective.[19] Livid American anti-abortion activists meanwhile threatened boycotts of any companies connected to the pill and organized theatrical protests.[20] On June 23, 1988, with the French government not yet having decided on the medication, Roussel-Uclaf executives dashed inside the company's Paris headquarters past protestors dressed in striped uniforms to mirror Holocaust victims, yelling, "You are turning the uterus into a crematory oven!"[21] It was Roussel-Uclaf's shareholder meeting. Protestors outside the company's walls called RU-486 a "chemical weapon" against the "unborn," ignoring that Baulieu, "father of the abortion pill," was a Jewish former French Resistance member.

These Holocaust references dredged up the not-so-distant, dark past of Roussel-Uclaf's parent company, Hoechst A. G. in Germany. Hoechst had been in a conglomerate of companies called I. G. Farben that profited from the poisonous gas Zyklon B that Nazis weaponized to murder millions of Jews in concentration camps.[22] Hoechst's genocidal complicity was now on public display, all over an abortion pill. The company's German-Catholic and anti-abortion CEO, Wolfgang Hilger, vehemently said that RU-486 defied Hoechst's values.[23] Besides, money was on the line. If these American anti-abortion groups' threats of boycotts against Hoechst spread, was an abortion pill worth that cash loss? Hoechst immediately pressured Roussel-Uclaf to withdraw the drug's French application.

Then in September 1988, China beat France to RU-486 approval.[24] China's government did not frame medication abortion access as an individual right but as a way to slow population growth.[25] The Chinese government's controversial one-child policy was already in place, and mifepristone was seen as another population control tool, not a means of feminist empowerment.[26] Despite China's approval of the drug, Roussel-Uclaf did not supply the country with mifepristone.[27] The company stalled. When France finally approved RU-486 later that September of 1988, Hoechst reiterated to Roussel-Uclaf that it wanted mifepristone scrapped anyways, that the pill should never be sold to anyone ever.

Baulieu, aware of Hoechst's aggression, still doubted Roussel-Uclaf would bend the knee. That seemed ridiculous. Rather than worry, he busily prepared for his upcoming talk later in October on a panel about RU-486 at the World Congress of Gynecology and Obstetrics in Rio de Janeiro, Brazil, where Bygdeman and Aubény would also speak.

But on October 21, 1988, just days before that conference, Sakiz held a secret meeting with Roussel-Uclaf executives to debate mifepristone. Baulieu was not invited or told of the Paris gathering. The only woman present among 19 men in a corporate boardroom was Dr. Catherine Euvrard.[28] According to Sakiz in a 1989 *New York Times* interview, Roussel-Uclaf's executive vice president had just announced that he, too, was against the pill, seemingly doing so to

THE MORAL PROPERTY OF WOMEN

curry favor with Hoechst and angle for Sakiz's job.[29] Sakiz panicked and called that emergency meeting. Almost all of the men there that day argued against RU-486, that an abortion pill would not make much money since developing countries would mostly order this pill at a low price per the 1982 WHO agreement. Besides, abortion was taboo. Sakiz then called a vote among the executives for Roussel-Uclaf to withdraw mifepristone entirely. Of the 20 people present, 16 voted to stop the pill, including Sakiz.[30]

Euvrard and Ulmann sat stunned; they were two of the four who voted that day to protect mifepristone.[31] Euvrard would later call her colleagues "male chauvinists" "afraid of controversy, afraid to fight. For them, it is always the problems of politics, money, and corporate image."[32]

What happened next had two conflicting accounts, one from Baulieu and Sakiz, the other Ulmann told me. According to Baulieu, Euvrard called his office in Paris after that vote and said Sakiz wanted to speak with Baulieu before his flight to Rio for the World Congress. It was only after Baulieu hung up the phone that another colleague hurriedly told him that Roussel-Uclaf was stopping RU-486. Baulieu, furious, left immediately to talk to Sakiz in person, finding the CEO "visibly shaken" in his wood-paneled office.[33] Sakiz proceeded to tell Baulieu in private that his hands were tied over mifepristone—but Baulieu, as an independent consultant and not as a company employee, could speak out against Roussel-Uclaf's decision while Sakiz, as the CEO, could not. Only Ulmann insisted to me that this heated exchange between Baulieu and Sakiz could not have happened because, by this time, Baulieu was already in Rio with Ulmann.

Against Sakiz's orders to not say a word of Roussel-Uclaf's decision to anyone at the World Congress, it was Ulmann who angrily flew to Rio and broke the news to Baulieu there. "I was about to be fired," Ulmann told me, calling Baulieu's version of events a "rewriting of history," one likely intended to massage Sakiz's public image given what happened later. In 1997, Sakiz became CEO of a new company, Exelgyn, to sell mifepristone after Roussel-Uclaf gave his company (and not Ulmann) that pill's worldwide patent rights (excluding the

US).[34] Sakiz made his career off a medication he once abandoned; it was not a good look. But Sakiz has since passed away, and Baulieu, in his late nineties, could not grant an interview with me to help verify which version of events was true.

However Baulieu found out what Roussel-Uclaf did, in late October 1988 at Rio's Hotel Nacional, hundreds of attendees at the World Congress erupted over Roussel-Uclaf's statement that a "polemic" against RU-486 forced them to pull the medication.[35] Bygdeman thought it scandalous. Aubény felt "completely devastated," she told me. "But personally, I couldn't believe it, and I didn't believe it. I wouldn't have thought that they could have stopped the trials to go on." French public opinion backed her, with an October 1988 survey finding 64 percent of the French people supported mifepristone.[36] "We are witnessing a return to morality," said the French minister of women's rights after Roussel-Uclaf's disastrous announcement. "And who are the victims of morality? Women. Always."[37]

The International Federation of Gynecology and Obstetrics (FIGO) had just released a study finding more than 500,000 women died of pregnancy-related causes a year, nearly all in the Global South, with unsafe abortion as one cause.[38] FIGO wrote a protest letter to Hoechst's CEO, who simply replied that abortion was immoral.[39] Feminists at the World Congress furiously organized petitions to both companies, all while Baulieu smiled at the irony: Roussel-Uclaf quietly withdrew RU-486 seemingly to avoid a fiasco yet created one.[40]

A few days later, Baulieu packed his bags to leave Rio for Paris when he got a call. A reporter asked him to comment on mifepristone.[41] Baulieu had spoken to the press dozens of times the past couple of days. What new was there to say? The journalist informed him that the French minister of health, Claude Évin, had stated, "From the moment government approval for the drug was granted, RU-486 became the moral property of women, not just the property of the drug company."[42] The French government, which owned 36 percent of Roussel-Uclaf, told the company that if it did not put mifepristone back on the market, the government would then strip Roussel-Uclaf of the pill's patent and hand it to another company, which French law allowed.[43]

Roussel-Uclaf caved. World Congress attendees burst into applause at the news. Bygdeman and Ulmann breathed sighs of relief. Baulieu and Aubény opened bottles of champagne. Yet outside Rio's Hotel Nacional, where one night's stay cost more than some Brazilians made in a year, women whispered to each other about that other pill sitting on shelves in pharmacies: a cheap tablet version of the prostaglandins Bygdeman had studied for decades.

Without rounds of applause or glasses of champagne, misoprostol arrived discretely. But trouble was not far. On October 29, 1988, the *New York Times* had a big, front-page story, "France Ordering Company to Sell Its Abortion Drug."[44] Next to that piece was another: "US May Allow Anti-Ulcer Drug Tied to Abortion," the article on Cytotec that Margareth Arilha read in São Paulo, all while the first reports appeared of fewer dead women in maternity hospitals.[45]

Later coverage on Cytotec's use for abortions stirred a storm in Brazil, as mentioned earlier in the book.[46] Word of misoprostol as another abortion pill spread and, by the early 1990s, reached the ears of European researchers like Aubény in France.[47] "We knew at that point that the Brazilians were already using misoprostol for abortions without a lot of complications, so then we started to adopt it like the prostaglandins," she told me of France's shift to combining mifepristone with misoprostol. "We owe a lot to the Brazilians, to a country where abortion was not legal."

CHAPTER 5

"OBSCENE, LEWD, OR LASCIVIOUS"

One January morning in 1989 in Paris, 45-year-old Faye Wattleton walked into Roussel-Uclaf's headquarters for a strictly confidential meeting (this secrecy was the company's idea, not hers).[1] American abortion clinics were under siege by then. But as soon as Wattleton, who did not know about misoprostol yet, heard the French minister of health's "moral property of women" line, she clocked RU-486's promise to dramatically expand abortion access in the US. She was the first Black president of Planned Parenthood Federation of America, the largest provider of abortions in the country.[2] And now that French women at last had RU-486, Wattleton wanted Planned Parenthood to lead mifepristone's clinical trials across the US to secure FDA approval of the pill for American women. Only Wattleton needed to convince Roussel-Uclaf's CEO, Dr. Edouard Sakiz, to work with her. That January 1989 would be her first of three trips in two years to plead with the company.

Around 1965 as a nurse-midwife, Wattleton herself needed an abortion beyond the law. She found a doctor, a man, who gave her no anesthesia during her procedure and scolded her. Abortion pills did not exist for her. "I am not ashamed to talk about it," she said of her abortion in a 2007 MAKERS interview. "I am ashamed to think, however, that if I didn't talk about it that some ground would be lost because women, young women, would believe it was all manufactured and it wasn't all that bad. It was bad."[3]

But Wattleton's abortion would likely have been legal about a century earlier. In America from colonial times until the mid-1800s, people could have legal abortions before "quickening," or when a pregnant person felt fetal movements, usually around 20 or 24 weeks, this authority remarkably resting with the pregnant person and their subjective experience.[4] The term "abortion" did not even refer then to a person ending a pregnancy pre-quickening, with "bringing on the menses" often used instead, similar to how some women in Brazil more than a century later would describe taking misoprostol to bring back a period.[5] Until the mid-1800s in the US, midwives, almost all women and some of whom were Black women, also typically performed abortions, which, when in skilled hands, tended to be safer than giving birth.[6] Yet American midwives would soon be smeared as immoral abortionists by their new competitors: white male doctors in the emerging field of gynecology.[7]

The American Medical Association (AMA) formed in 1847 and professionalized a male-dominated cadre of doctors, but midwives had already cornered a potentially lucrative market: maternal health.[8] With pre-quickening abortion legal at the time, providing abortions and offering birth control methods for a fee could be big business. Ann Trow Lohman discovered this in New York when fashioning herself as Madame Restell to sell "female monthly pills" and perform abortions, all while advertising as a "female physician."[9] At the AMA, Dr. Horatio Storer, credited as a "father" of obstetrics and gynecology, was aghast and launched "The Physicians' Crusade Against Abortion."[10] The AMA gave Storer a prize for his piece *Why Not? A Book for Every Woman*, in which he argued abortion evil and "quickening," by trusting a woman to know her own body, ludicrous: "If each woman were allowed to judge for herself in this matter, her decision upon the abstract question would be too sure to be warped by personal considerations, and those of the moment."[11]

The AMA anti-abortion campaign also aligned with that era's white supremacist, anti-immigration anxieties.[12] Women who could afford abortions (like those from Madame Restell) tended to be white, Protestant, and middle to upper class. Some white Protestant, middle- to upper-class men, fearing that immigrants and freed Black Americans would replace their whiteness, and that "their" women could move out of domestic spheres into public ones, viewed "their" women ending "their" pregnancies as "race suicide."[13] Then came anti-vice obsessive Anthony Comstock.

By 1873, Comstock convinced Congress to pass "An Act for the Suppression of Trade in, and Circulation of, Obscene Literature and Articles of Immoral Use," known as the Comstock Act, criminalizing mailing any "obscene, lewd, or lascivious book, pamphlet, picture, paper, print, or other publication of an indecent character, or any article or thing designed or intended for the prevention of conception or procuring of abortion."[14] A person breaking the Comstock Act could face imprisonment, fines, or both. In less than a year of enactment, Anthony Comstock, then a US postal inspector, was credited with seizing "130,000 pounds of books, 194,000 pictures and photographs, and 60,300 'articles made of rubber for immoral purposes, and used by both sexes.'"[15] More than half of the states swiftly passed so-called Little Comstock laws, and, by around 1910, abortion became a crime across the US.[16] Some states included exceptions for a legal abortion to save the pregnant person's life, with (white male) doctors deemed responsible for deciding which women counted for these exceptions.[17] As American University sociologist Dr. Tracy Weitz told me, "Abortion [in the US] was medicalized before it was moralized."

The Little Comstock laws in 1910s New York led to the arrest of Planned Parenthood's founder and one of Wattleton's predecessors, Margaret Sanger. A nurse and radical socialist, Sanger aggressively fought to make birth control available to women, including playing a key role in developing the first birth control pill, but even she opposed abortion. At her first birth control clinic, Sanger spread flyers that read, "Do not kill, do not take life, but prevent."[18] She incorrectly believed that if all women used birth control to prevent unwanted pregnancies, then no women would ever need abortions.

Some reproductive rights and justice activists today argue that the family planning field's historic framing of birth control use as "responsible" and abortion as a "failure," a perception Sanger helped instill, ended up stigmatizing abortion seekers. Sanger's position as a eugenicist later in life also left a troubled legacy. She advocated for segregating or sterilizing the "profoundly retarded," writing around 1919 in the American Birth Control League's journal that "the chief issue of birth control" was "more children from the fit, less from the unfit."[19] The rising American anti-abortion movement decades later would seize on Sanger's eugenic views to try to undermine the American reproductive rights movement's credibility—while the reproductive rights movement itself struggled to reckon with her complicated past.[20]

As Wattleton intimately experienced, criminalizing abortion in the US did not stop all women from having abortions but forced the procedure into the shadows. In 1966, the year Sanger died and just one year after the Supreme Court legalized birth control, Wattleton, who recently had her own illegal abortion, watched a poor teenager at a Harlem hospital die of an abortion that her mother tried to perform. Abortion was still a crime in 1970 in Ohio when Wattleton became president of a Planned Parenthood affiliate in Dayton. That Dayton clinic could not legally provide abortions but gave abortion-seekers a phone number to the Clergy Consultation Service on Abortion (CCS), a group connecting people around the country to doctors trusted to provide safe abortions for a fee.[21] Some CCS callers in Ohio were referred to an underground feminist group miles away in Chicago, a group known as the Janes.

Decades later in countries under abortion bans, the Janes would be a model of feminist, direct-action abortion care in which Jane members learned to safely perform procedures with no formal medical training. By the 2010s, feminist activists like Argentina's Socorristas en Red used mifepristone and misoprostol or misoprostol alone to support people through their abortions under bans, becoming Janes of another generation, as some activists in the US clandestinely do today with pills post-*Dobbs*.

The original Janes before *Roe* relied on mutual aid (donate what you can to pay for your care and to help those after you, and if you can't pay a cent, your care will be free). From 1969 to early 1973, the years in which Janes ran, the group provided an estimated 11,000 abortions with few complications and no known deaths.[22] Janes told each woman what to expect throughout her procedure, asking for her informed consent at each step, and did not scold her, unlike Wattleton's doctor.[23] A few members were eventually caught and arrested, but when the all-white, all-male Supreme Court decided *Roe* in 1973, legalizing abortion nationwide, their charges were cleared.[24] And the Janes, thinking their work beyond the law done, disbanded.[25]

Except *Roe* had problems. It centered the right of a doctor (presumed white and male) to privately confer with and care for a patient.[26] To some feminists, this reasoning was paternalistic and dangerously fragile. The American medical community that a century ago helped stigmatize and criminalize abortion was now implicitly expected to shield a woman's right to an abortion, one precariously placed under a right to doctor-patient privacy. *Roe* also only allowed a pregnant person to access an abortion until fetal viability, or when a fetus could survive outside a person's womb. In 1973 without advanced medical technologies, that vague viability line was considered around 28 weeks in pregnancy; today, it can be closer to 24 weeks. *Roe* additionally introduced into abortion law a trimester framework for pregnancies that barely existed in medical literature before. This framework defined in law how many weeks in a person's pregnancy a state could not restrict abortion (first trimester), could "regulate" but not ban abortion (second trimester), or could restrict or ban abortion (third trimester).[27] Such arbitrary lines carved around the pregnant body and into law had seismic, lasting impacts on women's lives.

In the US before and sadly after *Roe*, low-income women of color often grappled with broader complexities when seeking an abortion, as Angela Davis wrote in *Women, Race & Class* in the early 1980s: "When Black and Latina women resort to abortions in such large numbers, the stories they tell are not so much about their desire to be free of their pregnancy, but rather about the miserable social conditions which dissuade them from bringing new lives into the world."[28] Davis argued that the late 1960s, early 1970s US abortion rights campaign, with its majority-white leadership, seemed to assume abortion could solve systemic problems, "As if having fewer children could create more jobs, higher wages, better schools, etc., etc."[29]

Planned Parenthood's Wattleton, especially as a young Black woman, understood that criticism. But *Roe* swiftly brought a new problem: much of the abortion rights movement, including some of the Janes, thought hospitals, clinics, and doctor's offices would suddenly now provide legal abortion care.[30] Wattleton did not see that happen at her own clinic.

When *Roe* came, the Dayton clinic continued giving abortion-seekers that CCS number and, as Wattleton recalled, received no guidance from Planned Parenthood headquarters on what to do next.[31] Several doctors at the clinic vehemently refused to start providing abortions.[32] Many hospitals and medical schools across the country also largely ignored abortion care as if the law had not changed.[33] Independent clinics began opening in the mid 1970s to provide abortions and fill this abortion-access gap in mainstream medicine. This clinic model, however, contributed to siloing abortion, normalizing hospitals and doctors casting out a safe, simple procedure to clinics that would become easy targets of an increasingly aggressive anti-abortion movement that, just three years after *Roe*, had already seriously weakened the decision. Because in 1976, US Representative Henry Hyde of Illinois had an idea: "I would certainly like to prevent, if I could legally, anybody having an abortion: a rich woman, a middle class woman, or a poor woman. Unfortunately, the only vehicle available is the . . . Medicaid bill."[34]

The Hyde Amendment successfully banned federal funding of abortion for low-income people reliant on the state and federal health program Medicaid, doing so as an attachment to an annual Department of Health and Human Services (HHS) appropriations bill.[35] Wattleton was horrified. Given structural inequalities, she knew this ban would disproportionately harm Black women like her. But Planned Parenthood Federation of America seemed complacent to her in the immediate years after *Roe* while the NRLC expanded local chapters. When Wattleton became Planned Parenthood's president in 1978, she announced that she was "putting the world on notice."[36]

Planned Parenthood joined *Harris v. McRae* to argue that Hyde was discriminatory, but Wattleton recalled many Planned Parenthood board members threatened a no-confidence vote in her largely over her fight against Hyde.[37] The Supreme Court in 1980 upheld Hyde in *McRae* regardless.[38] As of this writing in 2024, Hyde has been renewed annually in Congress ever since and has morphed into a ban on almost all federal funding of abortion care.[39]

On the heels of the *McRae* decision, the election of Republican Ronald Reagan in 1980 ushered in an anti-abortion New Right that dominated national politics for the next decade, all as researchers in Europe tested an abortion pill. Wattleton meanwhile set up a DC lobbying office, and Planned Parenthood's total income leapt from about $104 million in 1977 to more than $300 million a decade later.[40] A militant anti-abortion faction, Operation Rescue (OR), entered the national stage around 1988 with its founder, Randall Terry, calling Planned Parenthood "the single largest child killer in the United States."[41] Yet by 1989, just 50 of Planned Parenthood's 178 affiliates were offering abortion care; of the 1.6 million abortions provided in the US in 1988, only 104,000 were at a Planned Parenthood clinic.[42] Independent clinics provided the bulk of abortions in the country amid OR's chilling slogan, "If you believe abortion is murder, then act like it's murder."[43]

OR arguably revealed discord in the American anti-abortion movement.[44] NRLC and Americans United for Life (AUL) pursued what legal scholars have called an incrementalist strategy: use the law to slowly chip away at abortion access, Hyde as one gash, until a Supreme Court one day reversed *Roe*. Terry thought this too slow if abortion was indeed murder. OR led abortion clinic blockades across the country, where hundreds of people (nearly all white) hurled their bodies at clinic entrances to intimidate patients and providers while attempting to shut down abortion care at that clinic that day.[45] Violence against clinics escalated. Between 1977 and 1988, 110 cases of arson, firebombing, or bombing were directed at abortion clinics in the US.[46] And by the early 1990s, 84 percent of US counties had no abortion services at all.[47]

This was the grim world in which Wattleton arrived at Roussel-Uclaf in Paris in 1989 and hoped that these pills, theoretically with any doctor able to prescribe them, might upend a crisis at home. An American taking abortion pills over the counter without a doctor was too radical—and far from reality in France.

When RU-486 first rolled out in France, Roussel-Uclaf and the French government required providers report each mifepristone pill prescribed.[48] Women needed to prove they had been a resident of France for at least three months before taking the pills. And since France approved this method only up to seven weeks in pregnancy, many women may not even know they were pregnant that early. A woman needed to go to a clinic four times to receive the pills, just like in Roussel-Uclaf's trials.[49]

At her first visit, she learned her abortion options (medications or procedure) and decided which was best for her as providers screened for contraindications. On her second visit, after a week-long waiting period, she took mifepristone in front of a doctor. About two days later, she came back to a clinic for a prostaglandin, initially an injection of sulprostone or a suppository of gemeprost. France stopped using sulprostone for medication abortions when a woman died in 1991 of a heart attack after receiving a far higher sulprostone dose than recommended.[50] Hers was one death in around 70,000 cases of people in France who safely had medication abortions with this combined method by then, which meant the drug had a 0.0014 percent mortality rate.[51] France then switched to pairing mifepristone with misoprostol, which was safer than sulprostone as well as cheaper and, as a pill, more portable than gemeprost (which needed to be refrigerated).

Surveys at the time found most women in France who had a medication abortion and aspiration procedure preferred the medications, saying they felt "less traumatizing," "more natural."[52] A medication abortion cost about 850 francs, roughly $140 in 1990, the same as an aspiration in France.[53] But women typically paid only 20 percent of that bill since the French state covered most health care costs, a major difference from the US.[54]

When Wattleton visited Roussel-Uclaf in 1989, she went so far as to pitch to Sakiz that Planned Parenthood buy mifepristone's US patent from the company.[55] She thought the pills could at least expand abortion access within the Planned Parenthood network. Hoechst, which still controlled Roussel-Uclaf, wanted nothing to do with Planned Parenthood. Besides, even if Roussel-Uclaf kept the US patent and ran US trials at Planned Parenthood sites, would the pill get a fair shot at the FDA? Reagan's anti-abortion former vice president George H. W. Bush had just entered the White House and appointed a secretary of the HHS, a role that oversaw the FDA, who was known to be anti-abortion.[56] Sakiz's biggest worry, however, appeared to be whether Planned Parenthood could guarantee that Roussel-Uclaf would not face boycotts if they supplied RU-486 for US trials. Executives anxiously asked Wattleton during her visit how Planned Parenthood would track mifepristone to prevent a "black market," a question Wattleton found insulting. "They seemed to worry about everything except the women who needed what the company had serendipitously discovered," she later wrote.[57]

Hoechst soon announced conditions a country must meet for the company to consider applying to sell RU-486 within that nation's borders, including that abortion be legal there and that the country have "a peaceful atmosphere" on abortion, the latter immediately ruling out the US.[58] In 1989, several anti-abortion US Congressmen, including Representative Henry Hyde of the Hyde Amendment, went further. They wrote to FDA commissioner Dr. Frank Young, urging the agency to ban RU-486 from an obscure loophole, one that let a person bring into the US certain not-yet FDA-approved medications for "personal use."[59] The FDA proceeded to update its "import alert" to tell US Customs and Border Protection to seize anyone who brought RU-486 into the US for their own abortion "because use of the product could present unreasonable safety risk," stated Young.[60] Meanwhile, unlike the US government, the Chinese government repeatedly asked Roussel-Uclaf to sell mifepristone in China. But the company stalled to the point that Chinese officials gave up and synthesized their own mifepristone, flouting patent laws.[61]

As for the "unreasonable safety risk" that the FDA's Young referred to when effectively banning mifepristone from entering the US before anyone even had a chance to apply to the FDA for the medication's approval, the University of Southern California's Dr. David

Grimes ran a study around this same time that found mifepristone's side effects to be as mild as Tylenol.[62] "We've got to get doctors and medical people out of the process," Grimes said in a 1990 *Los Angeles Times* interview, arguing RU-486 should be available over the counter one day.[63]

But Roussel-Uclaf cut off Grimes's supply of pills for his studies soon after the FDA's import ban on the drug went into effect. Scientists in the US struggled to access the medication even for nonabortion studies. The NIH had already been researching RU-486 as a contraceptive and treatment for endometriosis and fibroids, but those studies largely stopped.[64] Democratic Representative Ron Wyden at a 1990 Congressional hearing pressed FDA official Dr. Ronald Chesemore on this confusion, asking, "At the time of the issuance of the import alert, did the FDA have any evidence that a black market was developing on RU-486 in the United States?" Chesemore replied, "I do not believe that we had any concrete evidence."[65]

Wattleton meanwhile braced for the Supreme Court to end *Roe* once and for all. On July 3, 1989, the Court in *Webster v. Reproductive Health Services* gave states greater rein to make abortion access harder.[66] Justice Harry Blackmun, the author of *Roe*, wrote in dissent, "I fear for the future."[67] So did Wattleton. She and other Black feminists worried abortion-seekers themselves were sidelined, including in the reproductive rights movement, all while those in the US who had abortions shifted from mostly white women in the early 1970s to disproportionately Black women by the late 1980s.[68]

Wattleton post-*Webster* joined Black feminists in a manifesto, "We Remember: African American Women Are for Reproductive Freedom," demanding 11 rights that would become tenets of reproductive justice, including the right "to choose to have a child," all linked to Black American women's history.[69] "Brought here in chains, worked like mules, bred like beasts, whipped one day, sold the next—for 244 years we were held in bondage," read the manifesto's opening. "Oh yes, we have known how painful it is to be without choice in this land."[70] Black feminist Loretta Ross, who later co-coined reproductive justice, co-coordinated "We Remember," explaining to *NBC News* in 2019, "We, Black women, who have been very active in reproductive rights for a long time felt like we were leaders without a constituency."[71]

And in 1991 with *Roe* predicted to fall imminently, Wattleton visited Roussel-Uclaf for the third time to plead for mifepristone, now with the Population Council's president George Zeidenstein.[72] The council and the WHO remained the only entities in the world with a guaranteed RU-486 supply for studies. If Roussel-Uclaf refused to sell their US patent to or run trials with Planned Parenthood, maybe the company would cooperate with the council. But Sakiz punted the decision to Hoechst, which did not budge. "They were clearly under the gun of the Germans," Wattleton told me.

About a year later, disillusioned not with the Germans but Americans, she quit Planned Parenthood Federation of America. What pushed Wattleton to leave was ultimately a meeting with allied, "pro-choice" politicians in Congress over a drafted bill to codify *Roe*, only this bill (which never passed) outlined sharp concessions on abortion rights that enraged her. She could not stomach how her own side bargained over women's bodily autonomy. As she later wrote, "an era of battling was ending and one of accommodation was taking hold."[73]

Months after Wattleton quit in 1992, the Supreme Court did not end *Roe* as both the anti-abortion and reproductive rights movements expected, surprising the nation in *Planned Parenthood of Southeastern Pennsylvania v. Casey*.[74] The decision instead again made it easier for states to restrict abortion access.[75] To Wattleton, the country seemed numb to its own cruelty in this era of accommodation.

"I know it sounds reproachful or even rebuking, but I will accept that label because we did not get here because this was an act of God," Wattleton told me in 2023 of the post-*Dobbs* US. "We got here due to enormous complacency and neglect. Now it's a much harder task to restore a right that has been taken away. . . . And those who methodically restructured the federal judiciary against abortion are moving on to the subject your book is covering: access to pills. The irony is pills can be passed in the mail, which brings us back to the Comstock laws. Back to Margaret Sanger being arrested for passing out birth control leaflets. Back to the first quarter of the twentieth century."

CHAPTER 6

THE BELLY OF THE BEAST

On December 5, 1991, in DC, 46-year-old Dr. Beverly Winikoff testified about a pill she could not get out of her head. "I just want to stop for a moment and address the question about why one might *care* about how women *feel* about this alternative," she stated to the mainly white male politicians before her inside the Rayburn House Office Building.[1] A senior medical associate at the Population Council, Winikoff spoke at the second of four Congressional hearings on RU-486 that US Representative Ron Wyden led. She *did* care about how women felt about these pills, and she did not need someone on the Hill to tell her why their voices mattered. "I was so happy to be there," Winikoff told me more than 30 years later. "Because you were in the belly of the beast. It seemed like this was where you could make things happen."

What she wanted to make happen would take her almost four decades (and counting) to see come true. "It's impossible to stop this train," she told me in 2023 with abortion effectively banned in almost half of US states yet more pills flowing across the country than ever before. Winikoff looked at me then flung her hand in the air and curled it into a fist. "If I go like this, I could have a dozen abortions right there. . . . Pills have legs."

Abortion was not taboo in Winikoff's home growing up as a Jewish girl in Manhattan, though her mother's gynecologist was arrested before *Roe* for performing illegal abortions. That made Winikoff proud. In high school when a friend told her abortion should be banned, Winikoff was sincerely confused: "What do you *mean*? And let a pregnancy you didn't want ruin your life?"

Winikoff's mother, who was a stay-at-home mom, encouraged her daughter's ambition. As a kid, Winikoff announced to her mom one day that she wanted to be a nurse, only her mom asked why she didn't want to be a doctor. Winikoff had not even thought of that. When Winikoff later in college considered becoming an ambassador, her mother warned her against that path "because you're a woman and you're Jewish and you're not going to get far." Be ambitious, yes. But also, be strategic. Find where you can make change and do it. Winikoff eventually became a doctor in global health. The day the Supreme Court decided *Roe*, she stood up and cheered with classmates in her packed graduate school lecture. She had already finished medical school and was nearly done with her public health degree. Soon after *Roe*, Winikoff testified to Congress for the first time, not on abortion but breastfeeding. "Mom-and-apple-pie kind of stuff," she told me.

The council recruited her in 1978 to study breastfeeding as a possible contraceptive, a decision made under the nonprofit's new president, George Zeidenstein. He wanted the council to move away from its population control roots and towards feminism. For the first time, thanks to Zeidenstein, the council began researching abortion around when Winikoff joined the team.

Winikoff liked to remember women imagined abortion pills before they existed. In the late 1970s, a feminist gynecologist based in India visited her at the council's New York office to ask a question. Her patients were women in rural, poor communities, and they wanted to know why, if one pill can prevent pregnancy, another pill can't end a pregnancy. Winikoff thought this question brilliant, only she knew of no abortion pill. The doctor didn't believe her. *How is that possible? We need it.* Years passed until, in the mid-1980s, Winikoff heard a talk at the council with Roussel-Uclaf researchers from France presenting on RU-486. To Winikoff, this pill was pure magic. "You didn't need anybody to *do* anything to you," she said. "You didn't need to lie down on a table and have something inserted into you. You just could take a pill. That was revolutionary. And it meant this [pill] could go places where medical services didn't go."[2]

She befriended Roussel-Uclaf's Dr. André Ulmann, and they became close collaborators in researching RU-486 more. Ulmann did not have freedom at Roussel-Uclaf to do all the studies he wanted to do, but Winikoff, through the council, could pursue those avenues that he could not. Winikoff especially sought to know what women actually felt about their medication abortions in their own words, known as "acceptability" studies. She helped lead the council's early studies in India and Cuba asking women what their experiences were like, eventually bringing their voices into her testimony at that December 1991 Congressional hearing.

Among those joining Winikoff to testify that day were France's Dr. Étienne-Émile Baulieu and Sweden's Dr. Marc Bygdeman, the latter already studying RU-486 as a promising contraceptive. The spectacle of American abortion politics baffled the Europeans. "They didn't have the vicious antis we had here—and the huge pushback," Winikoff told me. "They were always very quiet in Europe. But part of that was because they kept [medication abortion] so sequestered. . . . They were very happy with the medicalization, and I was not very happy with the medicalization." Baulieu did indeed testify proudly at that 1991 hearing about France's four-clinic-visit model for pills, a model Winikoff hated.

When it was her turn to speak as one of the only female researchers present, Winikoff channeled her mother's strategic thinking to explain to the men in suits why these pills mattered to women. She did so by comparing abortion pills to none other than cars, that stereotypically masculine product. "One may ask, 'Why produce red cars when we already have very good blue cars?'" Winikoff testified. "'Why do we need medical abortion when we have a safe and effective technology in surgical abortion?'"

She proceeded to share the council's early findings that about 90 percent of women who had a medication abortion said they would choose the pills again. Of those who had an abortion procedure before, 83 percent preferred the medications, often saying this new method was more in their control. And so, Winikoff concluded, choosing between a medication or procedural abortion was not really like choosing between a red or blue car. It may be more like choosing between a small car to park in a tight space or a big car to fit a large family. Some preferred a procedure, others pills. Different people had different needs, and this method "fits a previously unmet need."[3]

Later that day, the NRLC's education director, Dr. Richard Glasow, testified on behalf of, in his words, "those innocent human beings whose life is threatened by abortion infanticide and euthanasia."[4] He argued that "proponents of RU-486 do not have a monopoly on scientific truth" but "an ideologic agenda that they cloak under the guise of science." Without evidence, he claimed medication abortions scarred women psychologically, then he needled at a favorite line in the press: this method was private and easy. But how were four clinic visits private or easy? (Winikoff thought the same, only with entirely opposite goals in mind.)

Glasow's point that a scientist can cloak ideologies in objective truth was not exactly wrong. Scientists were (and are) people with conscious and unconscious biases that can shape the questions they ask. In 1990, the General Accounting Office (today the Government Accountability Office) found the NIH barely included women in NIH-funded research.[5] But of course, the anti-abortion movement had been cloaking sexist, racist ideologies in objective truth repeatedly. When Wyden asked Glasow if the NRLC supported any testing of mifepristone, even for nonabortion uses, Glasow replied, "There is plenty of evidence that it is too dangerous to be put on the market anywhere." When Wyden asked for the NRLC's position on contraception, Glasow stated, "Sir, we take no position on contraception, period." Eleanor Smeal, president of the Feminist Majority Foundation (FMF), sat next to Glasow during this hearing and bolted upright, saying the International Right to Life Committee, an NRLC affiliate, opposed contraception beyond "natural family planning." She asked Wyden to ask Glasow why this contradiction. Glasow refused to answer.

RU-486 was still no closer to being offered in the US when the 1991 hearing ended, but both Winikoff and Wyden had hope that change was coming. "What I wanted from that hearing room was to make 'mifepristone' a household word," Wyden told me. "That was our lone star: to drive awareness." That "our" included an American coalition of around

40 reproductive health and rights leaders, almost all women (Winikoff among them), who had been strategizing about RU-486 since at least 1988 under the last days of the Reagan administration.

Marie Bass, then in her early forties, read in September 1988 about France approving an abortion pill and excitedly called her friend and business partner, Joanne Howes. Both thought RU-486 could end America's abortion conflict, or at least turn the dial down.

They ran a small, struggling consulting company in DC and were politically active. When Bass's other friend became head of the National Abortion Rights Action League (NARAL) in the early 1980s, she asked for Bass's help with their political action committee (PAC), a tax-exempt organization giving money to political campaigns. The NARAL PAC was flush with cash under Reagan as donors worried the end of *Roe* was nigh. Bass helped find political candidates this PAC should support and teach candidates, who were mostly white men (though she wanted far more women), how to talk about abortion. But over and over, candidates stumbled on abortion and lost elections.[6] Bass came to believe "mistakenly," she told me, that if abortion could be taken out of politics altogether, then the country could move on. "So, when we started hearing about RU-486, I thought that maybe, just maybe if women could put everything in their own hands, then that would do it," she told me. "Then that would mean [abortion] would not be this hot-button political issue."

Bass and Howes secured a small grant to start a DC advocacy group to bring mifepristone into the US. Abuzz on France's "moral property of women" line in late October 1988, they invited to an inaugural meeting what were then called women of color health groups, including the National Black Women's Health Project (NBWHP), alongside the larger usual suspects, like Planned Parenthood (still under Faye Wattleton) and the council (still under Zeidenstein). Yet to Bass's surprise, not everyone at the meeting greeted this pill enthusiastically. Mifepristone hit a nerve. "There was an old animosity between the people who were—and, frankly, in those days, a lot of the groups were—based around population control, and then there were the feminist health groups," Bass told me. One woman in the latter camp told her at the meeting, "You realize that women in rural India will bleed to death and die from this pill?" That image kept a horrified Bass up at night.

These old animosities stemmed from a knowledge gap on mifepristone and past scandals with reproductive health pharmaceuticals, including the council's Norplant, as mentioned earlier in the book. Feminist health groups were against population control, fearing the US would push RU-486 on largely poor women of color without vetting its safety and ethics thoroughly.[7] The groups with histories of population control asserted that RU-486 was indeed safe. The coalition did not come to a consensus on the medication that day, but everyone agreed they should keep talking. Then as more studies came out, anxieties dissipated. And the coalition, which Bass and Howes named the Reproductive Health Technologies Project (RHTP), began lobbying Congress, including Wyden.

While Wyden wanted to focus public attention on RU-486's potential nonabortion uses, Bass did not and, behind that 1991 Congressional hearing, urged him to listen. "I may have been wrong, but I came down on the side that this is abortion. We have to deal with this head-on and not try to say, 'Oh, but it's really this, it's really that,'" Bass told me. "We always used the term 'abortion.'"

So did longtime, wealthy abortion-rights activist Larry Lader, then in his seventies, who was not in RHTP and not exactly the lobbying kind. Lader wrote a biography of Margaret Sanger and, in 1966, a book titled *Abortion*, its first line reading, "Abortion is the dread secret of our society."[8] When women who read that book began asking him where to find a safe abortion pre-*Roe*, Lader became an activist and, in 1969, co-founded NARAL, which was then called the National Association for the Repeal of Abortion Laws and focused on a state-by-state campaign to legalize abortion. Supreme Court Justice Harry Blackmun would cite Lader's *Abortion* eight times in *Roe*.[9] But Lader, stunned at *Roe*'s swift victory, saw the abortion rights movement transform overnight, NARAL renaming itself the National Abortion Rights Action League and shifting strategies to broadening its base as well as lobbying Congress.

Lader felt the organization became more moderate after *Roe*, prompting him to leave NARAL in 1975.[10] By 1982, NARAL had more than 10 times as many members as when he left and a fleet of attorneys with a DC headquarters, "a luxury we never had," he wrote of their pre-*Roe* activism.[11] "But perhaps NARAL was right in surrounding itself in corporate trappings," he added. "It now had to be a key player on Capitol Hill."[12] Lader, however, did not have to be a DC player mingling with buttoned-up politicians; he could be more publicly aggressive than lobbyists on the Hill. He soon founded Abortion Rights Mobilization (ARM), a small leftist activist group, and wrote about mifepristone as critical to the country's future, even titling his 1991 book *RU-486: The Pill That Could End the Abortion Wars and Why American Women Don't Have It.*[13] In it, he wrote a plan to raise public outcry over RU-486, with Sanger in mind.

In 1933 in New York, a package of pessaries (a kind of diaphragm) arrived from Japan for Dr. Hannah Stone when Customs seized the parcel for violating the Comstock Act. This was a setup Sanger engineered, tipping off Customs to ensure an arrest and then force a challenge to an anti–birth control law in court.[14] In *United States v. One Package* in 1936, Stone won back the pessaries, a court ruling a ban on importing birth control devices did not refer to "things which might intelligently be employed by conscientious and competent physicians to promote the well-being of patients."[15] To Lader, why not do something similar with the FDA's 1989 import ban on RU-486? Why not make a media spectacle the new Bush administration could not ignore? "If US Customs seized the pills, the receiving doctor could go into federal court, as Sanger had done, to force the government to return the package to him or her," wrote Lader. "A victory would give enough legitimacy to the abortion pill to rouse the indignation of American women and to put considerable pressure on the White House and the FDA."[16]

But Sanger's *One Package* case needed tweaking for the 1990s. The UK had just recently approved mifepristone, so Lader could travel to London with an American pregnant person who wanted an abortion, surreptitiously pick up pills there, then the two could come back. ARM could tip off Customs to seize the pills at New York City's JFK airport upon return. Only this plan paid little attention to the abortion-seeker, as if she were a prop in a play. Lader, like Sanger, did indeed have a troubling side, the *Boston Globe* in 1997 noting "altruism and ego" seemed to drive him.[17] He also wrote of China's one-child policy ambivalently: "Yet with all these complications, the Chinese experiment provides a model that may have to be followed elsewhere, at least in part . . . a system of democratic punishments and inducements will have to be adopted in such countries as India, where population pressures are severe."[18] It was perhaps no wonder ARM had a hard time finding, in Lader's words, a "Jane Roe of the 1990s" to pull this plan off.

Yet in June 1992, Lader got a lead: Leona Benten, a feminist-anarchist in Berkeley, was 29 and about six weeks pregnant. She believed in bodily autonomy, queer liberation, and prison reform. She volunteered at a feminist clinic in Oakland and, when she went there for an abortion, the clinic director told her ARM's plan, asking if she was interested in helping bring attention to the abortion pill.[19] She wanted in. In 1983, Benten had an unsettling abortion procedure in a hospital. "I don't like surgery, I don't like hospitals, and I believe in self-determination," she told the *New York Times* in 1992. "So, I'd much rather take a pill than put myself in the hands of someone who's going to do a procedure on me."[20]

Lader quickly flew Benten to New York, where she arrived in jeans, without the polish he wanted for mainstream media appeal.[21] She borrowed a black skirt to wear at their eventual JFK press conference once they would fly back from the UK with the pills. ARM prepared statements to go out to the press, FDA, and Customs saying RU-486 was on its way. Lader and Benten flew to London on a Monday and arrived there on Tuesday, someone in the city anonymously handing Lader an envelope with RU-486 pills. The next day, the two sat on their return flight. Benten, pregnant and exhausted, wore that black skirt. Lader gave her mifepristone to hold and, when they landed, the two walked through Customs. When asked if she carried unapproved drugs, Benten said, "Yes," and gave the pills. She was not arrested.

Benten stepped into the JFK arrivals area to a media turnout bigger than expected. Lader was thrilled, only Benten, overwhelmed, cried. "I tend to go into things thinking I'll be O.K.," she told the *New York*

Times in 1992. "But it was very hard at the airport when they confiscated the pills, after I hadn't slept in three days, and hadn't been able to eat because I was nauseous from the pregnancy. And the hardest thing is feeling like a yo-yo, waiting as all these other people decide what's going to happen to me."[22]

Days later, Benten and Lader sued the FDA in *Benten v. Kessler* ("Kessler" for Dr. David Kessler, then FDA commissioner), arguing the RU-486 import alert illegal. A judge ordered the pills be returned to Benten.[23] But then a conservative court stayed that order before she could reclaim the pills. ARM appealed, and the Supreme Court agreed to hear the case, Benten still in limbo. The court decided 7–2 against Benten days later.[24] They lost. Except to Lader, they won anyways. They made it to the highest court in the country. The press was widespread. People asked President George H. W. Bush and competing candidate Democrat Bill Clinton about RU-486 weeks before the November 1992 presidential election, with Clinton pledging to help bring RU-486 trials to the US if he was elected president.[25] Didn't the plan work?

But what about Benten? She wanted pills to be the story, not her. Yet some reporters found her home address and hounded her, going through her mail.[26] A *New York Times* story dismissively described Benten as "the pregnant, unmarried 29-year-old," and a headline in the *Los Angeles Times* declared, "An Unorthodox 'Everywoman': Leona Benten was supposed to engender sympathy in her role as banner-carrier for RU486. But she proved to have a mind, and an agenda, of her own."[27] God forbid. The press met her unapologetic search for an abortion, let alone a second abortion, with open hostility as Benten publicly defied Clinton's campaign line that abortion be "safe and legal, but rare."[28]

However, Benten told reporters in 1992 she would do this RU-486 activism again if given the chance, only she "never wanted to be famous like this."[29] She reiterated that years later, how no one forced her activism. She believed in what she did, even if she hated how the press and some fellow reproductive rights activists treated her.[30] Today, Benten no longer speaks to reporters. And in 1992, after the Supreme Court decided her case and that yo-yo-ing over her body stopped, she walked into a clinic in Oakland and had her procedure.

Lader may have taken credit for pushing mifepristone into the American public eye, but he could not take credit for the 1992 election when Democrats, for the first time in more than a decade, won the White House. To Bass at RHTP and Winikoff at the council, Clinton's victory meant mifepristone finally had a chance. Clinton would appoint a new secretary of the HHS to oversee the FDA, replacing Bush's anti-abortion appointee with the first woman to hold the post, Dr. Donna Shalala. And FDA Commissioner David Kessler promptly wrote in December 1992 to Roussel-Uclaf's CEO Sakiz, formally inviting the company to file mifepristone's New Drug Application (NDA) to the FDA.[31] The agency could make no promises. But the letter, unlike the FDA's import ban on mifepristone a few years earlier, was an olive branch.

On January 22, 1993, two days after Clinton's inauguration and on *Roe's* twentieth anniversary, the new president wrote a memo instructing his new secretary of the HHS to "assess initiatives . . . [that can] promote the testing, licensing, and manufacturing of RU-486 or other antiprogestins."[32] Clinton told the press, "Here in the United States, RU-486 has been held hostage to politics. It is time to learn the truth about what the health and safety risks of the drug really are."[33] That truth had been learned with studies around the world, of course, just not yet for the FDA's review. The leader of one of the most powerful countries now urged one pharmaceutical company to relinquish one product.

Outside the White House that same day, thousands of anti-abortion protesters gathered in DC for the twentieth annual March for Life, the victory of pro-choice Clinton be damned. "We were not supposed to be here, according to the press," sneered Nellie Gray, the founder and president of March for Life, overlooking a shouting crowd of mostly white people. *Casey* had just been decided that summer, failing to end *Roe* and casting doubts on the anti-abortion movement's lasting power. "This movement was supposed to be dead. Are you dead? No! The movement is *strong*."[34] Gray, who dressed in all red that day to symbolize blood of the "unborn," believed abortion should be entirely, nationally banned and was known for her motto "no exceptions, no compromise."[35]

Byllye Avery was under no illusions that the anti-abortion movement was dead. She was not focused on mifepristone in 1993, however, but on ending the lingering Hyde Amendment. Now that Democrats had control of the White House and Congress for the first time since before Reagan's 1980 election, she wanted the party to move quickly to strike down Hyde's nearly two-decade ban on federal funding of abortion care.[36]

A longtime Black feminist health activist, Avery opened one of Florida's first independent abortion clinics in the 1970s when *Roe* came. But she noticed that most people seeking abortions at the clinic were Black like her while the pro-choice movement's visible leadership remained largely white. Something was wrong. In the 1980s, Avery pioneered health workshops run for, by, and with Black women, founding the NBWHP. She heard in Black women's stories far more complexity than she found in pro-choice messaging on abortion. To her, talking about abortion as an individual "choice" ignored a person's social context, overlooking structural inequities like racism and poverty, which all felt woefully out-of-touch with many abortion-seekers' lives: "To say to a person who feels beaten down and who does not have the means 'you have a choice' is nonsense."[37]

And so, when Avery was asked in 1993 if FDA approval of mifepristone would end America's abortion debate, she was emphatic: no.[38] She tried to return attention to ending Hyde. Avery did not see how a pill alone could change a social context in which an anti-abortion movement fought tooth-and-nail to control women's bodies, especially Black women's bodies, and a mainstream reproductive rights movement seemed to be siloing abortion while deprioritizing issues like Black maternal mortality disparities. In 1994, one of Avery's mentees, Loretta Ross, joined fellow Black feminists to abandon pro-choice language and coin a broader framework of "reproductive justice."[39] The term spliced reproductive rights and social justice. It was defined simply as: 1) the right not to have a child; 2) the right to have a child; and 3) the right to parent children in safe and healthy environments with dignity.[40] Hyde meanwhile remained.

CHAPTER 7

"THE PILL THAT CHANGES EVERYTHING"

D r. David Gunn parked his car outside Pensacola Women's Medical Services in Florida while trying to ignore the anti-abortion protestors hurling slurs at him. It was the morning of March 10, 1993. Anti-abortion crowds had been gathering outside the clinic for months, shaming Gunn and any women who entered for care. These crowds seethed and stewed, though there was a sense that they were waiting for something worse to happen. That day something did.

As Gunn stepped out of his car, preparing to start his job providing abortion procedures for the many people expecting this care, a young white man slowly emerged from the mass of protestors. Few noticed him at first. He was quiet. The man then raised a revolver and yelled, "Don't kill any more babies," shooting Gunn one, two, three times.[1] Gunn did not survive. He became the first person in the US to be murdered for providing abortions.

At a Florida rally the week before, Randall Terry of OR said, "We've found the weak link is the doctor."[2] OR distributed "(un)Wanted" posters of Gunn, with one line on the posters reading, "[Gunn] also kills children at Pensacola Medical Services 7100 Plantation Road Unit 3 478–2477."[3] Terry denied culpability in Gunn's assassination and was not arrested.[4] A decade of anti-abortion terrorism, with little accountability, was just beginning.

Gunn's shooter was handcuffed and, while sitting in jail before his trial, received fawning letters from a white OR member named Shelley Shannon.[5] Months later at another clinic in Kansas, Shannon took a gun from her white purse and shot Dr. George Tiller, one of the nation's few later abortion care providers and a longtime target of anti-abortion harassment.[6] Tiller survived Shannon's assassination attempt and, determined not to give up, continued to provide later abortions at that same clinic. When Shannon, too, was arrested, police found buried in the backyard of her Oregon home an explosive-making manual from the Army of God (AOG), an American anti-abortion terrorist group with white supremacist underpinnings. Investigators also discovered Shannon's diaries, in which she documented in gleeful detail her bombing spree at eight abortion clinics the year before.[7]

After watching an OR recruiting video in the late 1980s, Shannon enthusiastically joined clinic blockades, where she met extremist AOG members and rapidly turned to violence.[8] The signs of her dangerous descent were largely ignored by law enforcement. Between 1988 and 1993, as Shannon became more aggressive, police arrested her almost 50 times and charged her with a crime 35 times, usually simply sentencing her to community service.[9] Even the Office of the Attorney General, after discovering Shannon's AOG explosive-making manual, still authorized only one agent to investigate her links to anti-abortion terrorist groups nationwide.[10] A jury later convicted Shannon in 1994 of the attempted murder of Tiller and sentenced her to prison. More than a decade later when anti-abortion extremist Scott Roeder assassinated Tiller in 2009, shooting the abortion provider while he was in church in Kansas, investigators found Roeder had been regularly writing to Shannon in prison.[11]

In 1993, the year of Gunn's assassination and Tiller's attempted assassination, abortion clinics reported roughly twice as many bomb threats, pieces of hate mail, and harassing calls compared to the year before.[12] RU-486 amid this dramatic uptick in violence became even more of an imagined panacea for the country's abortion access crisis in the eyes of many feminists. A June 1993 *TIME* cover agreed, showing a woman holding up a mifepristone tablet beneath the bold headline, "The Pill That Changes Everything."[13] With RU-486, feminists hoped that more doctors across the country could prescribe abortion pills. That could make it even harder for extremists like Shannon to target all abortion clinics and providers. But rising violence also scared away US pharmaceutical companies from buying mifepristone's US patent, even if Roussel-Uclaf agreed to sell that patent.

Dr. André Ulmann remained an advocate for mifepristone within Roussel-Uclaf as the company, when it merged into Hoechst Roussel in 1992, became more dysfunctional under Hoechst's heightened control. The company now formally banned Ulmann from launching mifepristone studies, especially in the US, "where under no circumstances would they allow us to file an application," he later wrote.[14] Ulmann became convinced that only a single-product company dedicated solely to mifepristone could withstand anti-abortion threats. In 1993, the year Clinton entered the White House and called for mifepristone's release to the US, Ulmann and a few former Roussel-Uclaf colleagues formed a startup company to buy mifepristone's global patent from Hoechst Roussel. Yet Hoechst Roussel refused, speciously claiming that its former employees working at this startup could still expose Hoechst Roussel to liabilities.[15] Ulmann was furious.

That dead-end meant mifepristone's journey to the US would depend on the Population Council, the nonprofit that had been studying medication abortion for a decade by then. The council had a new president, Margaret Catley-Carlson, who seized the momentum of their prior president, George Zeidenstein, to do what no one else had: secure mifepristone's US patent, run US clinical trials, file an FDA application, and land the pill's FDA approval, all for this pill to reach American women. This ideally needed to get done before the November 1996 presidential election when, if Clinton lost, an anti-abortion president could stall the pill again. And this had to happen without anyone bombing or assassinating the council's members.

Only the council was not a business. They could do research, but a company needed to sell the pill on the US market if the medication did get approved. Hoechst Roussel in 1993, after much pressuring from the Hill and RHTP members lobbying, verbally agreed to let the council run US trials and sublicense the pill's US patent to another company.[16] Mifepristone could be on the market by 1996, even 1995. Except it took more than a year to finalize a contract. Hoechst Roussel sought impossibly extensive liability protections from the US government itself. "If the extremists decided to blow up the plant or shoot somebody, that they would be indemnified against anything that the fanatics . . . would do," said Eleanor Smeal of the FMF in the 1997 documentary *The Abortion Pill.* "[That was] simply something that the United States government could not sign."[17]

In May 1994, the company finally acquiesced and gave the council mifepristone's US patent entirely for free. Why? "Because they wanted to be completely out of any question of liability," Ulmann told me. He was convinced Hoechst Roussel tried its hardest to sabotage the medication's path to the US. Ulmann's startup, the same one Hoechst Roussel rejected, now bid to the council to be the company tasked with selling the pill in the US, only it was rejected again. "We understood that probably there was some, I would say, lobbying against our position from Hoechst, which did not want us," he told me. "Because they knew that if we were in the picture, it would come to the US."

Ulmann had slim competition in the US. No big pharmaceutical companies bid to the council; they were too frightened or apathetic or both.[18] The council instead chose another startup called Danco Laboratories, run by lawyer-entrepreneur Joseph Pike, whom the nonprofit had worked well with before.[19] It seemed a safe bet. Only that pick would nearly upend the pill.

The council's vice president of corporate affairs, Sandra (Sandy) Arnold, became the logistical captain of "the mifepristone project," overseeing media inquiries, FDA relations, and an eventual morass of litigation, all while, she was told, federal agents were assigned to protect her from anti-abortion extremists. "Everywhere along the road, it was handled with a great deal of sensitivity to the fact that it was a political time bomb," recalled the now late Arnold in a 2020 student interview. "My sense was if they're gonna shoot me, they're gonna shoot me. . . . I don't know why I was that gutsy. My life has not been characterized by being out there in any way. But I had just decided that this was an important thing, and I could do it."[20]

Weeks after the council secured mifepristone's US patent in May 1994, a white anti-abortion extremist man, who was a known AOG member, assassinated abortion provider Dr. John Britton and his body-guard Colonel James Barrett at another Florida clinic.[21] A few months later, inside two Massachusetts abortion clinics, a white anti-abortion extremist man murdered two women.[22] The council's US clinical trials had already started.

While Arnold sat on the managerial side of the mifepristone project, Winikoff sat on the research side, critically weaving acceptability studies into the trials. But the council's Dr. Wayne Bardin, who was more senior than Winikoff, was officially in charge. Bardin was a decorated scientist, having developed the council's controversial Norplant, and apparently had an ego to match.[23] Winikoff did not get along with him at all.[24] This was not just a clash of personalities but of vision. Bardin wanted more lab research on mifepristone. "And we wanted to get the damn pills out there and approved by the FDA," Dr. George Brown of the council told me. Brown, as a vice president of the council at the time, was the same rank as Bardin and supervised Winikoff—but he was clear to me that Winikoff, not he, played a major role in the medication abortion trials. He admired her for that. Winikoff firmly believed Bardin did not love these pills as much as she did, as if Bardin felt that working on abortion tainted his legacy, or he just did not understand how important these pills could be to women. But she did.

Winikoff and her direct report, a young Dr. Charlotte Ellertson, wanted to de-medicalize pills, to one day put mifepristone and miso-prostol in women's hands, not under the control of doctors.[25] They titled a 1997 co-authored paper "Can Women Use Medical Abortion Without Medical Supervision?"[26] But Ellertson and Winikoff were stuck fighting with Bardin over who should run each of the trial sites. He wanted the nation's highest-ranking gynecologists at top universities to do so, only those were mostly older white men. Winikoff and Ellertson knew as well that some of those men mistreated women. The pair did not want those men anywhere near the trials. Besides, they wanted more women in charge. They managed to make sure roughly half of the principal investigators were women, which Winikoff still thought too few.

Bardin also wanted to repeat the four-clinic-visit Roussel-Uclaf model, only misoprostol pills were now being used with mifepristone. With Winikoff's maneuvering, the council's trials instead required women to have three clinic visits, not four, though they still needed to stay for hours under "medical supervision" after taking misoprostol. Winikoff thought that overkill but better than what she saw in Europe. Years earlier, she visited a medication abortion study site at the University of Edinburgh led by Dr. David Baird with the World Health Organization (WHO). She was aghast to see rows of women in hospital beds, bleeding and cramping there while "under observation." A nurse (a woman) saw her and, referring to Baird (a man), quietly asked, "Will you please tell the professor that these women don't need to be in the hospital?" Winikoff understood.

"Women know how to bleed and know if something's not going right," she told me. "If it's a lot, they can figure it out. If it's painful and it shouldn't be, they can figure that out. But guys don't understand that. How many times do people have a menstrual period in their whole life? It's a lot. It's hundreds. And these guys never had one."

Just north of Seattle in 1995, a 34-year-old woman, whose pseudonym was Sheryl Knowlen, walked into Aurora Medical Services for her appointment. Her doctor performed a pelvic exam and ultrasound on her, checking how far along she was in her pregnancy. The doctor told her what to expect with a medication abortion, answered her questions, and asked how she felt. She swallowed three mifepristone pills there. Two days later, Knowlen came back to the clinic to swallow misoprostol pills and stay about four hours "under observation." Throughout, she noted how much she bled and when, how much she cramped and when, how nauseous she felt and when. The process did hurt and take time, but the experience was okay. She was okay. About two weeks after her first visit, Knowlen returned for a pelvic exam to be sure she passed her pregnancy. That was all.[27]

Knowlen, who had three abortion procedures before, was among the more than 2,000 American women in mifepristone's FDA application.

Seattle's Aurora was one of the council's roughly 17 trial sites across the country; each site offered a medication abortion for free. The council kept the locations of these sites a secret due to security concerns.

After Knowlen had her abortion with pills, Aurora staff asked if she wanted to be in a documentary, *The Abortion Pill*. The directors, Marion Lipschutz and Rose Rosenblatt, told her they interviewed people who had medication abortions in France, the UK, China, and India, even women who took over-the-counter misoprostol in Brazil (before the country restricted the pill). But they struggled to find Americans to speak on camera about their abortions with pills. Knowlen thought this was due to a "climate of violence" on abortion in the country.[28] Under a pseudonym, however, she agreed to be interviewed. "If abortion had not been legal when I first got pregnant, I might be dead now," she said. "So, I feel that going through these interviews and being public is part of the payback."[29] Because of that climate of violence, the abortion provider who ran Aurora did not show her face in the documentary, which also did not name Aurora. That provider, Dr. Suzanne Poppema, once had an abortion too.

In the late 1970s while a medical resident in Seattle, Poppema was 20 weeks pregnant and did not "notice quote unquote" her pregnancy sooner, she told me. If she became a parent at that time, she worried that she might never realize her dream to be a family medicine physician. She was also raised Catholic and wrestled with shame about abortion. Yet the male doctor who performed her abortion procedure told her gently as she sobbed on the exam table, "Suzanne, you need to understand that you will never be judgmental about other patients ever again." She thought, *That's true*. "I remember having a special kind of conversation with the embryo at the time," Poppema later wrote. "'I'm very sorry that this is happening to you, but there's just no way that you can come into existence right now.' It was so clear to me that I was doing the right thing."[30]

That clarity was how she felt about becoming a doctor. At Harvard University Medical School in the 1970s, Poppema was one of about a dozen women in her class. Sexism in medicine stunned her. Poppema found some reprieve in befriending feminists at the Boston

Women's Health Book Collective (who wrote *Our Bodies, Ourselves*). She learned more about abortion from them, not medical school. To many of these feminists, the white male-dominated OBGYN field was synonymous with patriarchy: a woman lying naked in stirrups, a man in between her legs in control of her body.[31] Only 16 percent of OBGYN residents in 1975 in the US were women (that shot up to 83 percent by 2015).[32]

Poppema chose family medicine because she believed it the "backbone" of health care. She became active on abortion rights a year after *Roe* when, in 1974, a Black medical resident, Dr. Kenneth Edelin, was arrested for performing a legal, later abortion procedure at Boston City Hospital.[33] An all-white 12-member jury convicted Edelin of manslaughter; nine jury members were men. Poppema was horrified that Boston City Hospital, "in its great stupidness, stripped [Edelin] of his residency until the charges were dealt with," she told me. She joined protests to push the hospital to return his residency. Edelin's conviction was later unanimously overturned on appeal. "That was a lightning rod for me," she told me.

After her own abortion a few years later, Poppema was determined to learn to provide abortion procedures herself, only no one in her residency could teach her. They did not know how. She found a physician at a family planning clinic who could teach her and did so. Poppema kept urging her residency program to teach abortion care, to no avail. When she opened a family medicine practice in a conservative area near Seattle, she told her colleagues that she would provide abortions. "One of them said, 'Over my dead body you'll be doing those here.' And I said, 'Well, that'll be sad because I'm doing them,'" she told me.

Some of her family medicine patients were strongly anti-abortion, though Poppema was still the person they called to deliver their babies. One such patient once asked her if it was true that she performed abortions. "'I said, 'Yes, and I know that's very difficult for you. So, I understand if you need me to help you find another doctor,'" Poppema told me. "And she never did because I wasn't the evil baby killer." Poppema believed convincing family medicine doctors to provide abortions could not only expand access but also destigmatize abortion. Because to her, good family medicine doctors were trusted community members and thus difficult to demonize.

Around 1982, she opened Aurora Medical Services and provided a range of reproductive care, including abortion, decorating the space with calm paintings and soft lighting (she called herself a "hippie doctor"). Some women apologized to Poppema during their abortion procedures, and she would gently say they were welcome to do so but did not have to. When she learned around 1989 of RU-486, Poppema was ecstatic. "This is totally it," she told me. "The Reagan years have happened. The poop is hitting the fan. This is going to free us from everything. Because anybody can be an abortion provider. You don't need fancy equipment. You don't need hospital privileges. You just need half a brain and a big heart." Then after the shock of Gunn's murder, Poppema began to wear a bulletproof vest each day to work while holding more closely that hope of pills freeing the country. As soon as she had a chance, she signed up to lead one of the council's trial sites. "And I told people, 'You'll see,'" Poppema told me. "'Before the end of this decade, it'll be approved.'" That did not happen.

Post-*Dobbs*, Poppema is today retired but kept her medical license to prescribe and mail pills to thousands of people in abortion-restrictive or ban states. She was one of the first American providers to send pills to people in the COVID-19 pandemic. When Texas's six-week abortion ban struck in 2021, she prescribed more pills. Friends advised her to not be public about her work, fearful she may be attacked. But Poppema spoke out because, at the end of her career, she could take risks many younger providers could not. She helped Washington pass a law post-*Dobbs* protecting providers from extradition if sued for prescribing pills to people in a ban state. She kept going. "And it's exhausting, but I can't, I can't give up. I just won't give up," she told me. "I'll go out kicking and screaming. But yeah, I'll be kicking and screaming about reproductive justice."

When we spoke in 2023, Poppema appeared deeply sad, bluntly calling her decades of reproductive justice activism "a slog against terminal depression, really," that ever since Reagan, "it's blow after blow after blow." Pills nonetheless continued to promise something to her. "I still hold mifepristone and misoprostol as our little shining orb that we're keeping close to us because we know, we *know* it's our key," she told me, then cried, surprising herself. "It's a home-free kind of talisman. And the more women know about it is what we need."

For years before medication abortion pills existed, Poppema traveled with a manual vacuum aspiration kit in her car, so that if a patient needed an abortion procedure, she could be there right away. Poppema now wanted every household to have an abortion-pills kit. Even if no one in the household used the pills, maybe a friend will one day ask for help.

After the council's trials finished in late 1995, the new Republican-controlled Congress wasted no time in aggressively passing a "partial-birth abortion" ban.[34] The NRLC coined the medically inaccurate term "partial-birth abortion" to shift public attention from more socially accepted earlier abortions (like when taking pills) to more stigmatized later abortions (like the abortion procedure Poppema once needed).[35] The life-saving medical procedure considered closest to a "partial-birth abortion" is dilation and extraction (D&E or D&X), one of the safest ways to end a person's later pregnancy.[36] Some people who need a D&E cannot safely carry a wanted pregnancy to term or they have received a fatal fetal diagnosis. Clinton vetoed this 1995 ban. But he was up for reelection in November 1996 against Republican Senator Bob Dole, who proudly said he did not support a national total abortion ban.[37] That hardly comforted Winikoff.

The council needed to file mifepristone's application to the FDA right away and, in March 1996, they did. The FDA's Kessler legally let the council refer to the Roussel-Uclaf trial data and file a preliminary analysis of the council's own data.[38] Before the FDA could approve the pill, a panel of independent experts on an FDA advisory committee would ask the council about their application in a public hearing, then vote on if the FDA should okay mifepristone. A "yes" all but assured FDA approval. Millions of Americans could soon get pills.

While Winikoff worried the committee would give the council "a hard time because of political things," she said, she knew the science was rock-solid.[39] On July 19, 1996, the day of that committee hearing, she walked into a Maryland hotel, surprised to see cops ushering her to an underground parking lot with unmarked buses idling. She and her colleagues stepped onto a bus, no one knowing where they were headed. The bus dropped them off in a field with guards around a large tent. Others there that day remembered a space that looked like an airplane hangar. Brown thought they may have been "somewhere on the NIH complex." When I asked Winikoff if she had any guess as to the location, she told me, "There was no location! The location was nowhere!" Marie Bass of the RHTP, also present at the hearing, used air quotes and shook her head when saying to me, "It was in an 'undisclosed location.' The FDA, they were nuts. You can quote me on that. They were so afraid."

No anti-abortion violence happened at the hearing that day. The security was more dramatic than the otherwise dry meeting.[40] Among the eight committee members, at least one, a gynecologist named Dr. Mary Jo O'Sullivan, had known anti-abortion views. But the committee mostly just listened closely. They needed to decide, based solely on the evidence, if the potential benefits of this medication outweighed its potential risks.

Winikoff shared her research, how more than nine in 10 women surveyed in US trials said they were satisfied or very satisfied with their medication abortion: "Women clearly value the control and autonomy offered by the method. 'It offers a lot more control,' said one explicitly. 'Your body does it itself,' said another."[41] Winikoff understood the players in this moment: the council cared about its reputation, Danco about its potential profit margins, the FDA about that risk-benefit calculus. "But there's this other constituency, which has very little power, which is all the women who would benefit from this and would really like it," she told me. "I was in a position where I could try to understand that more and use data, if we could create it, that actually showed people that this is something women would want."

At the 1996 hearing, gynecologist Dr. Elizabeth Newhall, whose independent clinic in Portland, Oregon, was a trial site, gave an emotional speech on the pills. More than a year ago, she had been named on an anti-abortion hit list called "Deadly Dozen."[42] The FBI offered her protection in the middle of the trials as her clinic was outfitted with bulletproof glass. At the hearing, Newhall painted a scene: women took mifepristone on Mondays, then misoprostol on Wednesdays, "where, in our erstwhile recovery room, we had folding cots set up in two facing rows, sort of M*A*S*H style, where anywhere from six to twelve women began their expulsions together. . . . They all just saw blood and blood clots. The women read books, they played cards, they talked about politics, they laid quietly and looked out the window at downtown Portland. . . . " She added "the reasons women have for choosing medical abortions are as varied as women are," noting pills could be particularly important to sexual-violence survivors, whose history of abuse "profoundly affects the comfort and trust around gynecologic procedures." The room applauded when she finished.

Without flourish, the WHO's Dr. Paul Van Look proceeded to share more than a decade of medication abortion research across five continents, close to 50 studies by then, all showing this method safe. The committee finally voted on the question: Did mifepristone's benefits outweigh the risks? Committee member O'Sullivan then asked, "Benefit to whom? . . . Because if you are talking about a woman, it may be a benefit to her, but it is certainly of no benefit to her baby whatsoever." The chairman calmly explained the benefit was indeed to the woman. Six of the eight committee members voted "yes" while the other two members, including O'Sullivan, abstained. Even O'Sullivan could not in good faith reject the pill outright, so she did not vote at all.[43]

Six out of eight votes were enough; mifepristone only needed a majority. It was a huge relief to Winikoff, Bass of RHTP, and the many others determined that this medication reach the American people. In September 1996, merely weeks shy of the Clinton-Dole election, the FDA sent the council an "approvable" letter saying, yes, the data on mifepristone was solid. Danco just needed to finalize the pill's labeling and manufacturing details to move "approvable" to approved.[44] They were inches away.

However, due to fears of anti-abortion violence, no FDA officer signed that "approvable" letter to the council in a highly unusual move at the agency.[45] This secrecy unfortunately helped feed some anti-abortion conspiracy spirals about the FDA and mifepristone over the years, even though anti-abortion violence in the 1990s prompted that secrecy in the first place. FDA officials monitoring mifepristone have remained anonymous as recently as 2016, largely for their safety.

I spoke to one such former FDA official, whom I call Dr. Z. From 2000 to 2016, Dr. Z was the primary medical reviewer for Mifeprex (mifepristone's US brand name post-approval). They had 25 years of experience as a board-certified OBGYN prior to joining the FDA. They wanted to make it clear to the public that the agency did everything by the book when vetting and then monitoring the medication. There were no conspiracies. "I don't have a secret trove of documents, I can tell you that," they told me. "I do as you do: I go to www.fda.gov/drugs." They asked me which names from the FDA, aside from that of the FDA commissioner, signed those public documents in Mifeprex's lengthy approval package, documents anyone could download from the FDA's website. I hesitated for a moment, then told Dr. Z that I could find no names. Was I missing something? "You won't find any names," they told me. But there were plenty of non-FDA names listed: those working on mifepristone at the council, especially Sandra Arnold, and the providers running each trial site, including Dr. Suzanne Poppema.[46] They could not hide.

Except when Dr. Z joined the FDA in 1997, there was something puzzling. The council, for all its earnestness to get the medication approved by the FDA once and for all, had not yet responded to the agency's September 1996 "approvable" letter. Mifepristone lay dormant—not because of timidity at the FDA but near-catastrophic drama at Danco.

All seemed fine between the council and Danco at first. Danco's founder and head Joseph Pike successfully courted investors, who insisted on confidentiality given anti-abortion terrorism.[47] To shield investors' identities, Pike nestled Danco inside of a Russian-doll-like maze of entities registered in Delaware and the Cayman Islands. Danco controlled one entity, which controlled another, and so on. Pike raised $13.3 million, close to his contracted goal with the council, when Catley-Carlson, the council's president, received a worrying call from an investor in March 1996, the month the council filed their FDA application for mifepristone. She learned that someone named Joseph Pike pled guilty to a misdemeanor charge of forgery tied to a 1985 real estate deal in another state, where said Pike had then been disbarred. The council asked their own Pike if he was that same person. He initially denied it, then admitted it was him. Pike claimed a disgruntled former client lodged the forgery charge and that he pled guilty to just make the charge go away (the ex-client claimed Pike misrepresented the truth).

The council's reputation-conscious board was outraged. They feared a whiff of scandal could taint this intensely scrutinized mifepristone project.[48] The council insisted that Pike sell his controlling shares in Danco immediately. He did not budge. Pike said that he had done nothing wrong and had secured millions for Danco already. To end their contract, the council sued Pike for fraud, alleging that he also did not fully account for all the money he raised.[49] Pike denied anything nefarious. When the news of this fiasco broke in fall 1996, just before the presidential election, medication abortion advocates were devastated.[50] What if this stopped mifepristone? What if the pill that could change everything never came to the US?

They were lucky that Clinton was reelected in 1996, buying at least another four years until the political pendulum swung again. But if Danco's investors pulled out, would four years be enough time to start a new company from scratch? Dr. Paul Blumenthal, an abortion provider who led one of the council's trial sites and was a member of RHTP, felt sure a Pike-less Danco would survive because, well, "there was money to be made here," he told me. The council and Pike settled in 1997 to undisclosed terms; Pike was out. The council allowed Danco's investors to pull their funds since the nonprofit could not guarantee whatever Pike had promised them. Many investors did leave, some questioning the council's business acumen.[51]

Also in 1997, the overseas manufacturer Pike found for mifepristone, Gedeon Richter, backed out of their contract with Danco and was now being sued too. Danco needed to find new investors (or get current investors to invest more) and a new manufacturer, all doing so secretly under continued threats of violence.[52] By fall 1997, at least seven lawsuits had spiraled out of the "abortion pill" venture.[53] Catley-Carlson told the *Washington Post*, "I now think I would do due diligence on my great aunt."[54]

The council had spent $12 million on the mifepristone project by early 1997, and the pill still had not been approved.[55] Catley-Carlson soon left the council, perceived by some to have taken the fall for the council's external lawyer mistakenly not vetting Pike enough.[56] Arnold became even more of the mifepristone project's captain in Catley-Carlson's absence. But with the council mired in litigation, another player reappeared in 1997, making mifepristone pills in a secret US location: Larry Lader's Abortion Rights Mobilization (ARM). "We're the only game in town," Lader told the *Boston Globe* in 1997.[57]

In the fall of 1992, after the Supreme Court's *Benten v. Kessler* ruling on RU-486, Lader called a young Columbia University chemistry professor, Dr. David Horne, to introduce himself and ask for a favor. He wanted to reverse-engineer mifepristone, in other words make a replica of the drug in the US, and Lader needed a chemist. At the time, someone could legally manufacture a patented drug in the US if they did not sell it for profit. A New York law at the time also let authorities in that state, rather than the FDA, clear a new drug within New York if "every ingredient in the pill" were "bought within the boundaries of New York," as Lader later wrote.[58] This was what he wanted ARM to do. ARM relied on donations and would not sell mifepristone. Horne believed in the right to abortion and agreed to work with Lader for free.[59]

Lader had a few mifepristone pills from China (procured through friends) and his London trip with Leona Benten. He wanted Horne to build a lab in a warehouse outside of Manhattan, to synthesize mifepristone using Lader's pills and Roussel-Uclaf's published patent application, which read more like a vaguely worded recipe than step-by-step instructions. Everything about this plan was hush-hush. Lader rented that warehouse as "ARM Research Unit," all so the word "abortion" would not appear in public records that could be traced back to them. If anti-abortion extremists found out about what ARM was doing and where, that warehouse would be a highly combustible target.

Weeks after Dr. David Gunn's murder in 1993, Lader announced to the press that ARM made 50 mg of mifepristone.[60] ARM secured a US manufacturer to secretly scale up making their pill supply for research trials, not toward an FDA application (seeing as the council was already doing that). The FDA okayed ARM's study protocols, and ARM's principal investigator was pediatrician and abortion provider Dr. Eric Schaff at the University of Rochester in New York.[61] Lader had a hunch that something could go wrong with the council, and he wanted ARM to be there just in case.

All this meant that, while the council's mifepristone project was stuck in limbo from 1996 to 2000, frustrating medication abortion advocates, ARM's research team kept building evidence for simpler, less painful, and better medication abortion regimens using mifepristone and misoprostol. One of their key findings was that women could safely take misoprostol at home on their own (what women in Brazil had already been doing without mifepristone).[62] By 1997, more than 1,650 women in the US got mifepristone for free through ARM's trials.[63]

The problem was the council, not ARM, still held that pill's US patent. Only they and Danco could bring mifepristone to not thousands but millions of women in the country.

CHAPTER 8

A FANTASY

The clock kept ticking. In June 1998, a Republican-controlled House voted 223 to 202 to block the FDA from testing, developing, or approving an "abortion drug," sticking the measure into an agriculture bill at the last minute.[1] It did not pass the Senate. Weeks later, another abortion provider, Dr. Barnett Slepian, was assassinated, this time by a sniper shooting through a window into Slepian's home in upstate New York, near where Dr. Eric Schaff led ARM's medication abortion trials.[2] Schaff was put under federal marshal protection until Slepian's murderer was identified (but not yet found). "We were pretty fearful," Schaff told me. Traumas piling up deepened some advocates' longing for the pills to diminish if not end this conflict. The FMF's website proclaimed that, with mifepristone in the US, "the number of abortion providers could double overnight."[3] But how exactly?

To a *New York Times* reporter in 1999, sociologist Dr. Carole Joffe likened this wishful vision of medication abortion to the legend of King Christian X of Denmark.[4] During Denmark's Nazi occupation, so the legend went, Christian X told all Danes to wear Stars of David to protect the Jewish people among them. If everyone donned a star, how could the Nazis find and kill all Jews? If every doctor in 1990s America prescribed abortion pills, how could extremists find and kill all abortion providers? Only Christian X never did tell all Danes to wear yellow stars.[5] It was a myth. That was Joffe's point.

Joffe had been studying abortion in the US for about two decades by then. She saw over and over how providers like Dr. Suzanne Poppema earnestly tried to normalize abortion into medicine but never succeeded. Joffe sincerely admired these providers. Yet this wasn't really working. Abortion was exceptionalized. Joffe painfully understood the source of this 1990s faith among feminists that these pills would somehow be a different story. "It was a decade of terror," she told me. "And so, there was this fantasy that [medication abortion] was going to solve the problem. I saw the hunger."

That fantasy was not wholly unfounded. Medication abortion advocates in the mid-1990s often cited a Kaiser Family Foundation survey finding that just 33 percent of OBGYNs provided abortions in the US but, when asked if they would prescribe medication abortions if approved, that number jumped to about 66 percent of OBGYNs.[6] At the National Abortion Federation (NAF), a well-respected professional association for abortion providers mainly in the US, several members excitedly referred to these figures. Joffe, who was on NAF's board at the time, listened yet remained skeptical. These were abortion providers talking among themselves about fleets of doctors across the country prescribing abortion pills one day. Where were these mythical people who were not providing abortions already and who now wanted to do so with pills? Joffe wanted to find them.

When Joffe asked reproductive rights attorneys what it would mean for doctors new to abortion care to prescribe abortion pills, the lawyers were abundantly clear: you cannot provide abortions legally *and* secretly. The two did not coexist in this country. That stuck with her. Whenever pills were preached to primary care providers at regional meetings, Joffe began to notice an eager audience nodding along until they learned that they, of course, needed to follow parental notification laws for abortion in their state, 24-hour waiting period laws for abortion in their state, and on and on. "I could see the bells ringing in people's heads, 'Oh my God, no way in hell I'm going to do that,'" Joffe told me. "And how the hell do you make [an abortion] known to your patients but nobody else?"

She searched high and low for nonabortion providers committed to offering medication abortion for the first time until she met two women who fit the bill. They ran a family medicine practice in rural Michigan in the late 1990s. Mifepristone was not available outside of trials yet, but they heard of methotrexate and misoprostol, another safe and effective medication abortion option for early pregnancies at that time. This method used two already FDA-approved drugs, only methotrexate was not a pill; a provider needed to inject that medication into patients.[7] The two doctors read the latest research and decided to bring this care into their practice. Shortly after they did so, one longtime patient, a conservative Christian, burst into their office one day and asked them, "Did you know they're talking about you on a Christian radio show? They're calling you both the Sisters of Satan."[8] This was what Joffe sadly anticipated. "Medically speaking, of course family practice people can do it," she told me of pills. "Socially, it's a whole different ball game."

Among many existing abortion providers, there was also a nagging ambivalence about pills. "With medical abortion, you feel a little bit less needed, because 'everybody' may end up doing them," said one doctor Joffe interviewed in the late 1990s.[9] Another confided to Joffe that "I'm not trained to watch people miscarry. When people come in miscarrying to the hospital, I'm trained to evacuate the uterus. . . . I think there's an underlying anxiety to [medical abortion] that is just not there when you do a [surgical] procedure and it's done in a few minutes."[10] They were comfortable performing procedures. Why fix what, to some, was not broken? One doctor grimly foretold mifepristone's "most optimistic scenario" for the country: that half of abortions in the US would be with pills "if the education was done right. . . . I'm looking at 25 years from now, realistically."[11] Indeed, more than twenty years after Joffe interviewed these providers, once the COVID-19 pandemic pried open legal telehealth abortion in the US, only then would at least half of abortions in the US be medication abortions.[12]

While Joffe unraveled that fantasy of pills, the tight-lipped Danco turned a corner. The company found a new mifepristone manufacturer around 1999, not revealing its name or location due to security fears. Danco stayed reclusive with an unlisted phone number and, on its office door somewhere in Manhattan, a different name.[13] By March 2000, Danco had raised roughly $34.7 million from confidential investors. According to internal Danco documents the *Wall Street Journal* reviewed in September 2000, the company had a more ambitious forecast for mifepristone than did those doctors Joffe interviewed. Danco predicted 29 percent of abortions in the country would be with pills within four years of mifepristone entering the US market.[14] And the company bet that sales of Mifeprex would reach about $34.2 million by 2004.[15]

There was still no FDA approval of mifepristone. Another presidential race loomed in November 2000, this time between Clinton's vice president, Al Gore, and Republican George W. Bush. Like his father, Bush unequivocally spoke against "the abortion pill," even saying on the campaign trail that he would "be inclined not to accept" an FDA approval of mifepristone.[16] The pill's advocates feverishly hoped that mifepristone would be okayed before this likely razor-thin election. Yet as approval finally neared, the FDA grew more terrified of anti-abortion violence. No agency record I reviewed nor former FDA official who worked on the pill at this time and whom I spoke to could confirm that the FDA received threats of violence regarding mifepristone during this time.[17]

In early 2000, the FDA's anxieties translated into actions: the agency stated it planned to approve mifepristone but place the pill under the "Subpart H restricted distribution provision."[18] This obscure regulation was generally considered the only legal tool the FDA had at the time to control the pill more tightly than most FDA-approved medications. The FDA had placed just a handful of drugs under that provision, including thalidomide, which caused severe birth defects if taken during pregnancy.[19] The FDA's "Subpart H restricted distribution provision" for thalidomide thus aimed to ensure that pregnant people in the US were not given that drug. However, mifepristone carried no such serious safety risks like thalidomide. The council and Danco repeatedly argued with the FDA that subjecting mifepristone to this restriction was wholly unscientific and unfair.[20] While they sparred behind closed doors, the reproductive rights movement had a messaging problem with the American public, embarrassingly evident during a largely empty conference the FMF hosted about mifepristone in April 2000 in DC.[21]

In the roughly 12 years since RU-486 burst into the American press, a hype around pills had tempered. Vicki Saporta, then head of NAF, told a room at the conference that mifepristone "won't end the abortion debate in this country."[22] FMF's website no longer stated RU-486 could double the number of American abortion providers overnight. Planned Parenthood representative Bonnie McEwan shared at the conference a survey the organization recently ran that found 30 percent of Americans had heard of mifepristone or RU-486 when, just three years earlier, 53 percent of Americans had heard of the pill. Why the drop? "I think it's because we waited and we waited, and we waited some more for approval of mifepristone," McEwan said to the room. "And while we were waiting, mifepristone sort of drifted off people's radar screens."[23] The same Planned Parenthood survey also found that people identifying as anti-abortion seemed to know more about mifepristone than did people identifying as supportive of abortion rights.[24]

Another hit came in June 2000 when someone "familiar with negotiations between the FDA and the sponsor of RU-486" leaked a bombshell to the *New York Times*.[25] The FDA wanted to require only doctors who already provided abortion procedures to prescribe mifepristone. "It kills the drug if it can't be used by primary care providers," Schaff told *The Times* that June.[26] The FDA's ostensible reasoning was that, at the time, about 4 or 5 percent of mifepristone patients may need an aspiration procedure after taking pills.[27] But that still didn't add up. "Your internist does not operate if you have a stroke as a result of the medication you're taking," sociologist Dr. Tracy Weitz told me. "There's no reason you have to be a surgeon to give this pill." The FDA did scrap that proposal after public outrage that June. Yet whatever slim leverage the council and Danco had to continue fighting the FDA on its other restrictions around the pill dwindled as the presidential election neared. Advocates knew FDA approval needed to be now or maybe never.

Weeks before election day, on September 28, 2000, the FDA approved mifepristone as part of a medication abortion regimen with misoprostol, allowing its use for people up to seven weeks pregnant. Millions of Americans could for the first time get mifepristone *and* misoprostol legally. Advocates were thoroughly exhausted but jubilant. Only they scratched their heads over the FDA's Subpart H rules on mifepristone until the reason behind them clicked. *Oh, so that was how they would control the pill.* "And of course, we were annoyed," Kirsten Moore, then head of RHTP, told me. "But we didn't think they would be that big a deal."

That was because the FDA's restrictions on mifepristone upon the pill's approval did not seem onerous to her at first. Doctors, for instance, would need to contact Danco to be certified to prescribe Mifeprex. Danco would then keep a confidential list of these certified providers. The FDA also put in place extensive "post-marketing surveillance" of the pill, and, in addition to "adverse event reporting" requirements applicable to every other drug that the FDA approved, the agency imposed a special "adverse event reporting" system on mifepristone, one that Danco would need to follow.[28] Under this special system, in which "adverse event" was broadly defined, even if a woman died of a gunshot wound the day after she took mifepristone, her death would need to be reported to the FDA as an "adverse event." Likely the most consequential FDA restriction, however, was that mifepristone be "dispensed" to patients from a clinic, medical office, or hospital, with the expectation that patients go to a clinic in person three times for a medication abortion.[29] When I asked a former FDA official closely involved in the pill's approval why the agency in 2000 put mifepristone under "restricted distribution," they did not wish to answer, though they did say, "If this drug had been any other drug than what it was, I think a lot of what was imposed on it wouldn't have been."

It appeared glaringly obvious to the advocacy community that these FDA rules were political. "What *is* this? Viagra just sailed through," Poppema told me of first learning about mifepristone's restrictions, her disappointment growing. Several advocates speculated that the Clinton White House likely pressured the FDA to restrict the drug so that the Democrats would not seem too lenient on the "abortion pill" and possibly jeopardize Gore's chances with swing voters. But there was no publicly known evidence of that, only rumors.

In a debate days after mifepristone's approval, Bush, when asked about the pill, stated he doubted that a president had the power to overturn the FDA's decision, though he added, "I hope the FDA took its time to make sure the American women will be safe who use this drug."[30] Gore replied, "Well . . . the FDA took 12 years. And I do support that decision."[31] Bush's campaign quickly stated after the debate, as if doing damage control with anti-abortion groups, that Bush would support efforts by Republicans in Congress to try to restrict mifepristone more.[32] Then in one of the closest presidential elections in US history, one that needed the Supreme Court to weigh in, Bush won the White House.

Advocates were right to insist on pushing mifepristone across the FDA approval finish line in September 2000, just under the wire. Yet they were wrong, as Bass of RHTP told me, to make that pill's FDA approval the finish line at all. "What we learned over the years . . . is don't make the goal FDA approval," she told me. "That's one step. But there is still a long way to go until you have a product that is available *and* accessible to women."

The 2000 Mifeprex label itself did not exactly help. ARM studies by then showed mifepristone and misoprostol safely ended people's pregnancies up to nine weeks, but the original, FDA-approved Mifeprex label told doctors to prescribe up to only seven weeks.[33] Since US doctors legally could prescribe a medication for off-label uses supported by evidence, a few did so from the start with Mifeprex, prescribing it up to nine weeks.[34] That slightly expanded access. But cost became another problem. Danco initially priced one mifepristone pill at $90, which Schaff and several advocates thought too high. And most clinics began charging patients about $600 for a medication abortion, the same as an aspiration, a price some believed too expensive for just pills and another blow to women.[35] Throughout the Bush years, however, advocates tread cautiously with mifepristone, fearing one misstep—or perception of a misstep—might pull the medication back all over again. That almost did happen.

In 2001, a woman died of toxic shock after she had a medication abortion, and a panicked Planned Parenthood supposedly briefly considered taking the pills out of their clinics.[36] The FDA and CDC investigated swiftly, as did the council, all finding mifepristone and misoprostol had not caused this person's death.[37] The woman had been infected with a rare bacteria called *Clostridium Sordellii* or *C. Sordellii*, found in the gastrointestinal tract and vagina of otherwise healthy people. *C. Sordellii* reappeared around 2006 when six women in the US died of toxic shock after they had medication abortions. The FDA and CDC investigated again, once more finding *C. Sordellii* infections, and independently determined that mifepristone and miso-prostol did not cause these women's deaths.[38]

Nonetheless, an anti-abortion Republican legislator led a Congressional hearing in 2006 calling for mifepristone to be nationally banned over these women's deaths, arguing without evidence that the FDA illegally rushed to approve the pill without vetting the medication properly.[39] Several Republican Congressmen that year asked the nonpartisan Government Accountability Office to investigate the FDA's approval and oversight of Mifeprex, and the office definitively concluded nothing amiss.[40] It even found the FDA took longer to approve Mifeprex than other Subpart H drugs—and almost three times longer than the average, non–Subpart H drug.

When the FDA then in 2008 created a Risk Evaluation and Mitigation Strategy (REMS) program, the restrictions on mifepristone's distribution that had been imposed under the Subpart H regulations were incorporated into the REMS.[41] This included the expectation that patients visit a clinic in person three times for a medication abortion. The FDA's public statements on supposed safety concerns around mifepristone, concerns the agency used to justify these restrictions, tellingly did not directly address the potential harm done to women who could not access an abortion. But Dr. Diana Greene Foster's groundbreaking *The Turnaway Study* traced over 10 years precisely that harm done to American women denied abortions, finding in 2020 that women resoundingly suffered worse financial, physical, and emotional health a decade after being turned away from an abortion compared to the women who accessed the abortions they sought.[42] Throughout that decade in which Foster followed women's diverging paths, mifepristone remained tightly controlled under the REMS, with misoprostol-only abortions in the US under the radar.

According to the FDA, about 5.9 million women in the US from 2000 to 2022 have used mifepristone for a medication abortion, only 32 of those women having died from an "adverse event" after their medication abortion.[43] Mifepristone or misoprostol did not cause any of those women's deaths.[44] That puts mifepristone's mortality rate at 0.000005 percent; a person's risk of death associated with giving birth in the US is shockingly about 14 times higher than that with abortion.[45] As a former FDA official who worked closely on mifepristone told of perhaps any drug that the FDA has approved thus far, that pill may be the most studied and the most monitored drug to also possess such a consistent, decades-long record of its safety.

Dr. Linda Prine intimately knew the harm done to those denied an abortion. She had two abortions before she went to medical school, which barely even mentioned birth control let alone abortion.[46] Prine joined a family medicine network in the 1990s in New York and, like Poppema in Seattle, took the initiative to learn to perform abortion procedures. Her family medicine office did not allow Prine to offer abortions there, however, even though they provided prenatal care and other simple, safe procedures. Prine needed to refer patients seeking abortions to a Planned Parenthood clinic, where she also worked and could perform abortion procedures. One day, a family medicine patient asked Prine for an abortion. The patient brought her one-year-old child to her appointment, and Prine noticed the child had rashes that looked like burns. She did as she usually did: referred this patient over to herself at Planned Parenthood. That patient never came. Months later, that patient reappeared at Prine's office, her pregnancy too far along for Prine to perform an abortion procedure. "And I said to her at the time, 'If I had been able to do this abortion for you in my own office back at the beginning, is that what you would have done?' And she was like, 'Yeah, of course.'"

Prine was furious and, along with colleagues, organized to integrate abortion care into their family medicine center. It so happened that mifepristone had also just been approved. Prine formed a nonprofit, the Reproductive Health Access Project, focused on bringing abortion pills into primary care. "And I thought in five years, we'll be done," Prine told me. But she didn't anticipate how hard it would be for primary care providers to navigate mifepristone's FDA restrictions.[47] Just that extra bit of red tape got in the way.[48] That wasn't the only problem.

The council's 1990s trial protocols with three in-person clinic visits largely became how American providers in the first decade of the 2000s and the early 2010s gave people pills, which made medication abortions burdensome to patients *and* providers. On top of that were dizzying state abortion laws and, as Joffe worried, that social stigma, a scarlet *A* of abortion. Even if a provider strongly supported abortion, their staff or neighbor or staff's neighbor might resolutely not and threaten to make their life hell if they prescribed abortion pills. The prospect of that happening, even if it never actually did, could be enough to spook providers. In 2001, Danco's then medical director, Dr. Richard Hausknecht, recalled the fervent wishes of a decade earlier that thousands of American doctors would provide pills. "Well, I can tell you that, as of today, that's not happened," he said. "They're afraid."[49]

According to the Guttmacher Institute, about 13 percent of all abortions in the US in 2005 were medication abortions, far lower than Danco's prior estimate of 30 percent by 2004.[50] This devastated Dr. Elizabeth Newhall, who consulted for Danco in the first decade of the 2000s and in the 2010s, knocking on gynecologists' office doors with medication abortion information. "I hate to be so simple as to say doctors were chickens," she told me. Newhall thought the FDA restrictions were nowhere near grueling enough to explain just how many doctors refused to provide this care. "You make one phone call. You fill out a piece of paper that says your name and your address and your [Drug Enforcement Agency] number and your license number. The whole thing takes under a day," she told me. "But it was having your name on that list." That confidential list of certified prescribers that Danco kept, which some doctors feared could end up in the wrong hands. Newhall believed a darker truth held other doctors back: "plain old apathy."

As for abortion-seekers themselves, women did not often know to ask their primary care providers or gynecologists for medication abortions. They, too, thought the abortion clinic was where to go. And many clinics, desperately trying to stay open amid anti-abortion onslaughts, were not quick to dispute that. Post-*Dobbs*, Newhall thought that women "hopping over doctors" to find abortion pills through networks (as described in later chapters) spoke as much to women's resistance as to the American medical community's failures.

"If I have a regret, it was that I tried so hard to bring [abortion pills] into mainstream medicine all by myself," she told me, then quietly began to cry. "And I went bankrupt."

In the first decade of the 2000s and in the 2010s, abortion pills stayed mostly confined to clinics that already performed abortion procedures.[51] But small, independent clinics like the one Newhall ran, which had once been a council trial site, struggled to combat what the reproductive rights movement called TRAP laws, or targeted regulation of abortion providers. These anti-abortion state laws, alongside the country's growing corporatization of health care, made clinics more expensive to run, pushing many to shut down, including Newhall's clinic, and all the while made it harder for people to access abortions.[52]

But with mifepristone legal in the US, access did expand in important other ways in the first decade of the 2000s and in the 2010s. Many Planned Parenthood clinics that did not offer abortions before abortion pills became available did so after, as Faye Wattleton once hoped. A few gynecologists and primary care providers that never performed abortion procedures did start to prescribe pills. And after the FDA in 2016 approved an update to several of mifepristone's restrictions to better align with the latest research, some nurse practitioners, midwives, and other licensed health care workers began offering medication abortions in states where they legally could.[53] "But the original fantasy of doubling providers overnight?" Joffe told me. "That was a fantasy."

Meanwhile, many abortion providers working in clinics when medication abortion rolled out tended to be content with aspirations and cautious with pills ("I come from a line of great worriers, not great warriors," Dr. Paul Blumenthal told me.). As Schaff told me, "Then the question is: who was advocating for medication abortion? It was mostly the feminist activists and the women who told their doctors, 'No, I don't want a surgical abortion. I want a medication abortion.'" Dr. Deborah Oyer, now a retired abortion provider who took over Poppema's clinic in Washington, was delighted at mifepristone's FDA approval. But it, too, took her time to understand why some people may prefer pills. *Why not do a five-minute procedure versus a several-day affair?* "Many of us felt that way," she told me of the abortion provider community. She noticed that some patients also did not know much about aspiration when they decided to try medication abortion. One of her patients once took pills that did not work for her after days of bleeding and cramping (which is rare but can happen). The patient then came back to the clinic for an aspiration done in minutes and told Oyer, "I did all *that* to avoid *this*?" There was indeed a long way to go to educate Americans on abortion in general, not only on abortion pills.

An ambitious vision, however, was already bubbling back in 1996 when the council's Charlotte Ellertson asked Blumenthal if he thought mifepristone could be over the counter. She had been making the rounds interviewing providers who ran the council's trial sites, Blumenthal among them. He paused at her question and said, "Well, yeah, why not? I mean, maybe not tomorrow." Ellertson looked surprised, as if most of her interviewees had not said that. She asked him to explain.

Blumenthal proceeded to think aloud how, in the simplest terms, four things were (and are) needed for a drug to be over the counter. One: Can you recognize your need to take this medication? Two: If there are contraindications, can you recognize them? "And in the case of mifepristone, there aren't many," he explained. Three: Is there potential for abuse? "And by abuse, the FDA usually meant one of two things," he told me as he did to Ellertson. "Can you kill yourself with this drug? Or can you get addicted to this drug?" The answer to both questions for mifepristone was and is no. Even with misoprostol, someone would need to take very large quantities of that medication to kill themselves, which, by that reasoning, someone could also do with aspirin, explained Blumenthal. "And the fourth criterion is really, are the instructions easy to follow?" Yes. Surely, if women can run companies and lead nations and fly planes and do surgeries, they can follow the instructions for a medication abortion. This conversation with Blumenthal likely shaped the 1997 article Ellertson co-wrote with Winikoff, titled, "Can Women Use Medical Abortion Without Medical Supervision?"[54]

Winikoff left the council in 2003 and formed Gynuity Health Projects, a nonprofit for global medication abortion research. While the American anti-abortion movement in the first decade of the 2000s and in the 2010s kept plotting to overturn *Roe*, a small group of researchers in the US, Winikoff and Blumenthal included, built evidence to convince the FDA to unravel mifepristone's restrictions and get pills into abortion-seekers' hands, legally. They now needed to disprove a negative: to show that changing one part of research-turned-clinical-guidelines for medication abortion did not cause harm. But the pills were so safe and effective "that you'd need thousands and thousands of patients in a study to disprove something that's not likely to happen," Blumenthal told me. Prove a pregnant person did not need a blood test before she took pills, did not need an ultrasound before pills, did not need to see a provider after taking pills, could pick pills up in the mail or (shock!) at a pharmacy. All to better meet the lived realities of millions of people. It took years and years.[55]

Winikoff all the while remained convinced that once more people in the US knew about abortion pills, then women would not give these pills up. "And I think that's what's happened," she told me in 2023, with bans in almost half the country post-*Dobbs* and reports of more people using abortion pills in the US than ever before, largely thanks to telehealth abortion (as will be discussed in a later chapter). She continued to believe that mifepristone and misoprostol would both be available over the counter one day. I asked her, however, about abortion pills failing to live up to that early 1990s fantasy of doubling the number of abortion providers in the first two decades of the 2000s, about all those hopes dashed. "But it didn't do it *that* way," Winikoff told me. "It did happen. All those things we thought [would happen] actually did happen. In the end." Then she sighed and added, "I shouldn't say 'the end' because it's never the end of this one."

Maybe that doubling, even tripling, of abortion providers happened if abortion-seekers themselves were their own providers, however pills found their way to them, bans or no bans, bringing that Christian X legend to life after all. Joffe in 2023 echoed that. "To all the naysayers or doubters like me, miffy [mifepristone] has said, 'Look, without me, you're nothing,'" she told me of a post-*Dobbs* country with more pills crossing borders and entering homes than anyone can possibly fully count. "That really is true," Joffe told me. "They can't arrest everybody."

CHAPTER 9

"THE MOST NORMAL THING TO DO"

A round 2001 in León, a city in the central Mexican state of Guanajuato, 30-year-old Verónica Cruz Sánchez learned about an abortion pill: misoprostol.[1] She was stunned.

A fast-talking social worker born and raised in Guanajuato, Cruz Sánchez believed that controlling one's body was a foundational, feminist freedom. But in 2000, before she knew about misoprostol, Guanajuato's legislature passed the worst abortion ban in Mexico at the time, one that outlawed abortion entirely and imprisoned for up to eight years anyone who had an abortion.[2] Guanajuato, one of the country's most conservative states, had at least allowed rape survivors legal abortions until then.[3] Cruz Sánchez organized immediately. "No. No, we are not going to allow it," she told me through an interpreter in 2023. "I don't know what we are going to do, but we are not going to allow that to happen."

Mexico's 1931 federal penal code criminalized abortion in almost all cases.[4] A person who had an abortion and anyone who provided one could be imprisoned for up to six years. There were exceptions for rape survivors and if a pregnancy endangered the pregnant person's life. Yet like the state-level authority in the US, each of Mexico's 31 states plus Mexico City (which was considered a federal district rather than a state) could pass its own abortion laws. For as long as Cruz Sánchez could remember, abortion had been difficult for people in Guanajuato to talk about in this overwhelmingly Catholic community that had been taught abortion was a sin—and where poverty was stubbornly high.[5] But parteras, or midwives, had long been quietly called to help a person who wanted to bring her period back.[6] Abortion had almost always been there.

Now Cruz Sánchez built a local coalition to pressure Guanajuato's governor to veto the state's new, total abortion ban. She and allies went door-to-door talking to people about abortion as a human right. Many women shared that they had been raped and could not access a legal abortion that they were entitled to even prior to this ban. Or they did not even know that, as a rape survivor, they had a legal right to an abortion. Cruz Sánchez and her colleagues also discovered that the rapist was often tragically the woman or girl's biological father. When these stories became public, people across Guanajuato were horrified and called on the governor to stop the ban, which he did. But Cruz Sánchez knew that would not be enough. Someone needed to at least ensure that anyone who had been raped could access a legal abortion in Guanajuato so as not to repeat past injustices.

That summer of 2000, she co-founded a feminist collective called Las Libres, or the Free Ones. Their budget was minuscule, and their office was inside a house in León.[7] Las Libres approached local doctors, finding those who agreed to provide free abortion procedures for rape survivors. They expanded their network to psychologists, attorneys, and people who could help in other ways, like driving someone to their abortion appointment, all agreeing to do so for free. In late 2000, Las Libres spread the word that anyone in Guanajuato impregnated from rape and needing help could come to them for free, safe, and legal abortions. Whomever showed up could, if they wished, be accompanied by a Las Libres member to their abortion appointment.

Feminist accompaniment models had long existed beyond abortion care.[8] In the US and much of Latin America, some queer and feminist activists learned to accompany gender-based-violence survivors to police stations or hospitals, supporting them in navigating legal and health care systems that could be discriminatory. With abortion, accompaniment essentially meant someone truly centering the person having an abortion, listening to them without judgment, and being fully present with an abortion seeker as their equal. It was while accompanying someone in Guanajuato during their abortion in 2001 that Cruz Sánchez heard of misoprostol.

A feminist gynecologist in the Las Libres network had recently attended a conference in Europe, where she learned about a safe abortion pill available in Mexico. This pill, misoprostol, technically required a prescription in the country. But unlike the high-profile mifepristone, which was registered and marketed as "the abortion pill" in countries like the US, misoprostol with its abortifacient "side effect" was nowhere near as tightly controlled. Over in the US, that pill did not have those FDA restrictions binding mifepristone (the agency still had not received an application to even consider approving misoprostol for abortions). Yet since studies in the late 1990s and first decade of the 2000s found that the use of misoprostol on its own for abortions was less effective than the use of misoprostol with mifepristone, providers in the US did not pursue misoprostol-only abortion care. Not until almost two decades later when new data would emerge from epidemiologists partnering with accompaniment groups would another misoprostol story unfold. But back in the first decade of the 2000s in Mexico, with no mifepristone available, when this gynecologist with Las Libres realized misoprostol's potential, she thought the pill was amazing.

She had previously been providing abortion procedures to sexual violence survivors whom Cruz Sánchez accompanied. "And because I was accompanying women to her office, I learned a lot medically about abortion," Cruz Sánchez told me. "And it was the gynecologist who told me that there was a pill. She started it. She said, 'Now we're going to do it with a pill because it's less invasive.'"

Some feminist gynecologists in Mexico already knew about misoprostol in the 1990s from conferences and papers, including medical articles on that medication's "misuse" among women in Brazil.[9] A few physicians secretly told their patients about misoprostol as an abortion pill that could be found in some pharmacies (if one knew where to look) despite the country's near total abortion ban. I spoke to one such gynecologist who asked not to be named since she risked losing her license for what she did decades ago. This gynecologist, whom I call Dr. T, worked in a public hospital's pediatric unit in 1990s Mexico, where adolescents and girls with unwanted pregnancies and painful stories frequently came to her. She wanted to help.

But it would have been too legally risky for Dr. T to perform an aspiration procedure in her office at that hospital; she and the patient could easily get caught. She could instead carefully write a patient a prescription for misoprostol to treat gastritis or stomach ulcers, something that would not catch attention. Dr. T first checked that the patient (who was often joined by their mother) understood that this medication seemed highly safe from what was known, but there were not many studies on the pill's use for abortions yet. Dr. T would be there if anything did go wrong. The women and girls were usually "very, very willing to accept, to try," Dr. T told me. "And I always thought, let's try . . . and in a way, we learned together."

Dr. T would closely monitor the patient as she took misoprostol, asking her how she felt, how much she bled, and if she had any other symptoms. If there were complications, Dr. T could tell the patient to come back to the hospital, where Dr. T could now legally perform an aspiration to complete what otherwise presented as a miscarriage. "And I think this was the story of most of us who were learning together with the women themselves," Dr. T told me. "We were learning how to use these beautiful drugs. It's really something we should protect."

When we spoke in 2023, Dr. T feared the American anti-abortion movement's attempt to ban mifepristone in the US post-*Dobbs* and worried misoprostol would be next. Mexico had not faced such aggressive legal attacks on either medication. "I have no words for what is happening right now in the States," Dr. T told me, calling women in the US "rejenes," or prisoners of war. "We are in a war. We must go undercover. But it will not last forever. . . . And a last reflection is probably this solution will come from the more marginalized women, the ones who even before the sentence of the [US Supreme Court] did not access legal abortion themselves. They could count on their networks, their knowledge, their friends. And white WASP women will have to learn from them."

In Guanajuato around 2001, Cruz Sánchez intently watched the gynecologist who had just told her about misoprostol, paying attention to the instructions the doctor gave to her patients on how to use the pills and what to expect. "And so, I learned with the first three, four, or five women that we accompanied with the pills, and then I said this is wonderful to see because doctors are usually the obstacle for women to access abortions," Cruz Sánchez told me. "With pills, you can do it. . . . If this doctor continues to do the medical supervision, we no longer need to ask anyone's permission, regardless of whether it is legal or illegal. If women do it with all the information, with all the support, it is extremely safe."

That doctor did remain as "medical supervision," as did others. Yet the "supervision" was usually not a doctor watching the person take misoprostol pills, as in the trials that the Population Council ran, but being on call if someone needed an aspiration, like what Dr. T had done. Since misoprostol could be less effective when taken without mifepristone, some people took misoprostol to start their abortion processes, which presented as miscarriages, then got an aspiration from an allied provider (as women in Brazil did years earlier). Over time, experienced acompañantes would know more than many doctors did about using misoprostol for abortions, discovering that these pills could work much better than researchers thought. Using mifepristone and misoprostol together was still considered the ideal. And suppliers of mifepristone were growing in the first decade of the 2000s, especially once more companies in India produced mifepristone.[10] But in Mexico, mifepristone could still be difficult to find even via informal markets.

Las Libres then started a bolder strategy. They learned to do as women in Brazil did: find friendly pharmacies that sold misoprostol over the counter without a prescription at all. A box of misoprostol usually contained 28 pills, more than the eight or so needed for one abortion, and one box cost around 900 pesos, about $85 at the time.[11] Las Libres realized that they could now accompany even more women with misoprostol.[12] What happened next grew organically. "For us, it was never an issue of whether it was illegal or legal," Cruz Sánchez told me. "We always positioned ourselves on the side of the right, on the fact [that abortion] is a human right of women. . . . And the second proposal of our model has always been that we are going to make [women] think of it as a right—beyond whether their family disagrees, whether society criminalizes, whether it's stigmatizing."

They pursued their second proposal by just talking openly with those they accompanied. They met women one-on-one before their abortions and asked questions. "'What do you think about abortion? Who told you that? Where did you learn that?' Because we found, on a case-by-case basis, that the stigma associated with abortion is mostly based on ignorance," explained Cruz Sánchez. "Most people don't know what abortion is." The biggest concern women shared with Las Libres was not that abortion was a crime (many didn't know it was) or, though most were Catholic, that it may be considered a sin. It was that abortion might kill them or make them infertile. Some would say to Cruz Sánchez, as she recalled to me, "I know I'm killing someone, but I have to do it because if my husband finds out, if my parents find out, if my family finds out that I'm pregnant, they're going to kill me." Cruz Sánchez assured them that they would be safe—and were not alone.

"We always publicly stated that we were going to do [accompaniment] because it is a woman's right," Cruz Sánchez told me. Some women came back to Las Libres after their abortions, saying accompaniment emboldened them and asking how they could help. They had leftover misoprostol pills and came up with an idea: keep the pills "because the next time the next woman comes, you are going to give her the pills, and you are also going to tell her about the experience," Cruz Sánchez told me as these women told each other. "And that's wonderful because everybody knows that it's not the same to be told about an experience as it is to be told about the living through that experience, right?"

Those women became acompañantes, learning from each person they accompanied how to care better for the next person.[13] "We don't even need money," Cruz Sánchez told me. In later years when they met women before their abortions, they gathered in groups in public to bring abortion out of the clandestine. People brought with them a friend, mother, sister, aunt. Person by person, year by year, a shift seemed to happen. "Accompanying didn't just mean saying, 'Here are the pills, go home, get an abortion,'" Cruz Sánchez told me. "But provoking that conversation so people would learn that this was the most normal thing to do." Soon people invited Las Libres to do workshops. Some told Las Libres they were opposed to abortion but still donated misoprostol to them and referred people there. Teachers told students about Las Libres and misoprostol. Wherever Cruz Sánchez went, she told people about these pills. "It is used like this, etc., etc."

As word spread, a few pharmacists in Guanajuato refused to sell misoprostol to women and girls who looked like they may be pregnant. But a trusted, postmenopausal woman or cisgender man could ask for misoprostol instead. Grandmothers, boyfriends, husbands, anyone who did not look like they could be pregnant then began giving the pills to granddaughters, daughters, girlfriends, wives, friends, anyone they loved. Some sent misoprostol to relatives in the US, where, despite *Roe*, their loved ones could not access or did not want an abortion in the formal health care system.

One of the first to write about Las Libres's accompaniment model was American sociologist Dr. Deborah Billings. She worked in Mexico at the time for a North Carolina–based nonprofit called Ipas, which focused on abortion and contraception access globally. Billings and Cruz Sánchez quickly became friends. They shared a quality: if a person told them not to do something, they wanted to do it even more. "But [Cruz Sánchez] will take it to the exponential, 20th degree," Billings told me, crediting her with "being so clear about what this was all about."

Billings published the first paper on Las Libres's accompaniment in 2004 without naming Las Libres or Mexico given security concerns, only stating that this model was in a Latin American country.[14] That paper alone was controversial within the global reproductive health field, Ipas's former executive vice president Ann Leonard told me, "because documenting a practice that's not legal carries its own risks." Ipas formed in the 1970s initially to integrate its patented manual vacuum aspirator (MVA) into health care systems around the world.[15] But in the first decade of the 2000s, the nonprofit began noticing and learning from grassroots feminist groups like Las Libres using misoprostol in creative ways under bans.[16]

Billings wished she had an acompañante for her two abortions in the US, one when she was a teenager and the other in her early twenties. "There was nobody there with me, and it was all hush hush," she told me. She eventually became an acompañante and felt the profound impact that accompaniment could have not only on the abortion-seeker but also the acompañante, nurturing a solidarity that she urgently sought to build in the post-*Dobbs* US.

When we spoke in 2023, Billings lived and taught in South Carolina, where, as of mid-2024, abortion was banned past six weeks in pregnancy and anti-abortion politicians controlled the state legislature.[17] Billings felt "overwhelmed," she told me. She and fellow reproductive justice activists had been pushing to expand the state's abortion protections. Repeatedly, she testified to politicians and judges about her abortion and miscarriage experiences, all in an attempt to be seen as a person. It was exhausting. Just before we spoke, Billings overheard a college student on campus say that she was nervous to take a pregnancy test, that it better come back negative. "If we continue to live in this bubble, then we're doomed," Billings told me, hoping the US could learn from Las Libres and Mexico. "We're just doomed."

Cruz Sánchez first began noticing just how far the mentality of Americans on abortion needed to change back in 2006. That year, in recognition of forming a network for rape survivors in Guanajuato to access legal abortions, Cruz Sánchez became the first Mexican to receive the Defender of Human Rights Award from Human Rights Watch, an international human rights research and advocacy non-profit.[18] She was then invited to the US to lecture on her activism. But these lectures could be strange experiences for her. When she explained to Americans how hard it was for sexual-violence survivors to access legal abortions in Mexico, her audiences seemed to voice relief that the US did not have such a problem thanks to *Roe*. Cruz Sánchez thought, *Well, not exactly.*[19]

Las Libres had contacts along the US-Mexico border, with Guanajuato home to many people who migrated to the US, and Cruz Sánchez heard how difficult abortion access could be in abortion-hostile states like Texas, especially if a person lived undocumented. She also thought that abortion pills in the US should be free for everyone. Yet

Cruz Sánchez believed Americans understood abortion as an individual right, not a collective one. That worried her. Americans at her lectures often asked her how they could help Las Libres, offering to donate money. That question, to her, assumed that Americans needed to help Mexicans (rather than the other way around) and that money was the best way to help. That bothered her. It was not money that went door-to-door in Guanajuato to form networks and engage with people's feelings on abortion, no matter how complicated those feelings may be. That was community.

Although there were Americans doing grassroots abortion-access work in the US, namely volunteers at abortion funds that first formed decades ago after the Hyde Amendment went into effect, the American reproductive rights, health, and justice movements did shy away from self-managed abortion (SMA), often defined as when a person took misoprostol only or misoprostol and mifepristone on their own to have an abortion outside the formal health care system. SMA was what acompañantes at Las Libres were helping people in Guanajuato do with misoprostol.[20] To Cruz Sánchez around 2006, Americans seemed ignorant about abortion pills, including that misoprostol-only abortions, with the right information and support, could be safe, even quality care.[21] Why weren't more Americans talking about these pills?

At least two criminal cases in the first decade of the 2000s explain some of that wariness around SMA, specifically with misoprostol, that Cruz Sánchez noticed in the American reproductive rights, health, and justice movements. In 2004, a young woman in South Carolina was charged with a crime after she took misoprostol pills for her abortion; she was a recent immigrant from Mexico.[22] Then in 2007, a Massachusetts teenager took misoprostol for her abortion and was arrested; she was a recent immigrant from the Dominican Republic.[23] Both women knew about misoprostol from family members in their home countries, where misoprostol use for abortions was spreading (and from where loved ones appeared to have mailed them pills). Even without a South Carolina or Massachusetts law criminalizing the use of misoprostol for an abortion, hostile or ignorant prosecutors wielded other laws to try to punish these two women. This connected to a pregnancy-criminalization trend in the US, one disproportionately targeting low-income people of color.[24]

A few US reproductive health and rights nonprofits, including Dr. Beverly Winikoff's Gynuity Health Projects and RHTP, formed the Misoprostol Working Group in 2004 to better understand and raise awareness of "self-induced" abortion with misoprostol pills in the US.[25] After the 2004 South Carolina case, *Mother Jones* reported on misoprostol as a secret abortion pill. "All of us kind of recognize that keeping it a little below the radar may be the best in terms of advocacy right now," said Silvia Henriquez, then director of the National Latina Institute for Reproductive Health (today the National Latina Institute for Reproductive Justice), in that *Mother Jones* article.[26] The 2006 Congressional hearing attempting to ban mifepristone shortly after its FDA approval also appeared to shape that hesitancy. But the Latina Institute did discuss misoprostol with Latinx communities because, as Henriquez explained in that same article, "We can't *not* provide people with information because of the possibility there may be [abortion] sanctions down the road."

Planned Parenthood did not publicly acknowledge misoprostol-only abortions at the time, though the NAF website linked to information about how to safely use misoprostol for abortions, still stressing that a person should have their abortion under medical supervision.[27] SMA was a murky area legally. RHTP and Gynuity led a 2009 conference on "legal issues surrounding women's use of misoprostol for abortion outside the medical system."[28] One attendee hailed from the National Advocates for Pregnant Women (NAPW), a legal-advocacy organization addressing pregnancy criminalization (today called Pregnancy Justice), and warned of fetal-personhood arguments being used in courtrooms to strip pregnant people of their rights. People in the US caught using misoprostol for their own abortions, especially if they were not white, could be criminally vulnerable like what happened to one Black woman in South Carolina in 2001.

This woman was low-income, young, and a sexual-violence survivor who used crack-cocaine while pregnant. She suffered a pregnancy loss and was then criminalized, becoming the first person in the US to be prosecuted and convicted for a stillbirth.[29] Prosecutors argued without evidence that her use of crack-cocaine caused her stillbirth, and they effectively deemed the fetus she carried and lost had greater rights than she did.[30] This fetal-personhood playbook chillingly stretched beyond the US. Cruz Sánchez saw it in Mexico.

In 2008, she discovered women had been imprisoned in Guanajuato for homicide after they, too, had pregnancy losses, not abortions. It had been one year since Mexico City legalized abortion in pregnancies up to 12 weeks, the most progressive abortion law in the country, and a backlash came swiftly.[31] Conservative lawmakers in Guanajuato and 16 states across Mexico tried enshrining in state constitutions protections for "human life" at "conception," or fetal personhood.[32] Such amendments would mean that women who had abortions or any pregnancy loss could be charged with murder. Las Libres found at least eight women already incarcerated in Guanajuato for pregnancy losses after being charged with homicide and sentenced to up to 35 years in prison. They were all low-income women, a few of them Indigenous women who did not speak Spanish fluently. In 2010, after Las Libres campaigned, these women were freed.[33] Las Libres became even more aggressive with their accompaniment networks while working with allied lawyers to combat the latest barrage of anti-abortion laws rooted in fetal personhood.

Las Libres organized some of Mexico's first accompaniment networks that expanded to states beyond Guanajuato. Accompaniment groups took off into the next decade across much of Latin America as part of the Marea Verde, or Green Wave, as discussed in a later chapter. While Las Libres has been credited with this blossoming of accompaniment networks in Mexico, there are currently countless networks in Latin America and today's post-*Dobbs* US. Some have just two people, others hundreds. Some are public, others clandestine. Each adapts to their local and national contexts, whether in Argentina, Ecuador, Brazil, Indonesia, Kenya, Poland, or Nigeria, to name a few countries. They have sophisticated strategies to try to keep each other and those they help safe in some of the world's most abortion-restrictive environments, all with pills as one tool.

———————

In late 2001, the same year Cruz Sánchez learned of misoprostol, another approach with that pill formed inside a public hospital in Uruguay, a small, Catholic-majority country in South America with a near-total abortion ban.[34] Gynecologist Dr. Leonel Briozzo at Pereira Rossell Hospital Center was at an epidemic's epicenter in a devastating recession. Many pregnant people were suddenly unable to afford to raise a child and were resorting to invasive, self-induced abortions that killed them.[35] The rich could pay for a safe illegal abortion; the poor could not. Briozzo's team created a harm-reduction model for abortion care under a ban amid this crisis, a model that they called Iniciativas Sanitarias. They drew inspiration from past harm-reduction models in other stigmatized and criminalized public health crises, like HIV/AIDS activists in the 1980s US starting safe needle exchanges.[36]

Through Iniciativas Sanitarias, women could speak confidentially to Pereira Rossell health care workers about abortion options, and the hospital promised not to report anyone to law enforcement. "I owed myself to them, not the police," Briozzo told me through an interpreter. If a woman decided to end her pregnancy, the hospital could legally give her relevant public information, like what antibiotics to take before a procedure, and encourage her to return after her abortion to check for complications. The hospital could not legally perform abortions. But then Briozzo learned about misoprostol around 2002. The pill blew his mind. He proclaimed to anyone he met that misoprostol was "the penicillin of the 21st century for women's health . . . because it attacked the two leading causes of [maternal] death: abortion and postpartum hemorrhage," he told me through an interpreter.

Mifepristone was not yet accessible in Uruguay, though, like Mexico, misoprostol was effectively over the counter. Iniciativas Sanitarias took that same harm-reduction idea but now told abortion seekers about this pill.[37] The hospital workers spoke to women strictly in the third person and would not say exactly where an abortion-seeker should buy misoprostol. "Why? Because we couldn't recommend misoprostol. Because if we recommended misoprostol, it was a crime," Briozzo told me. "What we could do was inform them that in order to have an abortion with less risk at that time in the places where it was done, they used misoprostol." The Spanish word for what the hospital workers could legally do was asesoramiento, which literally translated in English to "advice," though Briozzo told me that translation was not quite right. He believed that there may be no equivalent word in English. "Because *asesoramiento* implies information but without giving the steps of advice on use. *Asesoramiento* is the thin red line you can't pass because if you pass the other way, the team is exposed to committing a crime, and therefore the whole program collapses."

At Pereira Rossell, staying on the right side of that thin red line led to a sharp drop in women dying. More and more Uruguayans learned to safely use misoprostol for their own abortions. The Ministry of Health made "the Uruguay model" official by 2004, the approach spreading across the country and, additionally thanks to a growing feminist movement, slowly beginning to reframe abortion as a public health as well as human rights issue. In 2012, Uruguay legalized abortion in pregnancies up to 12 weeks with some exceptions for later abortion care.[38] Uruguay became a vanguard in Latin America, where almost all countries still had near-total abortion bans. Mifepristone was soon registered in the country, and about 98 percent of abortions in Uruguay today are done with pills.[39]

But the new law imposed an obstacle course for abortion-seekers, and it was still a ban, albeit a ban on pregnancies later than 12 weeks. Abortion stigma also remained among many health care workers, leading some abortion-seekers to report mistreatment when they sought care in the formal health care system.[40] Briozzo believed there was much more work to be done on equal abortion access and quality of care. And paradoxically, Uruguay's new abortion law made it harder for people to get misoprostol compared to when a near-total ban existed. Because in 2013, the Ministry of Health took misoprostol out of retail pharmacies, even though women had been safely using the pills on their own for a decade by then.[41]

"If you're 13 weeks pregnant or if you're a migrant woman who has been in [Uruguay] for less than a year, you technically cannot have a legal abortion," feminist researcher Dr. Lucía Berro Pizzarossa told me. "You should be advised on how to self-manage an abortion with pills. That's not happening. Harm reduction disappeared with the law. . . . We have this idea that the best quality abortions happen in the presence or under the surveillance of a doctor. But I think that is very questionable." She has studied global SMA feminist movements and abortion law in Uruguay, her home country, and finds these medications fascinating for what they can reveal about us. "Abortion pills live this double life, right? On the one hand, they are highly regulated, highly criminalized drugs," she told me. "On the other hand, they've been declared essential medicines by the WHO since 2005."

Early in the first decade of the 2000s amid that double life of abortion pills, the WHO created its first public, international safe abortion guidelines. The agency stated that abortion pills should only be used under medical supervision. Dr. Beverly Winikoff was shocked at the WHO's "very, very conservative" approach to these medications, she told me. "Instead of people being excited and saying, 'Yes, yes, we can do this all over the place,' it was always the same. It was, 'This is so scary.'" Those guidelines were done in 2000, but the WHO did not publish them for three more years, terrified of what the US government under the incoming Bush administration might do in response. Dr. Paul Van Look at the WHO later co-wrote that the guidelines had "an exceptionally protracted process of internal review," one traveling to the WHO's director general, who reportedly asked Chelsea Clinton, daughter of former US president Clinton and a WHO intern at the time, to "read the document and assess what the reaction of the US government might be."[42]

When the guidelines were published in 2003, mifepristone and misoprostol were named the gold standard for medication abortion, with misoprostol-only abortions included as an option if mifepristone was not available. But the agency had hardly any translations or distribution plans to bring these guidelines in front of communities.[43] "The WHO kind of washed their hands of it and walked away," Dr. Anu Kumar, Ipas's CEO, told me in 2023. "It really isn't until quite recently that the WHO has been brave enough to talk about these issues."

A global feminist SMA movement growing in the 2010s would eventually help convince the WHO to rethink abortion pills, challenging the global medical community's assumption that quality medication abortion care needed a doctor. An accompaniment network in Argentina called Socorristas en Red has been collecting anonymized data since at least 2015 on their work under bans accompanying people through abortions with pills, consistently showing their doctor-less approach's safety, long before the WHO accepted SMA in 2022, as detailed in a later chapter.[44] "The WHO is always late," sociologist and Socorrista Dr. Raquel Drovetta told me bluntly. "The thing is that scientific organizations find it very difficult to accept that this evidence is scientific because it is researched by feminist organizations. And at that point comes the struggle over who generates knowledge and who generates science. . . . Are we going to wait for the WHO to tell us what to do? No, we are not going to wait."

LOOPHOLES

On June 11, 2001, in the Dutch port of Scheveningen, 35-year-old Dr. Rebecca Gomperts stepped aboard a small boat called the *Aurora* and, with her nails bitten from nerves, gripped the ship's railing while trying to stop herself from imagining the many ways this trip could fail.

Gomperts and her crew had already checked their supplies on board: 1,000 condoms, 120 IUDs, 250 emergency contraception pills, and, a late addition, 20 abortion-pill kits, each kit with one mifepristone and four misoprostol pills.[1] Those kits would be enough for just 20 people to have their abortions on that boat. "When I started the ship campaign, [pills were] not on my radar at all because it was not the world where I came from," Gomperts told me two decades later. "I wasn't the traditional or longtime abortion provider." That was an understatement.

The Netherlands, where Gomperts grew up, did not legalize abortion in pregnancies up to 24 weeks until 1984, two years after Dr. Étienne-Émile Baulieu spoke of RU-486 to the French Academy of Sciences.[2] Gomperts was just a teenager at the time. After she later finished medical school, she interned at a hospital in Guinea, where abortion was almost entirely banned, and witnessed women "brought in half-dead," she told me, hemorrhaging from trying to invasively end their pregnancies. Gomperts was still an outsider in the abortion provider community. She joined environmental activists at Greenpeace around 1997 as their resident doctor sailing on another ship, *Rainbow Warrior II*, to protest whaling and nuclear testing around Central and South America.

Almost all the countries where she sailed to on *Rainbow Warrior II* had abortion bans, with Gomperts seeing more women dying of self-induced abortions in hospitals just like in Guinea. She had an abortion years ago and wondered what would have happened to her if she had been living under an abortion ban when she needed help. According to the WHO, about 78,000 women a year, or one woman every 10 minutes, died of an unsafe abortion in the late 1990s.[3] It infuriated Gomperts to see abortion bans continue to be ignored as causing a global public health crisis and violating a human right. She aired her anger one day on *Rainbow Warrior II* when the captain planted an idea in her mind. There may be a way for women who lived in countries with abortion bans to legally access abortions on a ship like that one. When a boat sailed about twelve miles offshore, thus entering international waters, it fell under the law of wherever the boat was registered. On a ship registered in the Netherlands, abortions then became legal on board when that boat was in international waters. Gomperts thought this brilliant.

One abortion boat could not solve a global crisis but could make a statement. Except she did not know much about abortion pills yet.[4] So, when back in the Netherlands after her time sailing with Greenpeace, she received a grant around 1998 to study maritime law while envisioning providing early abortion procedures, not pills, on board a ship.[5] She excitedly confided her plan to longtime Dutch abortion provider Dr. Marijke Alblas, who was roughly two decades older than Gomperts. Alblas was impressed. She also knew Gomperts had an abortion, as had she.

In the late 1960s in the Netherlands under an abortion ban, Alblas was in medical school when she found out that she was pregnant and, determined not to have a child at that moment in her life, needed an abortion. Terrified, she told no one. It took Alblas almost four months to find a doctor who, for a price, agreed to perform her abortion. "It was the loneliest period of my life," Alblas told me. That doctor (a man) refused to provide abortions past 12 weeks in pregnancy, so Alblas, who knew that she was at 16 weeks, lied to him. He started her procedure when she began to bleed. He yelled at her, then kicked her out of his office as she bled. Alblas finally told her medical school friends, who completed her abortion and saved her life. "It was all those years ago," she told me at age 77 in 2021. "And I still remember how I felt."

She illegally, openly provided abortions in the Netherlands a decade later after becoming a doctor. Today, she specializes in complex abortion care for patients later in their pregnancies.[6] Alblas in the late 1990s was one of the few people who did not immediately dismiss Gomperts's boat idea, though she asked her, "But where do you get the money?" Gomperts's eyes narrowed. She would find a way. "Rebecca is like that," Alblas told me. "When she has something in her head, it must happen."

Around 1999, Gomperts founded Women on Waves, a nongovernmental organization (NGO) for her boat campaign, and began fundraising in the US while the Population Council and Danco were in hushed talks with the FDA over mifepristone. Gomperts's boat idea baffled Americans who had been terrorized by murders of abortion providers and bombings at clinics. When did abortion doctors become swashbucklers? What if someone shot her on the boat? But Gomperts could be convincing (and she would not be sailing to the US). She secured enough funds from the FMF and others to rent a boat, the *Aurora*.[7] She found a crew, including Dutch gynecologist Dr. Gunilla Kleiverda, and planned to sail in June 2001 to a destination kept secret for security.[8]

Gomperts, still thinking they would only do procedures on the boat, applied for a Dutch license to be able to perform abortions on the *Aurora*. Licensing rules required that the ship have a gynecological clinic on board. Since the ship was a rental, that clinic needed to be portable.[9] It was logistically complicated. An artist eventually agreed to build them a clinic inside a shipping container that doubled as a work of art.[10] The Netherlands meanwhile just approved mifepristone in 1999.[11] As medication abortion rolled out in the country, it became obvious to Gomperts and Kleiverda that providing women abortion pills on the boat would be much easier and safer.

Their license application, however, languished. It did not worry the crew yet. "Previously in the Netherlands, you could do things, then ask for permission after," Kleiverda told me. "And we had good relations with the health inspector. But we didn't realize that the Netherlands at that time was busy trying to clean up its image as a drug country. They were not at all amused that we were exporting our abortion services."

The "abortion boat" already was getting extensive media coverage when another problem arrived in May 2001, close to the *Aurora*'s sailing date. A reporter broke the news that the boat was headed to Ireland, one of the few countries in Europe that almost entirely banned abortion.[12] Their leaked destination rattled Gomperts. Just weeks prior, the FBI arrested the American anti-abortion extremist who murdered abortion provider Dr. Barnett Slepian in New York—after FBI agents discovered that the extremist had been hiding in Ireland, likely with help from local anti-abortion networks.[13] Now the world knew the "abortion boat" was on its way to that same nation.

Months ago, Dublin feminists invited Gomperts's boat to Ireland, the invite letter signed by Dr. Mary Muldowney, an Irish oral historian who became head of Irish Women on Waves.[14] A Catholic-majority country, Ireland was about an hour's flight from England, where abortion was broadly legal. Abortion-seekers in Ireland typically traveled to England for their care, if they could afford the trip.[15] Misoprostol was not over the counter in Ireland, and mifepristone was not registered in the country given the abortion ban. For Muldowney, a highly publicized 1997 abortion story in Ireland pushed her into activism "out of sheer personal horror," she told me.

Known as the "C Case," this story centered on a 13-year-old, referred to as "C" in court, who was pregnant from rape and suicidal but could not legally get an abortion in Ireland, so she flew to England for care.[16] Muldowney, who had a daughter not much older than C, shuddered at Ireland's cruelty. When she heard Gomperts mention an abortion boat on a talk show in 2000, Muldowney listened closely: what a way to force Ireland to confront itself.

Just before the *Aurora*'s sailing date, a Dutch paper reported Women on Waves did not have a license.[17] Gomperts began biting her nails. She started to wonder if, since they were switching from aspirations to pills, the boat may not need a license. Besides, if she delayed, then the ship's rental fees would go up and topple Women on Waves over budget.[18] Gomperts took a chance.

On June 11 in Scheveningen, she checked those 20 abortion-pill kits on the *Aurora* when the ship's owner called her in a panic. He read about the license debacle and feared there would be lawsuits against his boat, telling Gomperts to leave now or he may change his mind and stop the boat. They set sail. "That call was my first indication that things were about to heat up," Gomperts told me. "When I started the campaign, I underestimated a little bit the impact it could have."

But surely, those 20 kits would be enough. How many people would step on a boat for an abortion in front of the world's media? Only emails hit the Women on Waves inbox immediately as women in Ireland asked for help while the boat was at sea. The team directed women to call their hotline for an appointment.[19] Yet in the Netherlands, a conservative politician, furious at this abortion boat, declared anyone who performed abortions without a license could be put in prison. Women on Waves was in trouble.

In a scene from Diana Whitten's *Vessel*, a 2014 documentary on Women on Waves, a distracted Gomperts listened anxiously to a journalist advising her to smile and wave at reporters once the boat entered Dublin. The *Aurora* soon docked in the city's harbor across empty lots. "It was deliberately off the beaten track," Muldowney told me. "I dare say that location was for security reasons, but it did mean that if you went down there, it was fairly obvious what you were there for." Aside from a few anti-abortion protesters, the crowds greeting the *Aurora* were mostly made up of reporters.

Gomperts nervously smiled and waved on deck, as she had been told to do, when a journalist asked, "Have you got a license to perform abortions?" She held the ship's railing tightly, hoping no one noticed her chewed nails. "We will have a press conference tomorrow to talk about it," she said. This aggravated some journalists who had flown into Ireland to cover what looked like a flop. "Tomorrow, I would very much like . . . ," said Gomperts, her voice trailing. "I would very much like to discuss tomorrow."[20]

While she stumbled above deck, two nurses below deck fielded abortion-seekers' calls. One nurse, Juul Böckling, asked callers if they were no more than nine weeks pregnant, the Dutch legal requirement for a medication abortion at the time, and booked their appointments. A mother confided to Böckling that her teenage son's girlfriend was pregnant and in desperate need of help. More stories came with each call. Böckling answered about 50 calls that evening.[21] "We never thought there would be more than five," she said in *Vessel*. "This is the real story." Yet the other story was what abortion seekers told Böckling that they wanted. "We have people asking, 'If it's only treatment with pills, why can't you just give me the pills? I'll swallow them by myself,'" said Böckling in *Vessel*. "But we cannot do that," the nurse added with a sigh.[22] Not legally.

Meanwhile, the Irish activists were aghast at the ship's missing license. "I think everyone was in a state of panic," Gomperts told me. "It was really difficult because all the activist groups were disagreeing with how to proceed. And it was scary. The government is threatening you." The activist groups decided together not to risk the Dutch criminal courts. That meant they would not provide any abortions at all, a decision that "felt terrible," Kleiverda told me. "Some people were shattered," Muldowney told me. "I, for one, was let down. . . . I felt like [the story] became more about Rebecca than about the women who needed help."

Gomperts tried to turn media attention to the 78,000 women a year who died of unsafe abortion around the world, speaking forcefully to the press, no longer bothering to hide her chewed nails. When a reporter asked if this boat was a publicity stunt, she fired back, "Do you really think that we would have put so much effort into a thing like that?" But one question threw her: "Have you ever had an abortion?"

"I—you know—I don't think that's an appropriate question to ask," she said in a scene in *Vessel*. "Abortion is one of the most common medical interventions in the world. But because it is about women, it is invisible. It is a silent suffering, one nobody fucking knows."

"Or some sort of personal exper—"

"No, don't try," said Gomperts. "No, it's too easy. Are you going to ask somebody working for Amnesty International whether they have been tortured? Come on. That's not the issue. The issue is do women have basic human rights to be able to decide what is happening with their own bodies." She left the interview to calm herself, though she blurted out, "Shall we go outside and hand over the pills [to the women]? I would really love to do that. Fuck that."[23]

About 80 people had booked abortions on the *Aurora*, but the nurses called them back to cancel their appointments. Some callers cried; some fell silent. Nurses gave them a number to the British Pregnancy Advisory Services, which provided abortions in England, and allied Irish groups raised money for callers' travel, lodging, and abortion costs.[24] "I still occasionally have disturbed dreams about that day," Muldowney told me. "It was a bit traumatic that we couldn't actually bring the women out on the boat." And those 20 abortion-pill kits wildly miscalculated the need. "Sometimes when I think about what we were planning to do and the size of the *Aurora*," Muldowney told me, "I realize we needed a much bigger ship."

By the 2010s, another generation of Irish activists in a global feminist SMA movement clandestinely did what the *Aurora* did not: give people in Ireland abortion pills beyond the law.[25] And in 2018, after years of grassroots campaigning, the people of Ireland overwhelmingly voted to at last repeal the nation's abortion ban.[26] Ireland legalized abortion in pregnancies up to 12 weeks with exceptions for later care. The new law remained restrictive, even criminalizing people providing pills outside the formal health care system.[27] To SMA activists, this showed that there was more progress to be made, but there had at least been movement.

Back in 2001, that failed abortion boat in Ireland crushed Gomperts until, months later, abortion-seekers around the world emailed her to ask when a boat would be coming to them. "What fascinates me is that nobody really remembered what happened, only that there was an abortion boat," she told me. "What's most important about activism is you go, you do it, and that in itself changes things. Because you're breaking through the self-censorship . . . even when things don't go the way you hoped they would go."

In 2004, after another abortion boat trip went awry, Gomperts flipped her focus from ships to pills. She was in Portugal, which banned abortion at the time, when the Portuguese minister of defense sent warships to stop a Women on Waves boat approaching the nation's shore.[28] Women on Waves pivoted.[29]

Mifepristone was not yet registered in Portugal, but Gomperts knew most pharmacies in the country sold misoprostol over the counter under the brand name Arthrotec. The WHO had just released its abortion guidelines that included instructions on how to have a safe misoprostol-only abortion.[30] What if Women on Waves turned their hotline set up for callers to book appointments on the boat into a resource where people could learn to use misoprostol?

"What we did in Portugal, when we put out the information with misoprostol on how to do an abortion yourself, that was very revolutionary," Kleiverda told me, stressing that this move came at the "very beginning" of medication abortion's journey around the world. Women on Waves quickly linked its website to those WHO guidelines and research on misoprostol-only abortions while Kleiverda began training a Portuguese activist, who was not a licensed provider, on what information to give hotline callers. Information also spread differently in 2004 (YouTube launched the next year). To reach people, Gomperts went on a live daytime Portuguese talk show that she knew many women in the country watched.[31] She brought a box of misoprostol pills on the show and dove in, speaking rapidly through an interpreter.

To have a safe abortion with misoprostol up to 12 weeks in pregnancy, find this Arthrotec packet in a pharmacy. One will need 12 pills, or 2,400 micrograms. Put four pills under the tongue or in the cheek to dissolve for half an hour, then spit out what remains. Wait three hours. Take four more pills under the tongue or in the cheek to dissolve for half an hour, then spit out what remains. Wait three hours. Take four more pills under the tongue or in the cheek to dissolve for half an hour, then spit out what remains. One will bleed and cramp. One may have chills, a fever, diarrhea, nausea, and vomiting. Seek medical help if (a) one has a fever over 39 degrees Celsius (about 102 Fahrenheit) for more than 24 hours (b) one bleeds more than two pads per hour for more than two hours (c) one does not bleed at all (d) one has extreme pain. If seeking medical help, one can tell a doctor they are miscarrying. There is no medical reason for a doctor to know one took misoprostol. The treatment is the same as for miscarriages, which is a legal treatment. No blood or urine test will show that one took misoprostol. Do not take pills vaginally because traces of the pills may be left in the vagina. Otherwise, a doctor will not know the difference between a person having a miscarriage and having an abortion with pills.[32]

Gomperts stressed these pills were an option if there were no other ways that a person could have a safe abortion. She told people to visit the Women on Waves website for more information and to call the hotline, which rang and rang. That Women on Waves page on misoprostol became their site's most visited page at the time.[33] It then dawned on Gomperts that neither boats nor pills were as important of an activist tool as the web.

She admired HIV/AIDS activists who, years earlier, found cheap medications online and, defying laws, shipped them to people living with a stigmatized illness.[34] What if abortion-seekers in countries under bans ordered abortion pills online that could be shipped to their homes? Her timing was ideal. Mifepristone's global patent (excluding the US) recently expired, ushering in affordable generics of the drug, and India, which sought to be a global pharmaceutical manufacturing hub, just approved mifepristone.[35] In 2005, Gomperts founded the world's first-known telehealth abortion platform, Women on Web (WOW), in the Netherlands (today it's headquartered in Canada).[36] WOW operated legally where it was based and where its doctors were licensed. People in ban countries filled out an online form with their relevant medical history and date of their last period.[37] A doctor screened responses and, if all looked fine, off mifepristone and misoprostol pills went, mailed from a pharmacy in India.[38] The abortion-seeker paid around $100 or whatever they could afford.[39]

A WOW help desk of around five staffers, almost all not doctors, answered people's emailed questions about pills.[40] If a person's question ever did require a doctor's response, the help desk flagged it to Gomperts or another doctor on staff and, in the rare case that something about the person's experience seemed medically concerning, they advised the person to seek medical attention near them.[41] Due to potential criminalization risks, they also advised that the person not tell their medical provider that they took pills, only that they were having a miscarriage. Staffers found that people tended to be much more scared about the illegality of having an abortion than about the medications themselves. WOW sent pills in discrete packaging. But depending on the context, a person taking pills under bans could be sent to prison if caught having an abortion. This was delicate work.

When WOW started, the NGO did not send pills to countries where abortion was legal even if access was a major issue (like the US). The provision of pills in such countries almost always legally required an in-person doctor's visit in the first decade of the 2000s.[42] A WOW-like service based in the US was believed impossible with that FDA restriction against mailing mifepristone to patients. Abortion providers in countries with more liberal abortion laws (like the US) also initially tended to see telehealth abortion as lower-quality care compared to in-clinic abortion. What could Gomperts really do if someone taking pills needed help? No doctor had mailed abortion pills directly to patients before, certainly not to patients a continent away. These were early days of telehealth anything.

Alblas applauded WOW's boldness while nonetheless asking Gomperts: "But who do you reach with that? Just women who had access to the Internet." She worried women using WOW were "not the poorest of the poor," Alblas told me. "They don't know about it. But that doesn't mean that [Gomperts] hasn't helped many, many women."

Equitable, global access to abortion pills via the internet remains a massive challenge, even as more people live online today, two decades after WOW's launch. Gomperts told me in 2022 that WOW's biggest hurdle "is how to find the people that don't find you." She thought that so much power concentrated in a few social media companies made this information gap even wider today than when WOW started.

Back then, WOW would be one of the first search results when people googled abortion pills.[43] But WOW first faced online censorship in 2012 when Facebook (now Meta) deleted on their platform a WOW image with instructions on using misoprostol for abortions.[44] Censorship only became trickier for Gomperts to detect once social media algorithms became more inscrutable. She told me that, in March 2020 at the COVID-19 pandemic's start, WOW lost about 90 percent of its traffic on Google. Gomperts still did not really know why.

She used to rely on the press to tell people about pills, like explaining how to use misoprostol on that Portuguese talk show. In the 2020s, hyper-personalized news feeds on sites like Facebook, Instagram, TikTok, and X (formerly Twitter) mean she has no idea what people see and don't see online. "The pills, the active ingredients, and the women are not the problem," Gomperts told me. "The problem is the pharmaceutical companies. The problem is the doctors. The digital spaces. All the other spaces where there's this imbalance of people that are in charge. Those who have power and control to mitigate information and access."

Gomperts was the first person known to start telehealth abortion. But she was not the first to launch a website to educate the public about abortion pills.

Around 2003, two Massachusetts-based research nonprofits, Ibis Reproductive Health and Cambridge Reproductive Health Associates, launched medicationabortions.com to share evidence-based information about mifepristone and misoprostol.[45] People around the world soon began emailing the site questions, mostly about misoprostol. The person who initially ran that site, a demographer, promptly responded to each question, doing so without considering possible liability issues in the US around what may be providing medical advice without a license. Once a reporter began poking around the site, that person got nervous and stopped answering the site's emailed questions altogether.

What *did* it even mean legally for a nonprofit incorporated in Massachusetts to give information on abortion pills to people across the globe? "It sounds ridiculous now, but this is back in 2005 to 2007,"

Dr. Angel Foster told me.[46] A medical doctor and professor at the University of Ottawa in Canada today, Foster took over that site after the first person stopped (the site is now dormant). "There were some very conservative approaches to this, feeling like [the site] needed to be informational, but it really couldn't be dynamic."

Foster would soon study offline, community-based distribution models of misoprostol for abortions in countries with near-total bans where mifepristone was not available. "I think that these models are going to look very different in different places if they're organic," she told me. "There's cookie-cutter models that can be done in lots of different places, but there's also tailored, adopted models." In the mid-2010s, her research while on the Thailand-Burma border reflected that. Maternal mortality from unsafe abortion was "astronomically high" there, Foster told me. But misoprostol was available over the counter on the Thai side of the border. One day in 2007, Foster led a workshop to border communities about using misoprostol to manage miscarriages and treat postpartum hemorrhage. An interpreter came up to Foster after, asking if these same pills could be used for an abortion, explaining that her friend needed help. Could she take misoprostol?

Foster invited the interpreter and abortion seeker for tea to talk about the pills. Through that interpreter, Foster asked the abortion seeker questions to rule out rare contraindications and estimate how far she was in pregnancy. Foster explained what to expect when taking pills, how the pills worked, and how to use them. The interpreter listened carefully since she planned to support her friend throughout her abortion with Foster on call as an allied doctor. After that one person's safe abortion, they designed together a program to train other lay people to do the same.

Over three years helping about 900 people, the program found a 96 percent efficacy for misoprostol-only abortions, much higher than the roughly 80 percent shown in most studies until then.[47] Critically, the women in the program overwhelmingly reported that they had positive abortion experiences.[48] Yet what struck Foster most was how this all began: "It came from an interpreter and participant in this workshop who connected the dots immediately and said, 'Wait a minute. I can see how this can be used.'"

———————

Around 2007, 23-year-old lesbian feminist activist Sara Larrea heard Gomperts talk about her abortion boats at a conference. Larrea, born and raised in Ecuador, worked in Quito at a human rights NGO, Co- ordinadora Política Juvenil por la Equidad de Género (CPJ).[49] This boat idea intrigued her.

Ecuador had one of the world's worst abortion bans. People who had an illegal abortion could be imprisoned for up to two years while anyone performing an illegal abortion could be imprisoned up to three years.[50] For a price, some doctors provided abortions beyond the law. When Larrea's best friend got pregnant and needed an abortion as a teenager, they called doctors for weeks for help until they found someone. But even then, Larrea worried that this doctor may not be safe or may mistreat her friend. Thankfully, her friend was okay.

Mifepristone was not registered in Ecuador, though misoprostol sat over the counter. Larrea had heard that misoprostol could be used for abortions, but she believed what doctors told her: it was only safe to take under medical supervision. "Because we, as a feminist movement, were thinking that the only way to make abortion safe at the time was to legalize it and put it in hospitals under the power of medical professionals," she told me. When Larrea then learned of Gomperts's boat, she thought that might open a conversation on abortion in the country.

In 2008, a Women on Waves ship sailed for Ecuador when a storm hit. There would be no ship, so CPJ activists improvised. Maybe they could tell callers how to take misoprostol like the hotline set up in Portugal did. But WOW existed now. Should they direct callers to or- der mifepristone and misoprostol online? Only pill shipments from India to Ecuador could take weeks. And not enough Ecuadorians had internet access or a credit card to buy pills online. Most did at least have phones. Larrea thought back to her friend. "Of course, I do not want other people to go through weeks and weeks of asking everyone [for an abortion] and receiving all this rejection and aw- ful discourses," she told me. Now two doctors, both Gomperts and Kleiverda, were saying to these young activists that they could tell people how to safely take misoprostol pills at home without a doctor present. That was a big deal. They decided to do it.

They named the hotline Salud Mujeres, or Women's Health, and operated under a legal protection to give and receive public information, one enshrined in international human rights treaties that Ecuador signed. But Larrea was still scared they might be arrested or that someone taking these pills might get hurt. Yet for people with unwanted pregnancies and nowhere to go for help, what other options were there? Women on Waves and CPJ unfurled a giant banner in Quito that read "ABORTO SEGURO" (safe abortion) with their hotline number.[51] The phone immediately rang.

When Women on Waves left Ecuador, Salud Mujeres stayed open and staffed from three to about 10 people, mostly volunteers working around the clock. More people learned to use misoprostol. Salud Mujeres's blog, which had misoprostol information, saw about 2.5 million visits between 2008 and roughly 2014.[52] And that police crackdown on the hotline never came. Only once in 2010 did a court order shut Salud Mujeres down for about a day.[53] Activists got a new phone number and restarted. It was exhausting yet satisfying to Larrea. Feminists like her aspired to grand ideals like the end of patriarchy. "But that is a very long thing. And this was very fast," she told me of Salud Mujeres. "We can do this, and, in a year, we will have thousands of women calling us, able to access an abortion."

Salud Mujeres became the first autonomous, feminist abortion-pill information hotline in Latin America and the Caribbean. Similar hotlines sprouted after Salud Mujeres presented their model in 2009 at a feminist regional conference, where attendees included Mexico's Las Libres. Larrea trained people to start their own hotlines adapted to their contexts. If this strategy worked in Ecuador under one of the region's worst bans, maybe it would work elsewhere. At least five feminist abortion-pill hotlines took off in South America afterward: two in Chile in 2009, one in Argentina in 2009, another in Peru in 2010, and one in Venezuela in 2011.[54] "And now I know that there are not a lot of moments in life where you can actually think something crazy and then do it and see it working," Larrea told me. "And that was one of those moments in life. And it was amazing."

One July 2009 night in Buenos Aires, a few lesbian feminist activists stared at billboards of smiling women selling products they did not need. The activists checked that no police were nearby, then took out from their bags glue, brushes, and posters with a message printed on them. One activist spotted the looming face of actor Johnny Depp in a movie ad, then gleefully glued by his lips a poster that read, "ABORTO / TU DECISIÓN / INFORMACIÓN EN," next to a phone number.[55]

These activists delighted in talking about abortion in a positive way in Argentina, which almost entirely banned abortion like in Ecuador.[56] They were part of Lesbianas y Feministas por la Decriminalización del Aborto (Lesbians and Feminists for the Decriminalization of Abortion), and Larrea helped train them. That July, they marched in Buenos Aires with about 100 people to announce their abortion-pill hotline.[57] The activists wore rainbow flags, linking destigmatization of lesbianism to abortion. These people were a fraction of the thousands who, a decade later, would protest in the streets of Buenos Aires in the Marea Verde, or Green Wave.

Outside Latin America late in the first decade of the 2000s and into the early 2010s, WOW and Women on Waves helped to launch misoprostol hotline strategies in parts of Asia and sub-Saharan Africa as well, training trusted community health workers in several countries that banned abortion but that sold misoprostol over the counter.[58] However, hotlines had limits. Salud Mujeres did not support someone throughout their abortion process, for one. Activists at Salud Mujeres in the early 2010s debated if they should give misoprostol pills to people who could not find the medication. But doing so risked putting these activists in prison if they were caught. Or should they physically be with the person in their home during their abortion process? These big questions brought up activists' varied risk tolerances but also views of the state. As Larrea explained to me, "Do we want to demand the state provide abortion, or do we want to do it ourselves forever?"

But by 2014 in Ecuador, misoprostol seemed harder for hotline callers to find, with some anti-abortion pharmacists catching on to what was happening.[59] There had also been an uptick in people in Ecuador criminalized for abortions, which had been rare when Salud Mujeres started.[60] In nearby Brazil, similar reports emerged of people being criminalized for taking abortion pills or ordering them online.[61] WOW stopped mailing pills to Brazil when officials began tracing a few packages back to abortion-seekers, alarming activists.[62]

With these dramatic changes, several Salud Mujeres members in 2014 broke away to form another model: an accompaniment network called Las Comadres, which operated similarly to Las Libres.[63] "We understood that although the information was important, it was not enough if there was no real access to medication and safe conditions for abortion," Stephanie (Stefy) Altamirano, a volunteer Las Comadres member, told me in 2023 through an interpreter. She accompanied people who had abortions with pills, doing so mostly over the phone with each person, and with allied doctors as well as lawyers on call just in case, all trying to lower criminalization risks for the abortion-seeker.[64]

At WOW, the same year Las Comadres formed, many staff, including Larrea, quit over disagreements with leadership. Larrea had been working from Ecuador on WOW's help desk. To her, Global North–Global South power imbalances went unresolved as on-the-ground security issues became more fraught. A global SMA movement also seemed to be outgrowing relying on one NGO for pill supplies. And what about the most vulnerable people whom WOW could not reach? In 2014, a few former WOW employees created another telehealth abortion NGO called Women Help Women (WHW), one that Larrea joined from Ecuador. Like WOW, WHW prescribed and mailed mifepristone and misoprostol to people in ban countries.[65] But WHW's partners in ban countries, many of them feminist collectives, "basically run the pills," as WHW co-founder Kinga Jelinska told me from her office in the Netherlands, describing her team's work as "decolonizing our minds" constantly. While WOW found legal loopholes to get people pills, WHW did not. "There are not enough loopholes here," Jelinska told me. "The loopholes keep shrinking every day."

Born and raised in Poland, Jelinska remembered when, as a preteen, her home country in 1993 became a nation that moved from broad legal protections for abortion to a near-total abortion ban (the US post-*Dobbs* would join that list). While a young person in Poland, Jelinska "popped birth control pills like candy," terrified of becoming pregnant under a ban. No one around her talked about abortion either. She migrated to the Netherlands in 2004 for job opportunities and soon found an opening at WOW, which groomed her. But her thinking on pills evolved over the years. These pills were so safe. Why did a doctor need to be involved at all if you did not want one there?

Jelinska has had three abortions with pills without a licensed provider in the Netherlands. Her abortions were technically illegal in the country since she took mifepristone and misoprostol pills outside of the formal health care system.[66] However, she told me that she spoke loudly about her abortions to expose the absurdity of laws in even progressive countries not aligning with scientific evidence that, by 2022, showed SMA was safe. Much of that evidence came from WHW partners like Argentina's Socorristas en Red, discussed in the next chapter.[67]

CHAPTER 11

QUESTIONING EVERYTHING, COMPLETELY

Late on August 8, 2018, outside the Palace of the Argentine National Congress in Buenos Aires, thousands of people stood in the streets wearing green bandanas, waiting. Lawmakers inside the Palace were debating a bill to legalize abortion up to 14 weeks in pregnancy. The lower House had already passed the measure, and, if the Senate did so next, the president promised to sign the bill into law.[1] It would be a landmark moment.

Abortion had been criminalized in Argentina since the late nineteenth century. The country's 1922 penal code provisions on abortion allowed legal care only if a person had been raped, if a doctor deemed a pregnant person's life or health at risk, or if a pregnant person had an intellectual disability.[2] Anyone who performed her own abortion could be imprisoned.[3] That August night in 2018 seemed to mark a new era after more than a decade of grassroots feminist organizing. Young women were dancing in the streets earlier that day, hopeful; one even dressed as a box of misoprostol pills. Yet as Senate talks stretched for hours into the night, the faces in the crowds outside turned distraught when, after midnight, the Senate rejected the bill. Abortion remained almost entirely banned. Rain fell onto the masses of people in green crying and screaming. Police in riot gear sprayed tear gas on them.[4]

Among these protesters in green were a few wearing fluorescent pink wigs and who called themselves Socorristas. Some identified as women, others as nonbinary. Many were proudly tattooed since, as one Socorrista told me, "We put our bodies in everything we do."[5] A group of Socorristas weeks earlier had been invited to testify to the Palace about abortion access under Argentina's ban. It had become impossible in the country to untangle Socorristas from the fight for abortion rights. Now, after this August 2018 defeat, Socorristas doubled in size, more and more people asking to join them, the bill's failure igniting a Green Wave unlike ever before.[6]

In 2001, when Verónica Cruz Sánchez heard about misoprostol in Mexico and Dr. Beverly Winikoff guarded mifepristone's FDA approval in the US, the year Dr. Rebecca Gomperts sailed from the Netherlands to Ireland with pills and Dr. Leonel Briozzo began a harm-reduction model in Uruguay, 35-year-old teacher and single mother Ruth Zurbriggen in Neuquén, Argentina, wanted to create a feminist space that did not exist. She had been steeped in Trotskyism for years until its orthodoxy and male-dominated leadership disillusioned her. Zurbriggen grew up the second child of eight, cooking and caring for her siblings.[7] She felt that these invisible labors like caregiving, which were gendered feminine, were undervalued. She was not alone.

In Neuquén, Zurbriggen met two women who were fellow teachers and all three were studying for a second college degree while itching to shape local politics for gender equity. The three co-founded a feminist collective called La Revuelta just as a 2001 economic and political crisis hit Argentina.[8]

With so many more low-income women dying from unsafe, invasive abortions under a recession and a ban in Argentina, similar to what Briozzo was witnessing in nearby Uruguay, Zurbriggen and La Revuelta members joined a 2005 national meeting with around 300 groups and no political party affiliation. It was time to talk about abortion rights. Until then, factions within Argentina's feminist movement had been distancing themselves from abortion in the Catholic-majority country. They all now formed the National Campaign for the Right to Legal, Safe, and Free Abortion, or La Campaña, agreeing on a single goal: legalize abortion.[9] How far such a law should go would later be contentious. La Campaña at this inaugural meeting in 2005 also agreed on a symbol: the green bandana.

Many Argentinian movements used bandanas to recall the white kerchiefs that the iconic Las Madres de la Plaza de Mayo wore. In the late 1970s and 1980s, mothers donned those kerchiefs while protesting "the disappeared," or the thousands of people the country's military dictatorship at the time kidnapped, imprisoned, or killed without acknowledgment.[10] Las Madres marched outside the presidential palace of Buenos Aires day in and day out, demanding their missing children.[11] Connecting La Campaña's fight to these mothers flipped an anti-abortion narrative that "good" mothers did not have or support abortions. As for La Campaña's decision that their bandanas should be green, that color represented life, not in an anti-abortion "pro-life" sense but in centering the life of the pregnant person, the woman. Their 2005 meeting picked a slogan too: "Sexual education to decide, contraceptives to not have abortions, and legal abortion not to die."

Years later, Zurbriggen and Socorristas strongly criticized that slogan, believing it to be stigmatizing of abortion and too conservative. Longtime Argentinian feminist scholar María Alicia Gutiérrez, a key player in La Campaña, told me through an interpreter that, yes, this "legal abortion not to die" message was not ideal. "But it was proposed precisely to put the axis on the public health problem because it was the axis that allowed us to attract more people and more possibilities for debate," she told me. "For me, the key axis was autonomy and freedom to decide about one's own body. But if we put that [as our slogan], half of the population wouldn't have joined us. If we put 'women are dying,' they were much more with us. Even if it seems tragic. Even if it's not the way I like it."

Gutiérrez, who was 70 years old when we spoke in 2023, was one of the first researchers to write about women clandestinely using misoprostol for their abortions in Argentina. Early in the first decade of the 2000s around when La Campaña formed, she interviewed young women in public hospitals who told her frankly that they had taken pills to start their abortion process, then, as in early 1990s Brazil, went to the hospital for medical attention. Gutiérrez would ask, amazed, how they heard of this pill, and the young women would look at her in even more amazement and say, "But how do you *not* know? Everybody knows about it. It's word of mouth." "Okay, but tell me specifically," she would ask again. "How did you learn this?" Then came stories. "One night, I went to a dance at a club, [my period] was late, I started chatting with some friends, and they told me, 'But buy this at a pharmacy, blah, blah, blah, blah.'" Some pharmacists started to realize that Oxaprost, the brand name for misoprostol in Argentina, must be used for something else given all these young women buying a pill "that's a remedy for stomach problems for people who are a little bit older," Gutiérrez told me with a smile. "[The pharmacists] start doing complicated things like raising the price, making it more expensive, or denying it." Yet like in Mexico, women in Argentina found "friendly" pharmacies and told each other where to go for the pills.[12]

Since Argentina's Ministry of Health commissioned Gutiérrez's research at that time, all while the country had a near-total abortion ban, her paper did not use the word "abortion," and she referred to this practice instead as "misuses of misoprostol." She understood "misuse" was far from true. Early in the first decade of the 2000s, she also interviewed people at another public hospital in Argentina that treated many Peruvian migrant women. "And they knew exactly how to do it," Gutiérrez told me. Take Oxaprost, go to a hospital, "and tell any story: 'I fell, and I got hurt. I am miscarrying.' Because they knew perfectly well the possible strategies to face the issues of clandestinity and illegality."

Meanwhile on May 28, 2005, La Campaña went public. The coalition handed Congress a petition asking the legislators simply to discuss the legalization of abortion. That did not happen, not as months, then years passed. "There was a feeling of failure because there was no possibility of debating the law," Gutiérrez told me. "And that was when different organizations or networks [for abortion pills] emerged. One of the first is Socorristas en Red, women who accompany women having an abortion. You talked to Ruth. She was one of the first."

Zurbriggen did feel failure by then. La Revuelta in Neuquén had already started a free legal advisory service and hotline, Socorro Violeta, to support women and anyone experiencing gender-based or intimate-partner violence. Volunteers were accompanying survivors through legal and medical systems. But survivors kept calling that hotline needing abortions. La Revuelta built a small network of doctors who agreed to provide illegal abortions for a price. Yet in 2008, a disturbing experience with one doctor forced Zurbriggen to reimagine abortion care entirely.[13]

A former student of a La Revuelta member had contacted the group for help that year. He was twenty years old and named Newen. His 19-year-old girlfriend, Ailén, was pregnant and did not want to be. They were too frightened to tell their parents. Ailén was pregnant past eight weeks, and La Revuelta did not know a doctor that provided abortions beyond that gestational age. Newen searched until he found a doctor who agreed to perform Ailén's abortion the next day. The couple asked if Zurbriggen could accompany them to their appointment.

When they all arrived at the doctor's office, the doctor, a man, acted brusquely and took Ailén behind a closed door without explaining why. No one knew what the doctor next did to Ailén, not even Ailén, who later told them, "He checked me and placed something [in me], but I don't know what else."[14] The doctor released Ailén, telling her to wait nearby for hours with something inserted in her vagina, then come back. He did not explain why she needed to wait, or why he placed something in her vagina. Ailén, Newen, and Zurbriggen found a hotel, scraping money together to afford a room, then waited with Ailén as she bled. She did not have any pads. The doctor had not told her to bring any, only 2,500 pesos.[15] They cried. Ailén hours later went back to the doctor for her procedure. She was in pain afterwards. Zurbriggen felt a "total abandonment by the state," as she later co-wrote, describing that day as a "scar" on their collective.[16] She did know about misoprostol pills before this experience. But she thought an abortion with a doctor must be better. Not anymore.

La Revuelta from then on accompanied people for free through their abortions with misoprostol, unless the person preferred or needed a doctor. Around 2010, they launched Socorro Rosa, an all-volunteer abortion-access hotline in Neuquén. They studied materials on how to use misoprostol correctly, drawing on WHO guidelines and a manual that Lesbianas y Feministas wrote after launching their hotline a year earlier in Buenos Aires. They arranged to meet callers at public spots, where they handed over pamphlets on how to use pills and names of "friendly" pharmacies to get misoprostol, doing so quickly, afraid of being seen. "Everything was still quite clandestine in that sense," Zurbriggen told me. La Revuelta presented Socorro Rosa to members of La Campaña as a "Plan B" for safe abortion access, as Zurbriggen put it, a just-for-now option until Argentina legalized abortion.

Zurbriggen saw Socorro Rosa in a lineage of feminist abortion care beyond the law, like the Janes in the US pre-*Roe*. But by 2011, their hotline got so many callers across the country that Socorro Rosa asked groups in La Campaña if any of them would start their own hotlines in their provinces. They soon did so. What became Socorristas launched with five groups in 2012, and many Socorristas once had abortions themselves. They decided to be open about their accompaniment "because one of the main purposes was to take abortion out of the clandestine and into public life," Zurbriggen told me, like Las Libres's journey.

This was a critical move. Socorristas existed in a legal gray area at best. It was not a crime to give public information on pills, yet it was a crime for someone to have or perform an illegal abortion. That meant these activists, whom the law may view as abortion providers, risked imprisonment, as did those they helped. Yet Socorristas were "contextually safe" in these years, Zurbriggen told me, surrounded by allied movements and supportive actors in universities, state sectors, and the medical community.

Socorristas documented their accompaniment as they went to learn how to provide better care. When they began, they urged people to have an exam with a doctor after their abortions. Socorristas were insistent on that partially because they were not as experienced with the pills yet. But they were also strategic. Finding doctors who agreed to provide post-abortion care built alliances between Socorristas and those within the health care system. If Socorristas were "Plan B" until abortion legalization, Zurbriggen explained to me, then who would be there to provide abortions within the health care system once a new abortion law came?

In 2014, Socorristas expanded to 10 of Argentina's 23 provinces. About 35 percent of callers had been referred to the activists by doctors, who were publicly crediting Socorristas with helping to lower the rate of deaths and complications from unsafe abortions.[17] Socorristas sought to one day be "articulated alongside" the health care system, not against it, Zurbriggen told me. With a rising demand for their care, however, Socorristas revised strategies. "We would have three, four, or five people who needed an abortion, and we realized there was an inherent power in doing it together," Zurbriggen told me. They now met people before their abortions in a small group, rather than one-on-one. "To talk about their processes and their decisions together."

Something surprising happened in these meetings. When they asked people why they came to Socorristas, abortion-seekers often told them in all seriousness that "having an abortion with us is 'the legal way,'" Zurbriggen told me with a smile. It was not legal, so what did they mean? They would explain that Socorristas "felt legal. . . . Because there was accountability, a phone number, names, volunteers, and it was public." Zurbriggen believed Socorristas helped "set the levels of legality" for abortion care in Argentina later, similar to how a few Janes after *Roe* worked at abortion clinics in the US, bringing aspects of their once-illegal care into newly legal spaces.

Within La Campaña, however, tensions bubbled up over what legalizing abortion meant. Socorristas wanted La Campaña to push for legal abortion throughout pregnancy, arguing any ban on this care at any gestational age discriminatory. More moderate members of La Campaña strongly disagreed. Despite their disappointment, Socorristas stayed in La Campaña "for the sake of the movement," as Zurbriggen put it, and with some naivete in retrospect. "We thought the law was going to fix all the problems. It was not long before we realized that was not going to be the case."

In late August 2018 in Córdoba, 29-year-old Lucía Baez, an English and sex education teacher, watched surging Green Wave protests in the streets, struck by people in pink wigs and tattoos who looked powerful. She wanted to join them. Baez knew Socorristas existed, yet it was not until after that month's failed Senate vote that they became more visible to her. "For feminists that were alone in the world, let's say, alone here in Argentina, the Green Wave gathered us," Baez told me.

Zurbriggen connected me to Baez, who told me Zurbriggen was simply "Ruth" among the roughly 400 Socorristas, as of 2023. Baez was part of a 21-person collective of Socorristas in Córdoba, which was one of the network's largest collectives, where each Socorrista accompanied three to six people's abortions each week. "I have always thought that if you know what's going on, you should do something about it because it hurts, right?" she told me. "Only to know and not do anything." When Baez was younger, before she knew about pills, she needed an abortion under Argentina's ban. "I remember when I had my abortion, I would rather die, and I had it very clear in my mind. 'I won't be a mother. So, if I have to die here, okay,'" she told me. "And a lot of women think like that. . . . 'I want to have an abortion, and I will find a way.'"

Baez had an abortion procedure at a hospital—and she hated it. It felt violating. That was why she joined a local Socorrista collective in 2018. She did not want anyone to experience an abortion like that. Socorristas trained her. She studied their materials on accompaniment, especially their 2018 book about supporting people through later abortions with pills, which the WHO abortion guidelines at the time did not detail.[18] From that book and the mentorship of more experienced Socorristas, Baez learned to accompany these particularly difficult abortion cases: people using mifepristone and misoprostol or misoprostol only to end pregnancies beyond 14 weeks.

Baez and I spoke in English, though the Socorristas' deep philosophies could be challenging at times for her to translate from Spanish to English. She remembered in late 2018 the first group meeting she supported, where people spoke about abortion before they took pills. They gathered at a law school, the location signaling that just talking about abortion was not illegal. Baez shared with the group her abortion story "to create some kind of other type of relationship with the people that were there also needing the same thing," she told me. "And that helped a lot back then because people were a lot more afraid than they are now about having an abortion. They were truly afraid of a lot of blood and of going to jail." Baez assured them that they would be safe, that they were using medications, and that their abortions would not be like hers. After, she felt "powerful, not because I had some information that they didn't have, that didn't make me feel powerful. But being able to speak publicly about abortion made me feel powerful. And I felt that I could give that to others."

Week after week until the COVID-19 pandemic, Baez ran these sessions, usually at that same law school, yet she slowly stopped sharing her abortion story. "It became useless to me," she told me. "My experience is not today's experience." An older generation that did not know about pills may relate to "that moment in which you are not in control of anything," she told me of her procedure. Baez began to heal. When she first accompanied people, doing so mostly over the phone, she became anxious if the person did not respond right away. But that drifted. She learned to trust herself and the other person, believing that trust was a form of love. "We are truly loving, and we give a lot of love when we accompany someone because we want to," Baez told me. "And it is another way of activating things in political matters, right? It's like, yes, love is important. Love is strong. And it is political."

Love to her was education as well. As Baez told me, Socorristas turned to pedagogy in "everything we do, even the ones that are not teachers." She spoke of "socorrismo," which I understood as active listening and asking questions without judgment. That can be challenging for Baez when asking about violence since some people do not realize that their partner hurting them was and is not okay. "And she's standing there, she's not even crying," Baez told me. "And you're making notes, and you don't know if you can look at her eyes, terrible things." Baez will gently say, "Did you know that is violence?" Then she will explain what violence can look like. "What motivates us to do this is the capacity for change we have," Baez told me. "Sometimes we don't see it, but some other times they tell us, the people who are accompanied. They tell us how important it was." Some people she accompanied will email her years later to thank her "because sometimes it takes time to realize something," she told me. "And we are telling you that your life is yours."

In February 2020 near Córdoba, 28-year-old Emilié Suarez believed that her Socorrista, whom she knew as Guadalupe, "was everything."[19] Suarez was pregnant and did not want to be. She was in an abusive relationship and did not know how to get out safely. She did not tell Guadalupe about her abuse, only that she needed an abortion.

About two months earlier, Suarez's head pounded. She went to a doctor, who thought her birth control pills may be the cause, so advised her to stop taking them. The doctor told her to get an IUD instead. Roughly two weeks went by between her birth control pills running out and her IUD insertion. In that gap, Suarez's male abuser refused to wear a condom when they had sex, even though she asked him to do so. Years later, she realized this was another violence. Suarez started feeling unwell, so went back to her doctor, who told her she was pregnant. Suarez knew "very clear in my mind," she told me through Baez as our interpreter, that she did not want to be a mother. "Not only because of my partner being a violent person, exercising violence on me, but I felt that I already had that wish beforehand." Suarez panicked.

She tried to hide her pregnancy from her abuser. She did not know if he would support her wish for an abortion or beat her. Suarez had already reported him to police, but no one had intervened. Her abuser controlled her phone. Her neighbors knew about her abuse because they heard her screams. She worked where her abuser worked: a hospital. Increasingly isolated, she broke down one day, telling her abuser about her pregnancy and that she wanted an abortion. At first, he supported her, then he became erratic. Frightened for her life, she told her father about her pregnancy and abuse. Her family was "very Catholic," believing abortion wrong, she told me. Suarez's Catholic faith stirred an inner conflict over abortion, yet she felt that having her abuser's child endangered her. He might kill her. Her father went with her to plead with doctors for an abortion, explaining that Suarez's life was at risk.

In early 2020, even under a near-total ban in Argentina, a doctor legally could have performed an abortion for Suarez—if a doctor deemed her pregnancy endangered her life. She had bruises. She filed police reports. But doctors refused, telling her an abortion was illegal, that her life was not in danger. "I felt alone in terms of systems, how the state should have helped me," Suarez told me. "Nothing was guaranteed to me. I felt I was getting punches from the justice system, from the healthcare system, and punches at home. . . . I isolated myself from family and friends. And the only person who was there for me was the Socorrista."

In searching online for help, doing so when her abuser could not see, she found Socorristas on Instagram. She reached out. The Socorrista Guadalupe, who was in Baez's collective, connected with her over the phone. Yet since Suarez's abuser controlled her phone, Suarez felt too scared to tell Guadalupe the full story. Guadalupe supported her over the phone patiently during her abortion with misoprostol. "I received love from her, from our collective," Suarez told me of Guadalupe. "I couldn't find that love in the health care system. . . . I couldn't find it from my partner, my relationship."

Once she had her abortion in February 2020, Suarez was still in that violent relationship as the COVID-19 pandemic hit a month later and Argentina went into quarantine. Suarez became more isolated. But she kept checking the Socorristas' page on Instagram when her abuser was not looking. She kept thinking of Guadalupe. She realized she wanted to do what Guadalupe did: be a Socorrista. She wanted this while still suffering abuse at home.

On December 30, 2020, people gathered outside the National Congress in Buenos Aires again, wearing green bandanas and, this time, green masks. The Senate that day did finally legalize abortion in pregnancies up to 14 weeks, ending Argentina's near-total ban.[20] The relief was palpable. But when the law went into effect in 2021, many La Campaña members asked if Socorristas were still needed. Socorristas decided to continue for two reasons: first, the value of their care; second, as Zurbriggen told me, because "the law was not the ceiling but just the starting point for our struggle." Socorristas sought total abortion decriminalization without any gestational age bans. With Argentina's new abortion law in place, they began to accompany people through the health care system and worked to improve the quality of legal abortion care.

For Suarez, the new abortion law came as her abuse worsened. In November 2021, her abuser beat her so badly that she needed to be hospitalized. The police issued a restraining order against her abuser. After her hospitalization, Suarez began to heal, becoming less isolated. She started to see friends and family again. All the while, she kept checking Socorristas' social media accounts to see if she could join that Córdoba collective. Then in August 2022, she saw a post: a Socorristas training. When we spoke in 2023, she had just started accompanying people.

Socorristas helped Suarez unlearn much in life, she explained to me, and abort many things, not only her pregnancy but her abuse and abusive thinking. She described "socorrismo" as "questioning everything, completely." Suarez felt that being with Socorristas was like when a loved one touched your hair softly. She never met Guadalupe in person or told her about her abuse. By the time Suarez joined the collective, Guadalupe had left Córdoba. But Suarez hoped to find her one day. "Perhaps Guadalupe doesn't even imagine everything she did for me," Suarez told me.

When we spoke, Baez cried, Suarez cried, and I cried. I emailed Suarez after to thank her for sharing, writing in high school–level Spanish, apologizing for errors. Suarez wrote back in English: "Thank you for your space, listen to me and write to me, I am here for whatever you need. Hug Rebecca," followed by a heart emoji. I felt like Suarez and Baez were accompanying me in simply writing this book, that I had been a part of something moving that I did not know how to name—nor did I wish to name it. And I realized these pills were not what mattered most to them. Their power lived not in these pills alone but in each other. And, yes, in love.

Since Argentina's ban on abortion in pregnancies later than 14 weeks went into effect, the country in late 2023 elected an anti-abortion, far-right president who sought to reinstate a near-total ban.[21] In

December 2022, a year after the new abortion law passed, police arrested a few Socorristas members and raided their homes. Their criminal cases were unfolding when I spoke to Baez and Zurbriggen.[22] No such arrests or raids had happened when Socorristas publicly accompanied people under a near-total ban for nearly a decade. They were in a backlash.

The law had not fixed their problems. It did say the abortion-seeker herself would not be criminalized if she self-managed her abortion outside the health care system. Yet the law left out protections for Socorristas, whose accompaniment risked being misunderstood and criminalized for practicing medicine without a license. This worried Zurbriggen for their movement. Some Socorristas left the network following the arrests, too scared to carry on. Others, like Baez, believed that fear was exactly what these arrests wanted to accomplish, and the arrests only confirmed to her that their work was not done.

Baez and I once spoke while she accompanied someone via text with timers set for when the person on the other end of the texts needed to take more misoprostol pills. Every now and then as we talked, Baez paused and asked the person if she had started bleeding and how she felt. This person got mifepristone and misoprostol legally for free through the health care system, but her doctor told her to wait a week before taking mifepristone to start her abortion. This infuriated Baez. There was no medical or legal reason to wait. The longer a person delayed taking pills, the more their pregnancy progressed and the more painful as well as less effective her abortion might become. Baez assured this person that she could take mifepristone followed by misoprostol whenever she felt ready.

What seemed most remarkable to me, however, was that Baez acted like the experience of her correcting doctors on the effective use of the pills happened often. "Physicians are paid because that's their job," she told me. "This is not our job. This is what we choose to do as feminist activists to change the world. Going one by one."

CHAPTER 12

UNAPOLOGETIC LOVE

I t took more than a decade for grassroots activists like Socorristas to be recognized in the global scientific community as experts on abortion pills. Around 2016, American activist Susan Yanow, co-founder of Women Help Women (WHW), introduced American epidemiologist Dr. Caitlin Gerdts of Ibis Reproductive Health, a US-based nonprofit for reproductive health research, to accompaniment groups, among them Ruth Zurbriggen of Socorristas.[1]

Yanow trusted Gerdts. But histories of colonialism and racism in Global North–Global South reproductive health research meant it took time for SMA activists to also trust Gerdts and fellow Ibis researcher Dr. Heidi Moseson. It was not long ago that Dr. Étienne-Émile Baulieu, the so-called father of the abortion pill, visited the original birth control pill trials in Puerto Rico, where women in those trials did not give their informed consent. These SMA activists wanted to upend such legacies and be seen for what they were: experts too. Their partnership with Ibis would help expand knowledge of pills and recast who counted as a researcher.

Gerdts realized these SMA activists, almost all volunteers and not doctors, knew more about abortion pills than most clinicians she met. They astonished her. But in the global health field of medication abortion in the 2010s, SMA landed in a harm-reduction narrative, presumed to be of lesser quality care than in-clinic care with a doctor.[2] Zurbriggen, Inna Hudaya of an SMA hotline Samsara in Indonesia, Sybil Nmezi of another SMA hotline in Nigeria, and fellow activists understood that their models were safe, effective, *and* quality care. They had been collecting data for years that had proven this. Since 2010, Hudaya at Samsara had been tracking such data after noticing that the WHO's abortion-care guidelines at the time left out people who used miso-prostol for abortions beyond 12 weeks in pregnancy.[3] Samsara callers, however, were safely taking misoprostol later in their pregnancies and completing abortions with the hotline's support, all under Indonesia's near-total ban. "So, I dig," Hudaya told me. "I dig deeper."[4]

Almost no one else in the world had this kind of data on SMA given abortion stigma and criminalization risks where these activists worked. Realistically, only these activists could prove to the WHO that SMA was safe and offered quality care because only they had the evidence. At Ibis, epidemiologists like Gerdts could help by rigorously analyzing this data in a way that the WHO and the global scientific community might take more seriously.[5] Hudaya and Gerdts in 2018 wrote one of the first peer-reviewed papers on women safely self-managing later abortions with pills in a legally restricted setting (Indonesia).[6] The WHO invited Hudaya to a meeting about abortion soon afterward, where Hudaya sat next to clinicians, a departure from that 1984 WHO meeting on RU-486 at an Italian villa with mostly white men.

Then came a bigger step. In 2018, Zurbriggen and Nmezi co-designed a study with Ibis researchers, Studying Accompaniment Feasibility and Effectiveness (SAFE). They went line by line together to decide what to ask those they accompanied who agreed to partic-ipate in this research.[7] Everyone agreed not to ask people why they wanted an abortion. Activists convinced Gerdts that simply by ask-ing people that question, some abortion seekers may feel judged, as if they needed to justify their decision. Besides, nothing about their care would change based on their answer. And many studies already existed on why people seek an abortion (concerns about money con-sistently rank as the most common reason).[8] Gerdts slowly found her perspectives shifting through these conversations, as if activists were accompanying her too.

In 2022, *The Lancet Global Health*, a sister of *The Lancet* that, three decades ago, had first reported on women in Brazil "misusing" misoprostol for abortions, published the SAFE Study, finding that abortions early in pregnancy using pills—misoprostol or mifepristone and misoprostol—and with accompaniment support were as safe and effective as abortions with pills in a clinical setting or under clinical supervision.[9] The co-authors were Gerdts and Moseson alongside Zurbriggen, Nmezi, and fellow activists. The meticulous SAFE Study gave the WHO bulletproof reassurance on what the field by then expected. For the first time, the WHO's 2022 guidelines stated that the abortion-seeker could safely be her own provider, and that lay providers (like acompañantes) could safely support people.[10] As American sociologist Dr. Tracy Weitz told me, it was about time. "You have millions of women around the world doing this," she told me. "We don't have an epidemic of poor outcomes. We have to acknowledge that this is clearly safe."

Yet one SAFE Study finding did boggle minds: people's misoprostol-only abortions with accompaniment were 99 percent effective, much higher than in prior clinical trials.[11] Ongoing research is trying to pinpoint why. The SAFE Study was not a head-to-head comparison between the combined method and misoprostol only, as Gerdts explained to me. Activists accompanying people under bans often had no choice in which regimen they used. The SAFE Study also did not fit many clinical trial norms because of what this was about: care *outside* a clinical environment and in a criminalized setting. Gerdts told me, however, that one possible reason for misoprostol's high efficacy may be that the SAFE Study had a longer, three-week follow-up time between when a person began their abortion and when they self-assessed abortion completion. With enough time, support, and information, a person's body usually could pass a pregnancy with misoprostol pills. Follow-up time in a clinical trial may be much shorter, just a few days or a week.[12]

Highly controlled clinical trials additionally do not typically let a person take more doses of misoprostol beyond whatever regimen was under observation. In SMA, with guidance from someone like Socorrista Lucía Baez and her timers, people could take more misoprostol pills until their body fully expelled their uterine contents. Care could be flexible. Intangible factors may be at play too. Gerdts noted that if someone decided to enroll in a clinical trial, they likely had an interest in being in a medical setting. They might be more likely to seek medical attention rather than, say, continue to bleed after taking pills without seeking help. Clinicians are then trained to offer procedural interventions to resolve whatever might be happening to a person coming to them for care. Yet with SMA, people may have many reasons to not want to be in a clinical system, even if that option existed for them.

And then there was something Gerdts struggled to name. "But I think you just can't underestimate what an impact this model has on people," she told me. The SAFE Study did not measure that depth of feeling and connection that I heard from Socorristas, that unapologetic love.[13] "The work that these groups have done in the face of incredible legal risk to their safety and well-being in current governments who have abdicated responsibility for providing a basic health care service is extraordinary," Gerdts told me. "They are truly the global experts in medication abortion. . . . Because they're just *there* for more of it."

The year the SAFE Study and 2022 WHO abortion-care guidelines came out was the year of the *Dobbs* decision in the US. Gerdts and I spoke months after *Dobbs* erased the national right to abortion, upending millions of lives as state bans swept half the country. "It's disheartening to say the least to see such baseless laws and see the direction that our healthcare system in the United States is taking that is just absolutely against all evidence," she told me. "And knowing that there are groups out there who have centered science, evidence, and best practice and invited some of us in to help document the work that they do is certainly something that gives me hope."

Yet she believed accompaniment models like Socorristas cannot be "cut-and-pasted" to the US. The American criminal-justice system is one of the most punitive in the world.[14] The criminal-justice systems in most countries where SMA flourished, like Argentina, cannot claim such a superlative. In ban states post-*Dobbs*, people providing pills or accompanying others face criminalization risks to an extent that Socorristas never did, in addition to a criminal-justice system disproportionately incarcerating low-income Black and brown communities.[15] To Gerdts, those facts did not mean these models should be ignored. "One thing we do really, really need to learn and have so much to gain is the creativity and focus on security, risk, privacy, and access in person-centered care these groups have brought," she told me. "The experience that people have with [them], even in the

absence of any option in the public health system at all, is just exceptionally good, well-supported, and holistic."

Not one country's laws as of late 2024 align with the 2022 WHO
abortion guidelines, which include that SMA be allowed and that
abortion be decriminalized as well as legalized without any gestational age bans.[16] Dr. Bela Ganatra, head of the WHO's Prevention
of Unsafe Abortion unit in the Human Reproduction Programme
(HRP), told me that stigma remained one of the greatest barriers to
changing abortion care around the globe. "It is just painful that this
is a simple enough intervention," she told me. "And yet some years
later, we just take one step forward, one step backward. And we're
still not able to take this for what it is." But when I asked Ganatra if
she had hope, she looked surprised. "If I didn't have hope, I would
be burnt out by now."[17]

Kinga Jelinska of WHW has guided hundreds of thousands of people through their abortions with pills. "Yet Rebecca, I cannot come to
you and give you the pills," she told me in 2023 as I sat in the US, she
in the Netherlands. "Whether we would get caught is another thing.
But it is an illegal thing still for you. It would be illegal to take the
medicine because you would be doing this outside of the institutional
health care system." It would be illegal for Jelinska, who was not a
licensed provider, to do so in the Netherlands as well, and she was
quick not to "over-romanticize" liberal regimes. "They all are fucked
up," Jelinska told me. The EU has become a patchwork of abortion
bans, one country with a 12-week ban, another a 24-week ban, Poland
a near-total ban, and on and on.[18] "Europe is such a mess, Rebecca,"
she told me. That mess, to her, was by design and about control. She
wanted abortion pills available over the counter one day, as Dr. Beverly Winikoff long envisioned.

But Jelinska understood people still knew so little about abortion
pills given pervasive stigma and criminalization fears. "We are not
there yet that you can just basically drop abortion pills and leave
people to their own devices," she told me. WHW received about
140,000 emails in 2022 from people asking for support with taking

the medications mailed to them. "And the support is now much more decentralized than it was a decade or two decades ago because there are so many collectives who are doing this," Jelinska told me, referring to the global feminist SMA movement. "But there is still this need, right? Because there's still the fear that it might be medically complicated."

After the WHO recognized SMA, Sara Larrea, formerly of Salud Mujeres in Ecuador, watched talk of SMA surge. "Now everyone is on board with this strategy. Every organization. Every activist. Everyone," she told me in 2023. "But at the beginning, there was a lot of resistance. And that resistance did have to do with medical power." Now, she wondered if that medical power might take another form. Larrea questioned if mainstreaming SMA would erase the feminist models that pushed this practice forward. Typically, she explained to me, when health care institutions created protocols, they prioritized institutional needs like efficiency and cost. Scrappier, early feminist models with abortion pills did not do that. Activists flexibly centered the abortion-seeker. That also could burden activists "always on the edge of burnout," as Larrea described of Salud Mujeres. She nonetheless noticed in 2023 that bigger, systemic inequalities around abortion-seekers' lives in Ecuador have not gone away. "And none of these strategies are able to solve it," she told me, not hotlines, accompaniment groups, or global telehealth abortion services. "And that's deeply concerning."

A little more than a year after Argentina transitioned from a near-total ban on abortions to a ban on abortions in pregnancies later than 14 weeks, Dr. Raquel Drovetta of Socorristas saw the *Dobbs* decision come down as the US moved in the opposite direction. She told me that, as an American, I will never understand nuances of the Latin American context. Socorristas openly defying the law in Argentina for years stunned many of her Global North colleagues, who asked her, "But how?" She explained the law in Argentina "is like chewing gum. . . . You do not have a strict limit to say this is legal and this is illegal. Here, there is a border, a gray area in which we have moved for a long time, in which we have moved for more than ten years," she told me. "What is not illegal can be legal. It is idiosyncratic."

But despite these differences, she thought that Argentina might need to urgently teach the US something about politics. Americans of privilege may not have realized a right won could be lost. To her, Argentinians knew this intimately. Recent dictatorships and state crises time and again have forced Argentinians to stretch that "chewing gum" of law to survive. "These decades have taught us that we cannot take any law for granted, even less in Latin America, where each government can change absolutely all the policies that were thought for a country," she told me. "Here, we are prepared for surprises all the time. We live like that."

Two years after *Dobbs*, I noticed a photograph of protestors by the US Supreme Court's steps in March 2024 on the day an anti-abortion case to dramatically restrict mifepristone access nationwide was being heard.[19] And I saw them: people wearing green bandanas and bright pink wigs. "Sometimes when everything is illegal around you, it takes a lot of courage," Baez told me of the US. "But you are courageous people. You will be able to do it anyway."

CHAPTER 13

"REALLY, REALLY, *REALLY* THIS MAKES NO SENSE"

Around 2013, Kinga Jelinska, after presenting on WOW to several members of the American reproductive rights and justice movements, felt frustrated. The idea of mailing abortion pills to people in the US, not just to people in ban countries, did not seem to resonate with her audience. "I saw this being ignored for like a decade or two, 'Oh, that's only the countries that don't have access,'" she told me in 2023. "But it was exotic right at that point. 'It's not for the U.S.' And here we go. What is happening?"

When Jelinska spoke a decade ago, her American allies were overwhelmed by a whack-a-mole clinic defense strategy and marginally legal abortion-care infrastructure. Democrat Barack Obama was president yet disappointed many in the reproductive rights and justice movements. In 2010, with Democrats in control of Congress and the White House, the Affordable Care Act (ACA) looked poised to help millions gain health care coverage. It also seemed like a chance to end the Hyde Amendment's near-total ban on federal funding of abortion care. But the ACA passed while the Hyde Amendment remained.[1]

Some reproductive rights and justice movement members were furious not just at the Democrats but at what looked to them like their own movement bargaining away poor women of color's abortion access. "I saw how the women's movement more broadly, but especially reproductive rights, was being treated like the Ladies Auxiliary of the Democratic Party," activist Erin Matson told me in 2023, reflecting on her work at the National Organization for Women (NOW) in DC during the ACA's passage. "We were expected to be cheerleaders. And for the most part, people were just doing it. . . . 'Abortion' was being whispered, if said at all, like a really dirty word."[2]

Democrats angered many in the movement again a year later over Plan B, or emergency contraception. The FDA decided in 2011, based on ample evidence, that Plan B was safe enough to be sold over the counter to minors (it could already be sold over the counter to adults). But Obama's appointed secretary of the Department of Health and Human Services (HHS), who oversaw the FDA, pulled a highly rare move at the time and overruled the FDA's decision.[3] The Obama administration had been preparing for a 2012 reelection campaign and, seemingly to win over swing voters, suddenly became skittish about appearing permissive of girls having sex if Plan B became over the counter to minors on Obama's watch. So, in the eyes of several reproductive rights advocates and many in the scientific community, the White House effectively exchanged girls' bodily autonomy for the Democrats' political gain.[4]

An altogether different story frothed on the right, where the anti-abortion movement surged with power in the Republican Party. Legal historian Mary Ziegler has argued how anti-abortion lawyers helped mastermind a 2010 Supreme Court case, *Citizens United v. Federal Election Commission*, that lifted key federal regulations on political-campaign spending.[5] A pro-life Republican candidate became a cash-flush ticket in the 2010s to more power. Factions of the party were increasingly exploiting white supremacist, misogynist roots of a nation reeling from the 2008 Great Recession. In the 2010 midterm elections, riding on ACA backlash and racist dog-whistles about Obama as the country's first Black president, the Republicans dominated statehouse races with anti-abortion groups in the wings.[6]

The anti-abortion movement's state-level legal strategy to chip away at abortion access went into high gear, all aimed at ending *Roe*. As discussed in a prior chapter, medically unnecessary state restrictions on abortion, which the reproductive rights movement called TRAP laws (targeted regulation of abortion providers), drove up the cost of running abortion clinics and shuttered many, making abortion care even harder for Americans to get.[7] In 2013, Texas's TRAP laws captured national attention when Democratic Texas Senator Wendy Davis stood in pink running shoes for a nearly 13-hour filibuster to try to block Senate Bill 5 (SB 5). The bill would, among other restrictions, require abortion providers to attain "admitting privileges" at a hospital within 30 miles of a clinic.[8] That would be logistically impossible for most abortion clinics in Texas at the time and would almost certainly force them to close.[9] Davis delivered her filibuster to cheers and applause with extensive media coverage, her shoes briefly becoming a feminist symbol in the US. But a similar bill in Texas soon passed.[10] More clinics folded. The news cycle moved on.

The American reproductive rights movement's decades-long, well-funded bet to build political power at the federal level and influence Democrats in DC, often deprioritizing grassroots state politics in the process, was floundering miserably.[11] What Dr. Raquel Drovetta in Argentina told me seemed to be true: the ones blinded by privileges in the American public and even within parts of the reproductive rights movement may not have fathomed a right won could be lost, a democracy seized and lit on fire.

Where did abortion pills fit? Francine Coeytaux knew where—and was angry. A longtime reproductive rights advocate and researcher who was nearly 60 years old in 2013, she had worked with the Reproductive Health Technologies Project (RHTP) in the 1990s to advocate for the FDA approval of mifepristone and then Plan B. When the FDA wrapped mifepristone in restrictions, what were then called the Risk Evaluation and Mitigation Strategy (REMS), she learned one hard lesson. When Obama in 2011 did an about-face on Plan B, she learned that same lesson once again.[12] Playing precisely and nicely by the rules did not make sense when those rules could be rewritten to screw you. She thought what WOW did in legal loopholes, mailing people around the world pills, just brilliant. She wanted a similar model in the US, knowing telehealth abortion could radically expand access in this country as clinics dwindled. Yet mifepristone's REMS, which did not explicitly allow providers to mail that pill to patients, stood in the way. Rules were rules. Or were they?

Coeytaux and two other reproductive rights, health, and justice activists, Amy Allina and Leila Hessini, ran an inner-movement meeting called Bold Actions in 2013 in DC to brainstorm about abortion pills.[13] Coeytaux represented the Public Health Institute, Allina the National Women's Health Network, and Hessini Ipas. Almost 30 advocates and researchers came, including Susan Yanow, then at WOW, who reported that more people in the US had been asking their site for pills. Only WOW did not mail pills to the US due to the notoriously litigious American anti-abortion movement.

More Americans, Bold Actions attendees discussed, seemed to be nonetheless finding abortion pills online from prescription-less sources, a few even having been arrested for doing so. In 2013, a woman of color in Indiana took pills bought online to end her 23-week pregnancy. She went to a hospital, where she was then reported to police, charged with child neglect and "feticide," and sentenced to 20 years in prison.[14] One of her charges would later be dropped. In 2012, a white woman in rural Pennsylvania bought pills online for her teenage daughter because they could not afford to travel to a clinic. The two did not know how pills worked, so when her daughter began to bleed and cramp, the mother rushed her daughter to a hospital, telling staff about the pills only to be reported to police. The mother was later convicted of child abuse.[15]

Coeytaux believed Americans had a dangerous knowledge gap on abortion pills. At Bold Actions, she and public health researcher Elisa Wells, who had also worked on Plan B, proposed creating an informational website for abortion-seekers that told them in plain language all about the REMS-less misoprostol. The pair floated a more daring idea as well, wondering if activists should form "links to prescribers or an underground network to supply misoprostol," according to the Bold Actions meeting notes, where some activists would openly link people to prescribers while other activists in these latter supply networks would be "underground to assist more women individually (like a Jane Collective 2.0)."[16]

But studies at the time still showed abortions with misoprostol on its own were less effective and more painful than when used with mifepristone. The SAFE Study did not exist yet. Even though people were safely managing abortions with misoprostol-only in countries like Argentina, accompaniment groups were also forming in those contexts to guide people through their abortions. Abortion providers in the US, however, were not familiar with this misoprostol-only care. What if people took misoprostol, were still pregnant, then needed care at a hospital or clinic? What if the wrong person found out that a patient had used misoprostol pills and reported the patient to police? Also, if providers prescribed and mailed patients misoprostol, didn't a state's abortion laws still apply?[17] Some states already banned telehealth abortion (the anti-abortion movement had been keeping an eye on WOW).[18] No one had done something like this in the US before. "You had some people in the meeting who were like, 'Be bold. Let's just do it. There's no law that says we can't,'" Allina told me in 2023. "And other people saying, 'Hey, the consequences of 'Let's fuck around and find out' are not the same for every person or every community.'"[19]

After Bold Actions, Allina, Coeytaux, and Hessini co-wrote a *Women's Health Issues* article in which they suggested finding providers willing to prescribe misoprostol, bringing misoprostol into the US from Mexico and Canada, and vetting online sellers of prescription-less pills.[20] "We realize just how audacious our proposal is," a final line read in that article. "However, women are paying the price for our current timidity." Almost a decade later, Allina heard in those words her frustration that not enough people took mounting abortion restrictions seriously, an anger not just at the movement but at Danco, the FDA, and the Obama administration, how "really, really, *really* this makes no sense to keep [mifepristone] so locked up," she told me. "If you won't let us do it with mifepristone, [then let us do it] with misoprostol. Because women are paying the price. People are having pregnancies that they want to end. And we could help them. And we're not."

The 2010s marked other inner-movement turmoil. Reproductive justice groups spoke publicly about what they saw as grave mistakes mostly white-led mainstream groups were making. Monica Simpson, executive director of SisterSong Women of Color Reproductive Justice Collective, made waves when she published an open letter to Planned Parenthood in 2014 in *Rewire News Group*.[21] In it, she responded to a *New York Times* article on Planned Parenthood leaving pro-choice messaging behind to instead reframe abortion as one aspect of a person's reproductive life, using a reproductive justice framework without crediting SisterSong and the women of color who coined it in the early 1990s.[22]

Planned Parenthood already had a shaky reputation among some in the movement. To Simpson, the giant organization for years had contributed to siloing abortion in damaging ways. Her open letter referred to how, in 2011, Planned Parenthood and SisterSong stopped a fetal personhood amendment in Mississippi, though failed to also try to defeat a voting-rights restriction on the state ballot. Loretta Ross, SisterSong's co-founder, argued at the time that this was a short-sighted strategy.[23] More Mississippians would now have a harder time voting, particularly Black communities, who disproportionately sought abortion care, and more anti-abortion lawmakers would then likely be elected. In her letter, Simpson reiterated Ross's point, calling for change. A decade later, Mississippi would be at the center of *Dobbs*.

It took Coeytaux and Wells leaving siloed thinking on abortion in the US to gain perspective. Around 2014, they studied community programs in Ethiopia that gave misoprostol to women to prevent postpartum hemorrhage, a major cause of maternal mortality in the country at the time.[24] Yet these programs were not scaling up quickly. Coeytaux and Wells noticed provider biases. Some community workers did not seem to believe that women could learn to take this pill on their own. Others worried women might use misoprostol for abortions or sell the pills. "There was not an iota of evidence that any woman who knew they were sitting on something that would save their lives when they delivered was going to give this to anybody else," Coeytaux told me. "Doesn't matter."

Something promising struck them in Ethiopia, though. Because once the country in 2005 moved from an abortion ban to legalization, albeit still with tight restrictions, combi-packs with both mifepristone and misoprostol pills rolled out across the nation.[25] Coeytaux and Wells could easily find the pills over the counter there for about $5, nothing like the cost of abortion pills at a clinic in the US. "We've got to do something in the US because it is so wrong that in a country like Ethiopia with such resource scarcity and health care infrastructure challenges, they are making [the pills] available despite that," Wells told me. "Everybody says abortion is legal in the US, and it is. But the restrictions are so severe that it's not."

Meanwhile, as abortion access worsened and mifepristone remained controlled, some American activists quietly ran misoprostol-only abortion trainings in Texas's Rio Grande Valley along the US-Mexico border. One person attending a 2013 training was then 22-year-old Nancy Cárdenas Peña.[26] "I don't remember exactly when I found out that miso was over-the-counter in Mexico," she told me in 2024. "But it was something that I long understood." First-generation Mexican American, Cárdenas Peña grew up in the valley without health care access, so she and her family often crossed the border for affordable care in Mexico. "It was very routine and normal to not rely on formal institutions for medical care." But she had the right documents to cross that border. If loved ones living undocumented in the valley needed cheap medications, people with the correct papers sometimes drove to Mexico, picked medications up, and brought them back. Then as more of Texas's abortion clinics shut down in the early 2010s, Cárdenas Peña wanted to learn how to have an abortion without a clinic at all. "I was kind of blown away," she told me. "That training actually gave me the tools to do my own self-managed abortion in 2017."

By then, she still lived in Texas and was deep in the reproductive justice community, volunteering with the valley's abortion fund, Frontera Fund. Cárdenas Peña knew who could help her travel to a local clinic. But she didn't want to go to a clinic. When I asked if she took misoprostol alone or misoprostol and mifepristone, she smiled. "Just miso," which she pronounced like miso, as in miso soup. Most American medication abortion researchers I interviewed pronounced miso as "my-so," a detail Cárdenas Peña likely knew when she then quickly added to me, "Or my-so. However you're supposed to say it. The point is it works."

There is no one SMA story. There are millions. Cárdenas Peña used misoprostol for privacy, control, "and also just going to a clinic and having people yell at you for your decisions was not the thing for me." Yet she thought her positive SMA experience may not be common in the US post-*Dobbs*. She understood what to expect when taking the pills and felt supported. Her SMA in 2017 was crucially a decision that she made when *Roe* existed, not while living in Texas under a ban. Cárdenas Peña wanted to be direct with me about how her abortion felt. She bled a lot. She cramped a lot. Her abortion process lasted days. "It felt incredibly uncomfortable," she told me. "It was very difficult. . . . Would I do it again? Absolutely I would. This was still the best decision for me."

She hoped that everyone would have the "full spectrum of options and information for them to be able to make those decisions." Cárdenas Peña in 2023 became director of a national SMA campaign, Abortion on Our Own Terms, and one of the first American reproductive justice leaders to speak openly of her SMA. Eager to do more cross-border organizing work post-*Dobbs*, she has since been learning accompaniment models from Green Wave activists, who have also been learning from her and fellow Americans about legal abortion-provision models in the US. But first, a rewind.

As US clinics held on for dear life in the 2010s, another legal way to get pills to more people in the US was through telehealth abortion studies. These studies could also produce more evidence to the FDA to support ending mifepristone's REMS and explicitly allow the pill to be mailed to patients.

The earliest US telehealth abortion study was published in 2011 with the first author listed as Dr. Daniel Grossman, then at Ibis Reproductive Health, and with a Planned Parenthood affiliate in Iowa.[27] That state required a doctor provide abortions, but there was a drastic shortage of those doctors in Iowa. Telehealth could make it easier for one abortion doctor in the state to see more patients. Iowa's abortion law still required a patient to travel to a clinic for an ultrasound and, per the REMS, pick up pills there. So, in this small study, a doctor sat at one clinic in Iowa while leading a video visit with their patient located inside another abortion clinic in the state. Compared to telehealth services today, this was rather cumbersome. But the study nonetheless found almost all patients were "very satisfied" with their telehealth abortion experience, which was safe and effective.

In 2016, Gynuity Health Projects began a larger telehealth abortion study, aptly called the TelAbortion Study, legally mailing mifepristone and misoprostol pills across five states to hundreds of abortion-seekers with early pregnancies. And in 2019, Gynuity also found this service safe, effective, efficient, and satisfactory to patients.[28]

Danco simultaneously worked to update the FDA label for mifepristone to reflect the latest research on pills and broaden access. In 2016, the FDA approved a revision to mifepristone's label, which included allowing people to use the pill to end pregnancies up to 10 weeks, letting certified prescribers (not just doctors) provide the pill, and doing away with the 2000 label's expectation that a patient visit a clinic in person three times for a medication abortion.[29] Yet the REMS remained, along with what the FDA called the "in-person dispensing requirement" for mifepristone. This meant that a patient technically still needed to pick up mifepristone from a clinic. Some FDA officials in 2016 disagreed with keeping the REMS, the pill's medical reviewer, Dr. Z, among them. It had now been 16 years since mifepristone's FDA approval, and the medication's safety record was stunningly strong. Only removing or keeping the REMS was not ultimately Dr. Z's call. To a handful of reproductive rights advocates, the Obama White House overruling the FDA on Plan B a few years earlier seemed to signal that abandoning the REMS on the "abortion pill" would not end well in another election year, this time with Obama's former secretary of state, Democrat Hillary Clinton, running for president.

Danco was very careful about publicly criticizing the agency that regulated them. The tiny company, with fewer than 10 full-time staff and fewer than 100 investors, needed a working relationship with the FDA to continue selling its sole product. Besides, it may not have been the FDA that needed criticizing so much as the Democrats. Among some in the reproductive rights community, however, Danco's secrecy and for-profit motives (it was a business after all) made the company easy to blame for failing to remove the REMS when the truth may have been harder to swallow: the American reproductive rights, health, and justice movements had hardly any political power. Danco could not fix that.[30]

Coeytaux and Wells still wanted a website for the American public to learn more about abortion pills, returning to that idea from the 2013 Bold Actions meeting. They soon co-founded Plan C, a nonprofit advocating for access to abortion pills, though they had no funding.[31] Amy Merrill, a Plan C co-founder and "millennial digital strategist," in Coeytaux's words, created Plan C's website for free.[32] But some lawyers warned Plan C to abandon the website. They worried that creating a website with information about abortion pills could be illegal. Coeytaux did not understand.[33] What was illegal about sharing information about abortion pills? They were not giving medical or legal advice without a license. Shouldn't the site be protected free speech?

When Plan C's site launched in 2016, the nonprofit used that freedom of speech legal protection to realize a riskier part of their vision: vet and publicly share information about online sellers of prescriptionless abortion pills that operated illegally. What if Plan C tested if the pills these vendors sold were real? Plan C themselves would not sell or distribute pills.

Some critics in the reproductive rights and justice movement, however, argued that the site, in connecting people to these vendors, could expose vulnerable people to criminalization risks. Wells and Coeytaux were white women living in California and Washington. Did they truly grasp these risks? Over time, Plan C tried to address these criticisms by putting on their site digital security tips and language about the potential legal risks, depending on the person's state and context, of buying pills online from illegal sellers. Others in the movement applauded Plan C for their courage. They were out there playing offense when so many in the movement seemed to them stuck in defense, a posture that appeared to only worsen after 2016.[34]

When Donald Trump, or "Orange 45" in Yanow's words, won the White House in 2016, Yanow knew *Roe* would end. She understood abortion pills would then be more important in the country than ever before. Yanow furiously built an informational website about the pills that would be a little like Plan C, though more digitally secure and a WHW partner. The site, Self-Managed Abortion Safe and Supported

(SASS), went live in early 2017. To contact the site, someone typed a question into the site's portal, received a randomized web link, and clicked that link to view the answer to their question; that answer automatically blanked out after a short while so as to leave no easily traceable digital trail of the correspondence.[35] It was a fortress. But SASS did not link to abortion-pill vendors nor, at first, to Plan C. "Everyone was scared to link to us," Wells told me.

Coeytaux and Wells were discovering more websites claiming to sell and mail people in the US prescription-less abortion pills, both misoprostol and mifepristone. From her Washington home, Wells went online one night and bought pills to see what would happen. Her phone blew up with bank fraud alerts. Weeks went by. "And lo and behold, I went to my mailbox, and there it was, a certain length of time later." A packet of abortion pills. Plan C and Gynuity soon after did a study to test these pills. Gynuity fortunately had access to a lab Danco used to test their mifepristone product. And so, weeks after Trump's 2016 election, Plan C and Gynuity ordered abortion pills online: 22 products from 18 sites with names like buyabortionpills.net.[36]

Of those products, 20 were combi-packs and two were just misoprostol pills. Combi-packs at the time cost up to $360, more than half the cost that a clinic in the US charged. Misoprostol products were even cheaper. Soon, 20 products from 16 sites arrived (two products ordered were never received). The study made a startling discovery. All these pills were real. Gynuity's Dr. Beverly Winikoff figured that made sense. Mifepristone and misoprostol were cheap to make, costing about $2 a pill wholesale. Why send fake pills when genuine ones cost almost nothing? There was something else. Of the 20 products received, five were shipped from India. But 15 were shipped from inside the US. Testing showed those pills shipped within the US were made in India. Winikoff realized what that must mean. "People are taking [pills] in suitcases, going through the border, and then fulfilling orders from the US to the US," she told me in 2023. "And I'm sure it's still happening."

Blocks from Gynuity's Manhattan office in 2016, a single parent ran one such site from a New York City apartment.[37] I call her Lisa, a pseudonym, to protect her privacy. She found pills online in 2012 during her frustrating search for an abortion. The price of abortion pills in a clinic was too steep for her. She could not take time off work easily to go to a clinic even just a subway ride away. And she did not want to dart past anti-abortion protestors outside a clinic. After persistent googling, Lisa came across the same abortion pills offered at a clinic but sold for half the cost online. She ordered a combi-pack; it soon arrived. She found instructions online to take these pills correctly. Her abortion process was not a pleasant experience. But it worked. Then she wrote on her personal blog about her abortion. She could not believe more people did not know about these pills. Comments poured in from people asking how they, too, could find pills. In 2016, when she needed extra money, Lisa remembered that need.

She started buying combi-packs online from a wholesale supplier in India. It was simple to find a supplier. The tricky, certainly illegal part was how Lisa, not a licensed provider, would mail pills to people. She used an online alias pretending to sell jewelry, and she stayed under the radar. No advertising. Lisa knew abortion-seekers in situations like she was in years ago would find her. When she mailed packages, she tucked next to pills necklaces as decoys. She charged $85 with expedited shipping, cheaper than a clinic and many illegal vendors. More than 2,000 people in two years bought pills from her. But what started as a side-hustle increasingly felt to her like activism. She felt it was not fair that people paid so much for pills at a clinic when so many struggled to even reach clinics.

In 2018, Lisa heard a knock on her door. About eight federal agents stood outside and proceeded to search her home. They took her computer and phone. They did not arrest her. They did shut her website down. The FDA seemed to have learned about her after a man in Wisconsin was arrested for allegedly slipping mifepristone into the drink of a pregnant person.[38] That man pleaded not guilty to attempted first-degree homicide of an "unborn child." The anti-abortion prosecutor in the case found the source of these pills: Lisa, whom the prosecutor called a "drug smuggler." She was fined $10,000 and placed on a two-year probation.[39]

Wells remembered Lisa's service from that study Plan C did with Gynuity, telling *Mother Jones* in 2019 that Lisa "appeared to be a woman helping other women, and not a commercial enterprise."[40] Around 2017, Plan C began linking to vetted abortion pill vendors and giving them "report cards," testing and rating their services based on cost, product quality, and delivery time. Lisa's service, when it existed, earned one of Plan C's highest grades. These "report cards" later became Plan C's state-by-state guide to abortion pills by mail. The guide initially only listed vendors that operated illegally since no other pills-by-mail players in the US existed, not yet.

Lisa did not speak to me on-the-record for this book due to security concerns. Post-*Dobbs* under state bans, people selling and distributing abortion pills without a license, as she did in 2017, face significantly higher criminalization risks today than when she was active almost a decade ago. But something also exists today that Lisa did not have: more company. Lisa acted alone. Isolation may be the most vulnerable place to be in the illegal pill-distribution landscape in the post-*Dobbs* US. Far more vulnerable may be an abortion-seeker under a ban who does not know where to go.

In 2018, the same year agents showed up at Lisa's apartment, Dr. Rebecca Gomperts from her office in the Netherlands created a new NGO, Aid Access. Through this NGO, Gomperts would use her Austrian medical license to legally prescribe and send pills from overseas to Americans. A thrilled Coeytaux included Aid Access on Plan C's guide online. Aid Access was not like the prescription-less vendors. It was a feminist nonprofit organization with medical oversight, and Gomperts operated legally according to where she was licensed. Aid Access technically was not illegal, using those loopholes like WOW did. But when she started Aid Access, Gomperts imagined it as "just a safety net," she told me, for people with nowhere else to go. She could not have predicted Aid Access for many Americans would be a post-*Dobbs* lifeline.

The combi-packs that Aid Access mailed to people in all 50 states came from the same pharmacy in India that WOW used. The pills could take two or three weeks to arrive from India to the US. Not ideal for a pregnant person. As discussed in earlier chapters, an abortion with pills can be more painful and less effective at later gestational ages. The earlier a person took the pills, the better. Yet almost 75 percent of people in the US using Aid Access said they used the service because of money: they could not afford clinic care, including taking time off work or finding childcare to travel.[41] And some just did not want to go to a clinic, preferring privacy at home.

But Gomperts may have underestimated the guidance some people in the US needed during their abortions with pills. Aid Access's small help desk soon became overwhelmed with emailed medical questions. Yet Aid Access's asynchronous model meant that doctors did not answer immediately. Even if they did, they did so through email exchanges. Some conversations needed a call. And for that, Aid Access sought help from licensed abortion providers in the US already searching in the Trump era to go on the offensive. In late 2018, Gomperts spoke to longtime American abortion provider and family medicine physician Dr. Linda Prine. What if Prine and her colleagues started a hotline where people who used abortion pills or miscarried in the US could confidentially, quickly speak to a doctor in their country and time zone? Prine liked the idea and, with allies, formed the Miscarriage and Abortion Hotline (M+A Hotline).

This hotline was not the same as those within a global feminist SMA movement because medical doctors staffed it. But for Prine and the American provider community still under *Roe*, the hotline was rather radical, so much so that several American reproductive rights lawyers repeatedly warned them not to launch it. Many thought the doctors on the M+A Hotline could be sued and lose their licenses. Prine believed this legal advice overly cautious. These doctors would not be providing people abortion pills outside the law. So, what exactly was illegal about this hotline?

An exasperated Prine and allies moved ahead regardless, albeit with little funding. They launched the M+A Hotline in 2019 with 12 providers, each person taking two or three shifts a month. The hotline was open 12 hours a day in all US time zones. That was plenty at first. Not nearly so after *Dobbs* when the M+A Hotline needed to scale up rapidly. "And now everybody treats us like we're a sister organization," Prine told me in 2023. "The lawyers are all very supportive now nothing has happened. And I feel like that was a big lesson learned about all this caution the lawyers have around doing anything."[42]

These anxieties were not all in lawyers' heads, however. In 2019, the year that the M+A Hotline started, the FDA sent Gomperts a cease and desist letter for Aid Access.[43] Gomperts, safely in the Netherlands, called chicken on the FDA. She posted the agency's letter on Aid Access's website and sued the agency, arguing that the FDA was attempting to deny American women's constitutional right to abortion.[44] But the FDA could not actually do anything to Aid Access or Gomperts since both were beyond their jurisdiction. And so, Gomperts's lawsuit was dismissed.[45]

The 2020 COVID-19 pandemic changed everything for abortion pills in the US. When the secretary of health and human services under Trump declared the pandemic an emergency in March 2020, the FDA allowed providers to waive certain REMS requirements for drug after drug, including some opioids—but not that in-person distribution rule for mifepristone.[46] Of more than 20,000 FDA-approved drugs, mifepristone was the one medication that the agency required a patient pick up from a clinic, hospital, or medical office yet let that patient take by themselves, without medical supervision, wherever they wished.[47] This disconnect infuriated the reproductive rights and medical communities. Anti-abortion attorney generals in a few states, including Texas, meanwhile declared abortion "nonessential" medical care, using emergency orders in the pandemic to temporarily close clinics, effectively banning abortion for millions.[48]

In May 2020, the American College of Obstetrics and Gynecology (ACOG), SisterSong, and others sued the FDA, arguing that forcing people to pick up mifepristone was discriminatory and dangerous in a pandemic, particularly harming low-income communities and communities of color already dying from COVID-19 at higher rates.[49] In contrast over in the UK, the National Health Service (NHS) pivoted almost entirely to telehealth abortion (or "pills by post") for early pregnancies, doing so to limit COVID-19 exposure.[50]

The UK was obviously much smaller than the US and, with a nationalized health care system, could make this switch rapidly all at once.[51] Through the NHS, researchers could now gather data on the telehealth abortion experiences of more than 50,000 people in the pandemic. They soon proved on a much larger scale what those in the medication abortion field already knew: that "no-test medical abortion" was safe, effective, and satisfactory.[52] People even got their appointments faster and had their abortions earlier.[53]

But telehealth abortion entered the US in stops and starts, not like in the UK. A lower court ruling in *ACOG v. FDA* the summer of 2020 temporarily let mifepristone be mailed to patients, including allowing pharmacies to send mifepristone to patients for the first time.[54] One of the earliest US pharmacies to mail patients that medication was Honeybee Health, co-founded by Dr. Jessica Nouhavandi.[55] US-based telehealth abortion services began sprouting, making abortion much cheaper, costing around $250 to patients.[56] Yet unlike Aid Access, these services did not mail pills to all 50 states seeing as some states still banned telehealth abortion. Several clinics started including telehealth abortion services, too, at least in states where they legally could.[57]

Then on January 12, 2021, six days after extremists stormed the US Capitol to try to usurp newly elected president Democrat Joe Biden and put Trump back in power, the Supreme Court decided on *FDA v. ACOG*, that case all about mifepristone.[58] Their decision arrived on a day with one of the highest US death counts from COVID-19 so far.[59] The Supreme Court's new conservative supermajority unsurprisingly voted to stop the legal mailing of mifepristone to patients, at least temporarily. A few weeks later, more UK and US research on telehealth abortion came out, continuing to show the safety of this care.[60] Only then, with a friendlier Biden White House and ample evidence, did the FDA explicitly allow mifepristone to be mailed to patients. The agency did so in April 2021 as a temporary measure in the pandemic and then, in December 2021, made that decision permanent.[61]

Telehealth abortion services in the US dramatically expanded. Plan C figured the more services, the better. "Because that is normalizing of this," Wells told me. "Also, there's protection in numbers." What Winikoff and others waited years to see in the US was at last beginning to happen. And in 2020, amid a loosening of the REMS, more than half of people who had abortions in the US formal health care system used pills, up from 39 percent in 2017.[62]

Except still not many Americans knew about mifepristone and misoprostol. A 2020 poll from *KFF* (a nonprofit, independent US health policy research organization formerly known as the Kaiser Family Foundation) found that just about 21 percent of adults in the US had even heard of mifepristone or medication abortion.[63] When I asked medication abortion researcher Dr. Daniel Grossman in 2021 for the likely reasons why that number was so low, he explained that, for one, most of the American public education system simply did not teach comprehensive sex education, let alone abortion care. He also believed stigma kept many people from sharing their own abortion stories in their communities. "Because they're worried that they will be judged," he told me, urging greater attention on ending abortion stigma. Sure enough, that same *KFF* poll found that six in 10 Americans personally knew someone who had an abortion, including themselves.[64]

CHAPTER 14

"WE ARE GOING TO LOSE OUR RIGHT TO ABORTION ACCESS TOMORROW"

In Texas's Rio Grande Valley in 2014, a year after state Senator Wendy Davis's filibuster, 19-year-old Cathy Torres found out that one of her friends was pregnant and did not want to be.[1] The valley had one abortion clinic left (and it, too, would close later that year).[2] An abortion with pills cost about $800 at that clinic, more than Torres's friend could afford. Torres balked at the price when her friend told her. "What!? It's *that* expensive?" Her friend desperately searched online for abortion pills (there was no Plan C or Aid Access yet). She came across a site that claimed to sell abortion pills for around $400, half of what the clinic charged but still a lot of money. She bought them. A combi-pack soon arrived at her home without instructions. Torres and her friend didn't know what to do, so her friend took all the pills at once. "It was like a punch in the gut," Torres told me. "Because they didn't take them the way it is recommended to be effective and a little more comfortable." Her friend cramped and bled and threw up over days. It was painful and scary. Yet the pills worked.

Torres was upset. Why did her friend have to go through this? It wasn't fair. She began to learn more about reproductive justice and started volunteering at the valley's tiny abortion fund, Frontera Fund, which did not exist when her friend needed help affording abortion care. At Frontera, Torres answered abortion-seekers' calls and gave them money for their abortions at clinics. Calls ballooned during the pandemic when Texas's attorney general declared abortion "medically unnecessary."[3] Abortion would be almost entirely banned a few days later, then not, then banned, then not.[4] Callers to Frontera were often scared and confused. This havoc around abortion care in Texas con-vinced Torres that something much worse was coming. She nervously watched the Republican-controlled state legislature in early 2021 in-troduce Senate Bill 8 (SB 8), a ban on abortion past roughly six weeks in pregnancy, or about two weeks after a missed period, before many women even know they are pregnant.[5] It blatantly violated *Roe*.

Under SB 8 in Texas, as soon as a pregnant person's ultrasound de-tected a "fetal heartbeat" of an "unborn child," then abortion became illegal.[6] In reality, no "fetal heart" existed that early in pregnancy; an ultrasound instead picked up electrical activity from cells.[7] SB 8 also allowed people past around six weeks in pregnancy to have abortions only in "medical emergencies," without the bill clarifying what that meant.[8] Yet what made SB 8 especially pernicious was that the state would not enforce it. Civilians would.

Rather than criminalizing a person in Texas who has or seeks their own abortion beyond six weeks in their pregnancy, SB 8 allowed anyone else to sue someone who "aids or abets the performance or inducement" of another person's abortion past six weeks, possibly winning at least $10,000 in "damages" in court.[9] It was draconian and deliberately confusing. "We, as in all the Texas abortion funds and anyone who did repro in general in Texas, were like, 'Hey, this is very real. It's probably going to pass. We need to sound the fuck-ing alarm,'" Torres told me. "And the response was always, 'They'll never get that far. . . . This is insane.' And then fast forward, they did."

When SB 8 became law in May 2021, scheduled to go into effect on September 1 that year, advocacy nonprofit Plan C did a Texas road trip to make sure people knew about ordering abortion pills online, regardless of the looming six-week ban.[10] Almost 30 million people lived in Texas.[11] Plan C knew not every abortion-seeker in the state could possibly travel out of state for care, no matter how much money they had. The nonprofit commissioned a van to drive around Texas with a glowing billboard that read: "Missed a period? There's a pill for that." Even under a ban, people in Texas would be able to order pills in the mail.[12]

In the valley, Torres at Frontera quickly prepared for SB 8, know-ing that the number of callers who would need to travel out of state for abortions at clinics would skyrocket once that six-week ban came. Frontera usually saw about 400 callers a year, maybe eight of those needing to travel out of Texas, typically for later abortion care outlawed in the state.[13] But no one knew if a court might stop SB 8 as soon as that law went into effect. Texas abortion funds' attorneys mostly advised these nonprofit funds to avoid publicly advocating for pills-by-mail options in the state. Under SB 8, it was unclear if funds in Texas could be sued for even paying for a person's out-of-state, legal abortion care, let alone for sending someone in the state a link to Plan C to find pills. Torres worried, too, that the most marginalized people taking abortion pills in Texas under SB 8 could still be criminalized. Sure, SB 8 did not technically criminalize the person having their own abortion. Yet in the heavily surveilled valley, with border checkpoints every few miles, and amid a racist carceral state, Torres doubted that exception in SB 8 would be enough protection.[14]

On the morning of September 1, 2021, Torres was at an SB 8 protest when her phone for Frontera rang. The caller was seven weeks pregnant and "freaking out," Torres told me. A Texas abortion clinic had just turned her away because she was now more than six weeks pregnant. The clinic referred her to Frontera. Her nearest out-of-state clinic was in Kansas. But the caller had no money to fly there. What was happening? Torres almost cried. This was real.

Less than 24 hours later, the Supreme Court, in a measly three-page document, decided 5–4 to refuse to block SB 8 and to instead let the six-week ban stand.[15] The five justices, three of whom were Trump appointees, stated SB 8 raised "complex and novel antecedent procedural questions."[16] Justice Sonia Sotomayor wrote in her dissent, "Today, the Court finally tells the Nation that it declined to act because, in short, the State's gambit worked."[17]

"And then that was it," Torres told me in early 2024. "That was the beginning of the end, honestly. Not the end of us. We're still here and loud and aggressive, but just another inch towards a total ban." Frontera jumped from funding eight out-of-state travelers' abortions a year to 15 to 20 a month under SB 8—until a post-*Dobbs*, total abortion ban a year later.[18] There were more than 50,000 abortions in Texas's formal health care system in 2021.[19] Under Texas's post-*Dobbs* abortion ban, this would drop in 2023 to a startling 62—in a state home to roughly 10 percent of women of reproductive age in the country.[20] These figures did not include how many people in Texas were self-managing abortions with pills.

Among those ordering pills at home, Aid Access witnessed a staggering 1,180 percent increase in traffic during the first week of SB 8.[21] Aid Access started to offer advance provision of pills, where people could order pills before they may need them, just in case.[22] Plan C's site traffic leapt from about 500 visits a day before September 2021 to more than 25,000 a day after, with about 30 percent of visitors based in Texas.[23]

But Texas abortion funds continued to largely not publicly direct people to pills online given the legal risks to their organizations. A few voices in the reproductive rights, health, and justice movements argued this approach was overly cautious in a crisis. Yet to Torres, that criticism missed nuances. "It was a time where we were all in fight or flight," she told me in early 2024, continuing:

> And it can be argued that we still are, right? Let's get people the care that they need. And yes to all that. We're aware of that. But it's easy for someone to say if they are not a Texan. And if they're not doing work in Texas. That's even easier for someone to say if they're not from the border. They're not brown. Their organization is not femme and queer led. They are not fat. . . . I think it's very easy for people to assume the worst or scream into the void and wonder, "Why do I feel so alone in this?" And it's because laws like this, state governments, conservatives, the other side writes legislation and uses language to make you feel alone and isolated.

Across the US-Mexico border, Verónica Cruz Sánchez of Las Libres in Guanajuato saw SB 8 chaos descend the same month that Mexico's Supreme Court unanimously decriminalized abortion, a landmark ruling on the heels of Argentina liberalizing abortion more.[24] The Green Wave rose while the US retracted.

Volunteer community networks in Texas began coordinating with accompaniment groups in Mexico, Las Libres being one such group, to send people in the state free pills.[25] For almost two decades, Mexico's networks had operated safely under bans, with misoprostol over the counter in much of the country. Arms of the reproductive rights and justice movements in the US were developing their own SMA strategies and growing resources, which they had been preparing for this moment. Since 2018, If/When/How: Lawyering for Reproductive Justice had been offering free, confidential legal services to people about abortion, SMA included, through their Repro Legal Helpline.[26] After SB 8, the Miscarriage + Abortion Hotline (M+A Hotline) received more calls from people taking pills in Texas on their own and needing free medical advice.[27]

Texas's community networks secretly giving abortion pills to people took on the greatest legal risks. They could be sued, maybe imprisoned. Since Cruz Sánchez was more protected in Mexico, she spoke publicly about these networks, though not in detail, while her US partners remained quiet. People were not alone, if they knew where to look.

But in April 2022, what Torres in the valley feared came true: someone was arrested in Texas after taking abortion pills.[28] This person, who was Latinx, did not seem to have been accompanied. It did not shock Torres that the first person criminalized for an abortion under SB 8 was a woman of color who lived in the valley. What did surprise her was the murder charge. SB 8 and Texas's murder statute explicitly exempted women and pregnant people from being prosecuted for having an abortion.[29] Yet it happened. When this person went to a hospital after taking misoprostol pills, health care workers reported her to law enforcement.[30] The Starr County Sheriff's Office charged her with murder for "intentionally and knowingly causing the death of an individual by self-induced abortion."[31] This was a case of fetal personhood.

Torres at Frontera, Nancy Cárdenas Peña (then at the Latina Institute for Reproductive Justice), and South Texans for Reproductive Justice worked for two harried days to help release this person from jail. National attention fueled public outrage. Even a Texas district attorney admitted there was no legal justification for the murder charge, the state then dropping the case.[32] This tumult signaled to legal scholar Mary Ziegler that the American anti-abortion movement, long in lockstep to end *Roe*, may be fracturing in this new era.[33] What had once been fairly predictable anti-abortion maneuvers—target abortion clinics and providers—now turned unwieldy under SB 8.

On the night of May 2, 2022, the internet all but exploded when *Politico* published a leaked draft of the Supreme Court's *Dobbs v. Jackson Women's Health* decision.[34] Republican-appointed Justice Samuel Alito wrote smugly in the drafted majority opinion, "We hold that *Roe* and *Casey* must be overruled."[35] He argued the nation's "history and tradition" demanded such, a history that he falsely claimed was unblighted by abortion (one where slaveholding Founding Fathers instead forced women to give birth, though Alito did not mention this). "The Constitution makes no reference to abortion, and no such right is implicitly protected by any constitutional provision," Alito continued, "including the one on which the defenders of *Roe* and *Casey* now chiefly rely—the Due Process Clause of the Fourteenth Amendment."

The Fourteenth Amendment passed just after the abolition of slavery, when all women in the US still could not vote and Black women had only barely ceased to be the legal property of white men. Although the amendment stated people in the US had "equal protection under the laws," the country at the time this amendment passed thus already excluded women, who won the right to vote as late as 1920.[36] Now it seemed to Alito that "unborn human beings," not women, were people.

Alito in the leaked draft of *Dobbs* wrote that "far from bringing about a national settlement of the abortion issue, *Roe* and *Casey* have enflamed debate and deepened division."[37] That was fiction. For decades, most Americans consistently said that they want abortion legal in "all or most cases," according to Pew Research Center.[38] Alito also repeated "unborn human being" and "unborn child" four times in a single sentence, women and pregnant people nowhere to be found, all while insisting it was democratic for this unelected Supreme Court to "return the issue of abortion to the people's elected representatives," notably not to the people.[39]

On the night of the leak, many abortion providers and researchers were returning from a NAF conference in Florida. It was the first time most had seen each other in person since the pandemic. NAF was a close community, where providers asked each other if they still wore a bulletproof vest. They all knew something terrible with *Dobbs* was coming. But they thought they had a few weeks more until the Supreme Court finished its term in June. Sociologist Dr. Carole Joffe was on a plane that night, flying from the Florida conference to her home in California, sitting next to providers she had known for decades. On that plane, with a darkening sky outside, one provider checked their phone, and there it was. Whatever hope any had that this would end differently dissolved. "There were tears on that airplane," Joffe told me.[40]

They knew the ramifications would be horrific. In Mississippi, the state at the center of *Dobbs* and one of the poorest states in the country, the State Department of Health found that, between 2016 and early 2020, before the pandemic and *Dobbs*, an astonishing 80 percent of pregnancy-related deaths were preventable.[41] Black people made up about 38 percent of Mississippi's population, and yet this report found Black women in Mississippi in 2020 were four times more likely to die of causes directly related to pregnancy than white women. The authors wrote "a substantial portion of this care is being shouldered by smaller hospitals with limited resources, many of whom are facing possible closure and limiting or discontinuing the provision of obstetrical services, further increasing the burdens borne by the individuals and their communities."[42] It was bad—and about to worsen.

The night of the *Dobbs* leak, my friend in Kansas anxiously asked me if Aid Access was real. She worried about waking up in a few weeks in a state banning abortion. We were the same age, both in our early 30s, and she knew I was writing this book. She had scoured Plan C, her eyes widening in anger and panic when reading how to set up a PO box in a less-restrictive state to mail abortion pills there. She downloaded digital privacy tools, terrified of surveillance. *What the fuck is happening?* I told her Aid Access is real, abortion pills are safe, these are other trusted resources, and yes, this is fucked up. "I didn't realize my country hated me this much," she told me. We were now doing what many people I interviewed around the world had been doing for decades. Keeping each other safe.

Torres and fellow abortion funds in Texas immediately met with their attorneys after the *Dobbs* leak. The state's near-total abortion ban would go into effect 30 days after the Supreme Court officially overturned *Roe*. According to that ban, a pregnant person could only have a legal abortion in the state to save their life. But who decided what counted as a lifesaving abortion? It was effectively a total ban. Like SB 8, the ban did not explicitly criminalize a person for having an abortion in the state, nor criminalize someone paying for another person's abortion in another state that legally protected abortion. Yet under this ban, anyone who provided an illegal abortion in Texas could face up to 99 years in prison, the loss of their license, and at least $100,000 in fines per abortion performed.[43] These were even harsher punishments than in pre-*Roe* years of abortion criminalization.[44]

Attorneys advising Texas funds in this quickly moving crisis thought funds had a 30-day runway after *Roe* fell and before that trigger ban took effect, a tiny window in which funds could keep paying for out-of-state abortions for anyone past six weeks in pregnancy, per SB 8.[45] But paying for people's orders of pills *within* the state—like via Aid Access—potentially risked opening the funds to a lawsuit. It was confusing. It became even more confusing when allied attorneys then realized Texas clinics and funds might need to shut down entirely the day *Roe* fell due to a broadly worded, unrepealed abortion ban in Texas that dated to the Comstock Act era from about 150 years ago.[46] That older ban went defunct under *Roe*, but it might be resurrected with *Dobbs* to prosecute people, which Texas's anti-abortion attorney general loudly threatened to do.[47] Torres braced herself.

On Thursday, June 23, 2022, Torres felt in her gut that tomorrow would be the day. The day that *Roe* fell and Texas banned abortion and Frontera closed, possibly forever. She confided this to an out-of-state clinic manager and asked if anyone who booked an abortion there needed money that day. It may be the last day Frontera could help. Three people in Texas did. Torres called them.

One picked up with a worried voice. She was at a family dinner and rushed to a bathroom for privacy. "I know that you need help,"

Torres told her. "And I have to be honest with you. It has to be now." Torres sent her money and answered questions, telling her to take notes "because I will not be able to help you tomorrow." The caller was confused and scared, then Torres finally told her, "We are going to lose our right to abortion access tomorrow. . . . I just, I just know it. I know I'm some stranger. But please trust me." The caller did. She told Torres that she had never been on a plane before. She was anxious about flying alone for the first time to get to a clinic for her abortion. What if someone at the airport in Texas found out where she was going? Would she be arrested? What should she tell her family? What would happen to her when she got back home? They talked until around 3 a.m. When they hung up, Torres cried. "Because I realized I just funded my last abortion."

Torres could not sleep that night. The next morning, she got in her car and drove to "just be in my thoughts." While she was driving, her phone exploded with texts: *Dobbs* happened. She pulled over, called her mom, and they both sobbed. "I couldn't believe it, but I could, you know? . . . I don't think I'll ever forget that day."

The Supreme Court had a pattern of releasing seismic abortion rulings at the end of its term in late June or early July: *Webster* on July 3, 1989; *Casey* on June 29, 1992; and, on Friday, June 24, 2022, while one abortion-seeker in Texas stepped on a plane for the first time, gripping her seat at take-off, and another abortion-seeker ordered pills online under a ban, praying no one would find out, *Dobbs* came. The 6–3 decision overturned nearly five decades of a national right to abortion.[48] Republican presidents had appointed the six justices behind *Dobbs*.[49] Alito worded the majority opinion almost exactly as in the leak.[50] Nearly every person I interviewed for this book, almost 200 people across 12 countries, had a visceral, powerful reaction to *Dobbs* the day it happened, as if time stopped.

In January 1973, Dr. Beverly Winikoff and her graduate school classmates burst into applause when the decision in *Roe* was announced. Faye Wattleton in July 1989 stood on the brink of burnout outside the Supreme Court when *Webster* whacked at *Roe*, with the Hyde Amendment already in place for more than a decade. Around 1993, reports of women in Brazil using misoprostol for abortions surfaced while, in the US, the Population Council sparred over mife-pristone's patent. Advocates toasted that pill's FDA approval in 2000, hopeful it would solve the American "abortion wars." Late in the first decade of the 2000s and into the 2010s in mainly the Global South was the advent of feminist accompaniment networks, hotlines, and, in the Netherlands, telehealth abortion, with activists spreading pills within, outside, or in between the law. A pandemic burst telehealth abortion open in much of the US, and, in a worsening crisis, Texas's SB 8 led to expanding accompaniment networks across borders. The day after *Dobbs*, Plan C's site saw almost a quarter of a million visitors on that day alone, with around two million total visitors to the site throughout 2022.[51]

While this book does not extensively detail the post-*Dobbs* landscape, these final chapters underscore the increasingly pivotal role abortion pills play, though with a caution Susan Yanow summed up to me well.[52] When I told Yanow in early 2023 about a few of the US groups I interviewed regarding pills, asking if there were others, she nodded and said, "There's other groups. But they're clandestine. I think the challenge at the moment we're in now is you've got all these groups you named, including SASS, that are the public face of self-managed abortion, and then a lot of the people doing the real work who are, uh, being careful."

Those doing "the real work" with pills were in harm-reduction mode. "Because we can't really undo the total [harm] the Supreme Court has done," Yanow continued. "There are going to be lots of people who don't know about these pills and don't travel. And there will be people who have a child they don't want or didn't want. There will be people who die in pregnancy. And it was an unwanted pregnancy. I don't want to sugarcoat it. These are not a silver bullet." She continued to hope, however, that, out of this misery, a vision of abortion pills available over the counter one day would happen, even if she might not live to see the day.

CHAPTER 15

"THIS LAWSUIT IS FRIVOLOUS"

It had been nearly a month since *Dobbs* when 36-year-old reproductive justice activist Renee Bracey Sherman nervously held her written statement. In her mind, she recited words that may soon stun her audience but that she planned to say anyway.[1] She stepped inside DC's Rayburn House Office Building, where Dr. Beverly Winikoff had testified to Congress on mifepristone more than three decades ago. Bracey Sherman would testify, too, sharing her abortion story.

This House hearing on July 19, 2022, had a resigned title: "Roe Reversal: The Impacts of Taking Away the Constitutional Right to an Abortion."[2] *Impacts?* Bracey Sherman thought. *How about "Roe Reversal: This Is What the US Government Is Doing About It."* Democrats had the White House and razor-thin Senate control.[3] Two weeks after *Dobbs*, Biden issued an executive order on abortion that, among other points, directed his HHS to, within the next 30 days, "take additional action to protect and expand access to abortion care, including access to medication."[4] Except this order did not say how HHS would do that.

To Bracey Sherman, Biden was neglecting to use executive powers to meaningfully help millions of people living under state bans who needed abortions right now.[5] Biden barely even used the word "abortion" in public.[6] Weeks after the *Dobbs* leak, Bracey Sherman joined private talks with "pro-choice" Congressional members who told her their plan was to vote, vote, vote. It may have been the stupidest thing she had ever heard. The least that Democrats could do at that very moment, she thought, was tell those millions of people under bans the facts: abortion pills existed, and SMA was safe.

Bracey Sherman had long been critical of how some of the leadership in the American reproductive rights and health movement for years decentered, even stigmatized, people who had abortions, particularly people of color.[7] A Black activist herself, she thought the movement had not reckoned honestly with its own history of classism and racism. Bracey Sherman in 2016 founded a reproductive justice organization called We Testify for the leadership and representation of people who have abortions, especially people of color. She hoped that people telling their own abortion stories would empower them and destigmatize abortion. Like Kinga Jelinska, Bracey Sherman also believed abortion pills could blow open old dynamics that, to her, have held this movement back.

"I feel so lucky that when I was 19, my Abortion Care Network clinic was ten minutes from my home, and an Orthodox Jewish nurse held my hand, and she did so because her faith called her to," Bracey Sherman began in her testimony that July day. "But that almost wasn't my story. Shortly before my appointment, I didn't know if I could hold on. I didn't think I could be pregnant for another moment. I hoped it would all go away. And when it didn't, every day I considered throwing myself down the stairs, as I had seen in movies and in history books. One night, I drank an unsafe amount of alcohol, believing it would cause a miscarriage. It did not. Thankfully, I went to my appointment and received my abortion. That was when it was legal in every state. Now, it is not."[8]

Her voice cracked in sorrow and outrage. She had never before publicly shared her story of trying to unsafely self-induce her abortion. "And I know some will try the methods that I did. And I want them to know that there are safe methods to self-managing their abortions, according to the World Health Organization." She suddenly spoke quickly, veering off-script and raising her hand, a green bandana around her wrist, while counting: "It is one mifepristone pill followed by four misoprostol pills dissolved under the tongue 24 to 48 hours later. Or a series of 12 misoprostol pills, four at a time, dissolved under the tongue every three hours. There is no way to test it in the bloodstream. And a person does not need to tell the police what they took. I share that to exercise my right to free speech because there are organizations and legislators who want to make what I just said a crime."[9]

In her written testimony submitted to Congress before this hearing, she left out those words about how to take pills, worried she may be censored if she included them. But those were the words she had been steeling herself to testify. Those were the words she wanted most to say.

Bracey Sherman became the first person to put SMA protocols into the Congressional record.[10] She tipped off a reporter in advance, so her words went beyond the Hill. For her 19-year-old self in the first decade of the 2000s growing up in the Chicago area, it was abortion stigma that hurt her most. That included the stigma of being a young, single Black mother if she did not get an abortion. Even though her parents supported abortion, she was too scared to tell them of her abortion at the time. Once she finally did years later, her mother gently told her that she, too, had an abortion, then went on to nursing school, married a fellow student, and had a child: Bracey Sherman. "Renee, I chose you," she told her.[11] The more Bracey Sherman voiced her story, the more she learned those around her had abortions, amazed they had all held this secret for so long.

That summer, some activists took to task Supreme Court Justice Samuel Alito's demand to return the "issue" of abortion to the states. Kansas in August 2022 became the first state post-*Dobbs* with a successful ballot measure campaign that directly asked voters to stop an abortion ban.[12] Kansas had a Republican legislature. Yet in 2019, the state Supreme Court enshrined the right to abortion in pregnancies up to 22 weeks with exceptions for lifesaving care. Kansas was home to just four abortion clinics, one of which provided later abortion care in Wichita, where Dr. George Tiller worked until his assassination in 2009.[13] Would Kansans act now or stay home?

Nearly 60 percent of Kansans rejected the abortion ban.[14] Since then until November 2024, as of this writing, similar ballot measures to protect or expand abortion rights have won in 13 states, failing in three states.[15] Lifting abortion rights out of polarized partisanship seemed to be working—but the anti-abortion movement's attempts to confuse voters and restrict voting rights also gained ground.[16] Reproductive rights and justice activists at the same time were debating how far abortion protections should go.[17] *Roe* was not enough, so why not fight for more? To legalize abortion throughout pregnancy and to rest that right with the abortion-seeker, doing away with the decades-old doctor-patient framing. But others in these campaigns argued that, in particularly bright-red states, if they pushed that far that fast, they would lose.

The anti-abortion movement, watching state-level defeats and massive attention on pills, pushed further faster regardless. In November 2022, an anti-abortion coalition, Alliance for Hippocratic Medicine (AHM), sued the FDA to effectively ban mifepristone nationwide.[18] In *Food and Drug Administration v. Alliance for Hippocratic Medicine (FDA v. AHM)*, AHM erroneously argued that the FDA wrongly approved mifepristone in 2000 and that the pill was dangerous.[19] Millions of women in the US had safely used this pill for more than two decades, and more than 100 scientific studies spanning decades and continents time and again proved that this medication was safe.[20] More than 90 countries had also approved mifepristone by then, the pill possessing a remarkably consistent, strong global safety record.[21]

But this case's plaintiffs included anti-abortion OBGYNs who speciously argued their consciences may be harmed if they were forced to provide an emergency abortion to someone who took mifepristone and then needed their care. AHM referred to the unrepealed Comstock Act, one potential way to nationally ban abortion pills—as well as ban birth control and any "instrument" used in abortion.[22] Such a broad ban could even be used to gag miscarriage and obstetrics care, likely killing more women and pregnant people.[23] One AHM plaintiff, the American Association of Pro-Life Obstetricians and Gynecologists, had testified at the 2006 Congressional hearing on RU-486 to pressure the FDA to revoke its approval of the pill.[24] It did not work then, even under a Republican White House with the Bush administration. Now emboldened at the end of *Roe* and outraged at people using abortion pills despite bans, the architects of this AHM case appeared to be stirring more chaos.

AHM's far-right lawyers were part of Alliance Defending Freedom (ADF), a conservative legal organization the Southern Poverty Law Center named a hate group.[25] Some ADF lawyers were behind *Dobbs*, alongside gender-affirming-care bans for minors in several states.[26] "If you look at the anti-choice movement, they're very clever," longtime medication abortion researcher, abortion provider, and gynecologist Dr. Mitchell Creinin told me.[27] "This is a syndicate."

While working as one of Danco's medical consultants, Creinin helped the company write the 2016 FDA-approved label for Mifeprex. He ran one of the Population Council's clinical trial sites for mifepristone in the 1990s as well as contributed to the Abortion Rights Mobilization (ARM) trials. He has also been closely tracking anti-abortion claims about medication abortion. In 2019, he attempted to study one such claim of an "abortion pill reversal treatment," which anti-abortion groups stated worked if a person early in their pregnancy took progesterone shortly after taking mifepristone so as to halt their abortion and continue their pregnancy.[28] Creinin wanted to know if that regimen was even safe, let alone true. But when Creinin began a small study to test "abortion pill reversal," he shut it down over safety concerns after enrolling just 12 of their planned 40 patients.[29] Too many patients at the study's start had hemorrhaged. As I write in 2024, no rigorous research exists proving the safety or efficacy of "abortion pill reversal," yet some anti-abortion state laws mandate abortion providers tell patients about this supposed treatment.[30] It made Creinin furious. When we spoke in 2023, with AHM now attacking mifepristone, he called that case "the biggest bullshit, as we all know."

"This lawsuit is frivolous," Greer Donley, University of Pittsburgh law professor, told me in 2023, having extensively studied mifepristone's US legal history with the FDA.[31] But AHM filed that "frivolous" suit in the tiny town of Amarillo in Texas, a few hours' drive from Kansas, Colorado, and New Mexico, islands of in-clinic abortion access for people traveling there from ban states. Why Amarillo? One judge decided federal civil cases there. And that judge, Matthew J. Kacsmaryk, a Trump appointee, was openly anti-abortion.[32]

Dr. Heather Skanes, a Black female gynecologist, did not leave her home state of Alabama after *Dobbs*.[33] She left the state once for medical school, then returned to be an OBGYN there because of Alabama's stark maternal care disparities, especially for Black women like her. Now under Alabama's post-*Dobbs* abortion ban, Skanes believed those disparities would undoubtedly widen. Who would be there to care for birthing Alabamians? Who would provide emergency abortions to people near death? Who would at the very least tell pregnant Alabamians compassionately and honestly all their options, including an abortion with pills?

In Alabama pre-*Dobbs*, more than a third of counties had no hospitals with labor and delivery units or obstetric providers.[34] Alabama's maternal mortality rate pre-*Dobbs* stood at 64.63 deaths per 100,000, nearly double the national rate of 34.09 (Canada, by comparison, had around 8.6 deaths per 100,000).[35] For Black women in Alabama, that rate was a shocking 100.07 deaths per 100,000, easily one of the worst rates in the country.[36] Alabama also had one of the highest US poverty rates.[37] On the day of *Dobbs*, Skanes's home state added another superlative: one of the country's harshest abortion bans.[38]

There were no exceptions for survivors of rape or incest to get abortions under Alabama's ban.[39] A physician could legally provide an abortion only to save the pregnant person's life, though the ban did not explain what that meant while referring repeatedly to "the unborn child."[40] Those who illegally provided an abortion in Alabama committed a Class A felony and, as such, could get life imprisonment.[41] Those who attempted to illegally provide an abortion committed a Class C felony—and could be imprisoned for up to 10 years.[42] Like in Texas, Alabama's ban did not explicitly criminalize a pregnant person having an abortion.[43] It tried to isolate her.

Skanes worked at a Birmingham hospital when the ban went into effect. That hospital handed her their new abortion policy "copy-and-pasted from Alabama law," Skanes told me in 2024. "Alabama law is not medicine." Terms like "unborn child" written in the law made no sense to physicians who, at that very moment, were caring for pregnant patients miscarrying, bleeding, suffering. "But you're setting me up," Skanes told the hospital. "Because you haven't given me clear guidelines as to what we can and cannot do."

She witnessed hospital doctors, fearful of prison time for abortion care, wait until a pregnant person went septic before intervening. What could have been a simple, safe procedure or prescribing mifepristone and misoprostol to treat a miscarriage could then turn into a Cesarean section, or major abdominal surgery. Skanes became one of the few physicians at that hospital who did not wait for her patients to go septic before treating them. She prescribed mifepristone and misoprostol in emergencies. But before she could do so, this hospital required her to find one other doctor to sign off on her prescribing these pills for each patient. She then needed to tell a C-suite hospital administrator that she would be giving a patient these medications. Why? The patient's chart at the hospital would already state they were given these pills. To Skanes, this extra surveillance only delayed urgent care as a patient's life was on the line. She worried as well that this hospital over time would see that she was one of the only doctors providing these pills. As also one of the only Black doctors at that facility, she feared the hospital would target her, maybe report her to police. What use would her skills be to Alabamians from prison?

Under an abortion ban at a hospital, she believed any doctors' racist, sexist biases against pregnant people would fester. Skanes felt that even doctors in Alabama who supported abortion could find themselves facing intense pressure and confusion over what they could legally do, then hesitate to act, harming the pregnant person. Skanes left that hospital. When we spoke in 2024, she ran Oasis Women's Health, a Birmingham clinic known among locals as a safe place for pregnant people, particularly Black women.

Raised in a conservative Christian church, Skanes had her own abortion baggage growing up. But she was curious as a medical resident and did a rotation at an abortion clinic. Skanes realized every patient had their reason for an abortion. "And whatever that reason was, it was good enough," she told me. The heaviness of their stories overwhelmed her. Many were parents and could not afford another child.

One confided that her partner abused her. Another had a later, wanted pregnancy diagnosed with fetal anencephaly, which meant her baby (for she thought of what she carried as her baby) had no skull and no chance of survival. Some of Skanes's patients cried during their abortion procedure, not because they were uncertain or in physical pain, but because they felt like they were bad people. Or that if their lives had been different, they may have wanted this pregnancy. As Skanes told me of these patients, "It was a very, very powerful experience about the strength that it takes to do something that people don't agree with."

For those in Alabama not experiencing medical emergencies in a hospital and who needed an abortion once *Dobbs* fell and the state ban became real, there were hardly any local places to turn to for help. Alabama's attorney general threatened post-*Dobbs* to criminalize anyone in the state who paid for people's abortions anywhere in the country.[44] As in Texas, in response to these threats, Alabama's local abortion fund and reproductive justice organization, Yellowhammer Fund, shut down its direct abortion access work temporarily when *Dobbs* came. Yellowhammer, on advice from their lawyers, stopped paying for people's abortions within and even outside of Alabama in states where abortion remained legal.[45]

Yet Yellowhammer drew from global feminist SMA movement strategies under bans to, at the very least, carefully share with people public information about abortion pills under their constitutional right to free speech.[46] Yellowhammer trained 25 trusted community members, which the organization referred to as fellows, in just about everything there was to know on SMA and movement resources like the Miscarriage + Abortion Hotline (M+A Hotline). These fellows had contacts to allied, local doctors who would not report to police anyone who came to them for legal miscarriage or post-abortion care—after these patients may or may not have taken abortion pills. One such allied doctor was Skanes.[47] The fellows' names and locations were not made public given security concerns. This secrecy, however, was an obvious weakness: How did Alabamians know whom to ask for help? The most vulnerable could still slip through.

Pills were nonetheless flowing, if not to everyone equally. Plan C in 2023 could not keep up with how many prescription-less vendors were asking them to be vetted and listed on their website.[48] Some vendors' sites were sketchier than others. One vendor sent pills to Plan C's mystery shopper that arrived crushed in the mail. Plan C did not list that vendor, Elisa Wells told me, and used their leverage to demand better. "Because our listings are such powerful marketing for that," Wells told me. "And we list people for free."

Plan C told vendors they would prioritize testing sites that (a) sold pills plus shipping for under $250, (b) included extra misoprostol pills, (c) delivered to people within seven or fewer days of ordering, and (d) offered at least some digital security to abortion-seekers. Most vendors, Wells told me, did drop prices to $99, provide more misoprostol, and improve their ship time, though digital security on several sites was still lacking. One vendor Plan C listed turned out to be a "disaster," Wells told me in 2023. That site was supposedly accidentally sharing buyers' personal information, a serious vulnerability for abortion-seekers. Plan C hurriedly removed that seller from their website. Some actors in the reproductive rights and justice movements that had long been wary of Plan C were furious. But Plan C could not ultimately control what vendors did. For people trying to buy prescription-less abortion pills, Wells suggested they focus on their own digital security. It was an overwhelming landscape for many abortion-seekers to navigate.

There were meanwhile SMA information-sharing sessions underway in parts of the country. In 2023, I joined one workshop at a college in New York, where students whom Susan Yanow's SASS had trained were walking the participants through how to take pills safely. They explained what to say to a provider in the rare event someone needed medical attention. They spoke in the third person, "one would do this," so as not to be mistaken for providing medical advice without a license (similar to Dr. Leonel Briozzo's team in Uruguay speaking about misoprostol pills in the third person to abortion-seekers a decade ago). SMA activism in early post-*Dobbs* months tread cautiously, allied lawyers routinely vetting language on

SMA that activists shared publicly. Movement arguments arose over how much caution was too much.

Dr. Linda Prine of Aid Access and the M+A Hotline told me in early 2023 about another strategy with pills: a proposed telehealth abortion shield law that she had been urging legislators to pass in New York, where abortion remained broadly legal. If that proposal became law, then abortion providers licensed and located in New York would be able to, at least according to New York law, legally prescribe and mail abortion pills to people located in ban states. When Prine and I spoke, it had been seven months since *Dobbs*, and no US-based providers during that time could legally send pills to people in a ban state without risking imprisonment, potentially for life.[49] Prine was Aid Access's provider for New Mexico, which had abortion-protective laws, so she could legally send abortion pills to people in that state. She did not touch ban states like Alabama with dogged anti-abortion prosecutors.[50] "I'm not crazy," Prine told me. "But I think that we need to use what systems we can, and we need to use them urgently because things are really bad in these red states."

People in those states called her and the M+A Hotline nearly every day. The hotline that began with 12 providers in 2019 jumped to more than 70 providers by early 2023. Half of callers wanted to know how to get pills. The other half tended to be people in ban states, miscarrying or taking pills later in pregnancy, terrified. Pre-*Dobbs*, Prine remembered only one person who took pills later in pregnancy, around 18 weeks, and called the hotline. *Oh, my God, I didn't know somebody could do this*, Prine thought at the time.

American providers were generally not trained to support people using abortion pills past 10 weeks in pregnancy; the standard for later abortion care in the US was for specially trained providers to perform procedures. But, as with this pre-*Dobbs* caller, not everyone could access or perhaps wanted a procedure. Shocked at that hotline call, Prine spoke to doctors in other countries that did have experience supporting people's later abortions with pills (either with mifepristone and misoprostol or misoprostol alone). When we spoke in 2023, I mentioned to Prine the 2018 book Socorristas wrote about accompanying people through later abortions with pills. She eagerly asked me for a copy. She wanted to learn from them. Because now people nearly every day post-*Dobbs* were calling the M+A Hotline after taking abortion pills at 13, 15, 18 weeks in pregnancy.[51] According to Prine, these callers usually did not know what to expect, how taking pills at a later gestational age was not the same physical experience as taking pills earlier in pregnancy. They would likely be passing a recognizable fetus, which might be jarring for them if they were not emotionally prepared, and their abortion process would physically hurt more and take several days. All under criminalization fears, stigma, and secrecy. "People are very scared," Prine told me. "And they shouldn't have to be going through that experience."

Prine believed that New York's telehealth shield law could get people in ban states these pills faster, earlier in pregnancy. Without this law, if someone in a ban state ordered pills from Aid Access, for example, the pills were shipped from India, not the US, and could take weeks to arrive. "It's really dire, every day what people are going through," Prine told me. "I'm not sympathetic with folks who are saying [these telehealth shield laws] are really risky, that I don't think you should do this. Yeah, we'll see."

Three law professors—David S. Cohen, Greer Donley, and Rachel Rebouché—wrote a paper published in 2023 with their first draft put online in February 2022 that outlined this shield law strategy as a possible way to help protect abortion providers and patients in a shield law state from another state enforcing its anti-abortion laws beyond its state borders.[52] Shield law state officials and agencies, for example, could agree to not cooperate with an anti-abortion state's investigation into abortions provided within that shield law state. As Prine had explained to me, a telehealth-specific shield law would also allow licensed providers in that telehealth shield law state to prescribe and mail abortion pills to people located in ban or severely restricted states. This would work somewhat like how Women on Web (WOW) used legal loopholes to ship pills across national borders to people living in countries under bans. But some within the American reproductive rights movement were worried that telehealth shield laws could break interstate cooperation norms within the US and thus may not be protective enough. Also, even with telehealth shield laws in place, the ban or restricted state where the patient would be located would still consider the activity to have taken place in their state and therefore be illegal.

Back in Texas's Rio Grande Valley, Frontera Fund and other abortion funds in the state reopened in February 2023. They had gained some clarity in court following their post-*Dobbs* lawsuit against Texas's attorney general.[53] Texas funds were now paying for people's abortion care and logistical support, if people traveled to states where abortion was more protected. This included paying the costs of care, travel, lodging, and childcare (since most people who have abortions in the US are parents), which could easily add up to more than $2,000.[54] The funds still did not pay for people's abortion pills bought online within Texas given potential legal risks to fund staff living in the state. In July 2023, Yellowhammer and allies in Alabama similarly sued Alabama's attorney general for clarity that they, too, could at least pay for people's out-of-state abortions, where legal.[55]

Clinics operating in states with more legal protections for abortion were already surging with patients as travelers and state residents competed for appointments, often leading to delays in care.[56] A person who sought an abortion while 12 weeks pregnant suddenly may not receive care until 15 weeks, driving up costs for already-burdened abortion-seekers. This tumultuous and fragile infrastructure of clinics in the months after *Dobbs* frustrated Plan C and several activists. To them, pills by mail, particularly through telehealth shield laws, could not be more urgent. But after Prine and I spoke in February 2023 about the proposed telehealth shield law in New York, it still took months for that law and similar ones in a few other states to pass and go into effect, all while the AHM case to ban mifepristone worked—briefly.

CHAPTER 16

"I FELT LIKE I WAS ABANDONED"

In April 2023, Judge Matthew Kacsmaryk in Amarillo, Texas, did what a year prior would have been unthinkable: effectively, he nationally banned mifepristone.[1] His written decision brazenly repeated "unborn human" and stated lies about the pill.[2] Kacsmaryk argued the FDA did violate the dormant Comstock Act by allowing the sale of mifepristone.[3] He also stated the restrictions that the FDA put on mifepristone in 2000 proved that the pill was dangerous, and he argued that the agency negligently rushed to approve mifepristone.[4] This, of course, was not true.[5]

Beneath Kacsmaryk's nose in Amarillo, at least a few people were taking abortion pills anyways. I spoke to a couple of them, who could not be named due to security concerns. On that flow of abortion pills defying bans, Dr. Beverly Winikoff put it bluntly to me: "The antis can't stand it." That evidently included Kacsmaryk.

When Kacsmaryk's ruling fell to clamorous headlines, Danco came out to protect its sole product—and defend the FDA's decisions on mifepristone. Danco and GenBioPro (the company approved to make a generic version of mifepristone for the US in 2019) would be expected to pull mifepristone from the US market if Kacsmaryk's decision stood—since those companies were the nation's only two approved sellers of the pill. As mifepristone's original sponsor in the US, going back to the mid-1990s, Danco was best positioned to argue that the 2000 FDA approval was indeed lawful. Danco and the US Department of Justice under Biden swiftly filed an emergency motion with the US Court of Appeals for the Fifth Circuit to stay Kacsmaryk's decision.[6]

Except the Fifth Circuit was made up of three conservative federal judges, two of whom were Trump appointees.[7] In a 2–1 decision, the judges essentially watered down Kacsmaryk's extremism. The court argued they could not revoke that 2000 FDA approval because it was past the statute of limitations, so they instead effectively banned telehealth services for mifepristone by ruling the FDA return the pill to its stricter, original 2000 label.[8] The decision's one dissenting judge, James Ho, went so far as to write that a doctor may suffer "aesthetic injury" from mifepristone: meaning that if a pregnant person took that pill for their abortion, then sought medical attention, their doctor's sight of an "unborn patient" would be too "aesthetically" jarring to that doctor, depriving these physicians of the "delight in working with their unborn patients."[9] As if pregnant people were decorations.

Danco and the Justice Department appealed *that* ruling to the Supreme Court, which agreed to hear the case and, until they would make their decision, paused the Fifth Circuit's telehealth abortion ban.[10] All this happened in days.

The Supreme Court a year later would weigh the decision to ban mailing mifepristone to patients, a decision that could devastate dwindling abortion access. The stakes went far beyond abortion, however. If judges could overrule FDA decisions on a pill with a robust safety record, what did that mean for any drug on the legal US market? Or any federal regulatory authority? Several former FDA officials who worked on mifepristone filed amicus briefs in support of Danco and the FDA against AHM.[11] I spoke to many of them. They were adamant that this case was groundless. *How could it even get this far?*

A very faint silver lining may have been that in April 2023, with wall-to-wall press on this fiasco, "mifepristone" became one of Google's most-searched news topics in the US.[12] But social media censorship on pills reportedly spiked in the US post-*Dobbs*.[13] And the Amarillo havoc temporarily confused many abortion-seekers, who could still, for the time being, get mifepristone and misoprostol from providers on the legal US market in the states that did not ban abortion—or from vendors and community networks beyond the law, as well as from Aid Access in legal loopholes.

———

Throughout 2023, the first full year post-*Dobbs*, news stories emerged of women with wanted pregnancies who lived under bans and almost died or did die after they were denied emergency abortion care or received delayed emergency abortion care. Many of these women were in their early 30s, about the same age as me. Their stories were like those of women around the world who nearly lost their lives or died under abortion bans.[14]

In the US like elsewhere, these harrowing stories, while critical to share, do not today represent most people who have abortions. Several American reproductive rights and justice activists for years criticized outsized focus in the mainstream media on people who have wanted pregnancies and need emergency abortions, arguing that when those voices become the only ones heard, the millions who have abortions outside of those truly horrific circumstances go neglected and possibly stigmatized. At the same time, all abortion stories were why people in the reproductive rights and justice movements told me they fought to provide pills within, in between, or beyond the law.

In March 2023 in *Zurawski v. State of Texas*, five women who needed abortion care in medical emergencies joined two OBGYNs to sue Texas to clarify the state ban's exceptions for abortion care when their lives were on the line.[15] These five women in the case carried wanted pregnancies that turned life-threatening in Texas, then were denied abortions and forced to give birth, suffering serious harms to their emotional and physical health. More women with stories like theirs, 20 women in all, joined *Zurawski*.[16] Samantha Casiano, one of the women, spoke in tears in later testimony about how she was mistreated when she learned her pregnancy was not viable. "The case worker came in, and they handed me a brochure that said 'funeral homes' on top of it. . . . I felt like I was abandoned."[17] She threw up on the stand. The Supreme Court of Texas rejected *Zurawski* in May 2024, refusing to clarify the ban's exception.[18]

In September 2023 in Ohio, where abortion was still legal in pregnancies up to about 22 weeks at the time, Brittany Watts, a 33-year-old Black woman, was 21 weeks pregnant when her water broke, too early for the fetus that she carried to survive.[19] She needed urgent miscarriage care. Watts went to a nearby Catholic-affiliated hospital that refused to provide abortion or miscarriage care until a hospital "ethics" committee deemed a woman near enough to death to intervene. Watts did not know this protocol. She waited hours at the hospital, then left, returned, waited again, no one telling her of this "ethics" committee. A provider technically could have legally prescribed her mifepristone and misoprostol to safely manage her miscarriage. No one did. Watts went home a second time and, days later, passed her pregnancy in her bathroom, then returned to the hospital. Only then a nurse called the police to search Watts's home for the "baby."[20] Police found a miscarried fetus in Watts's toilet, removed the toilet, and charged her with "abuse of a corpse." An Ohio grand jury declined to indict her. A CBS News reporter later asked the soft-spoken Watts why she thought that she had been treated this way, and she replied: "Because of my skin color."[21]

In December 2023 in Texas, Kate Cox, a 31-year-old white, married mother of two with a wanted pregnancy, asked the state to block its ban for her care.[22] Her pregnancy at around 20 weeks had been diagnosed with Trisomy 18, meaning the fetus she carried had almost no chance of survival.[23] Cox also had two prior Cesarean sections and underlying health issues. If she were forced to give birth, she risked serious complications, including possible infertility. Her attorneys and doctor argued Cox fell under the ban's exception. A sympathetic court agreed.[24] Texas's attorney general, Ken Paxton, did not. He sent a letter to the hospitals involved in Cox's care, warning of prosecution if they helped with her abortion.[25] He appealed Cox's case to the state Supreme Court. An exhausted Cox could not wait any longer for the courts to decide her case while her body carried her "baby," in her words.[26] She went to a New Mexico clinic for later abortion care. The state Supreme Court overturned the lower ruling in the meantime, deciding Cox not sick enough. "It was crushing," she told CBS News in a TV interview in January 2024.[27]

Yet not all pregnant people, not all women, were seen equally, if at all. Around January 2024, as Cox's interview aired, the New Yorker reported on 27-year-old Yeniifer (Yeni) Alvarez-Estrada Glick, a Latinx woman with a wanted pregnancy who lived uninsured in a maternal care desert in rural Texas.[28] She grew up wanting to be a scientist. Maybe she would have surpassed biochemist Dr. Sarah Ratner, who found prostaglandins a century ago. But she turned down scholarships; she did not have a Social Security number.

Born in Mexico, Alvarez-Estrada Glick moved to the US at around three years old with her family. When in early 2022 she became pregnant under SB 8, she had hypertension, diabetes, obesity, and a history of pulmonary edema. Her wanted pregnancy was high-risk. The closest hospital was in a Catholic-affiliated network that avoided emergency abortion and miscarriage care, a situation Watts would face in Ohio. Alvarez-Estrada Glick turned to providers there early in her pregnancy. They could have legally told her abortion options and that her pregnancy might endanger her life. She technically met the six-week-ban's exceptions. If she consented to an early abortion, a provider could have prescribed her mifepristone and misoprostol— or referred her to another provider in Texas who would do so, even another provider in a state without SB 8. But no provider reportedly breathed a word of this to her.[29]

She likely did not know about the Miscarriage + Abortion Hotline, about Las Libres, or about Frontera Fund. Instead, she continued her pregnancy and, on July 10, 2022, days after *Dobbs*, her pregnancy went very wrong, very fast. She died. Her story received little attention compared to Cox's interview. She was not a blonde white woman. How many more stories like hers existed?

The state bears a particular cruelty on those whose names we may never learn. This is not a uniquely American story. Yet our willful regression is. This book began three decades ago with a story that started in the opposite direction: fewer women dying at Brazilian maternity hospitals despite a national abortion ban. Women learned to save their own lives with misoprostol. Then the Brazilian government restricted that medication. Brazil's maternal mortality rate went back up after its brief dip when the pill was effectively available over the counter. The country as of 2024 continues to have a near-total abortion ban. But from 1990 to 2019, the maternal mortality rate in Brazil, though perilously high, declined while, in the US, that rate skyrocketed, jumping nearly 60 percent in roughly the same time span.[30] Brazil also has universal health care that the wealthier US does not.

In Texas alone, amid high rates of uninsured people, that maternal mortality rate between 1999 and 2019 more than doubled, acutely felt in Black and Latinx communities.[31]

There is hardly any question among medical and public health experts that *Dobbs* will worsen a national maternal mortality crisis.[32] The infant mortality rate in Texas already shot up 12.9 percent after SB 8, the study's authors attributing SB 8 to this rise.[33] But in May 2024, Texas's Maternal Mortality and Morbidity Review Committee appointed anti-abortion OBGYN Dr. Ingrid Skop to its board.[34] Skop previously signed an affidavit saying Cox did not qualify for an abortion in Texas. She testified to Congress in 2021 that rape and incest survivors as young as nine could potentially carry pregnancies to term. And she was in AHM's lawsuit against the FDA to ban mifepristone. This committee was responsible for recommending to the Texas legislature ways to prevent maternal deaths, ways to save pregnant people's lives. The ACOG strongly condemned Skop's appointment.[35]

After the devastation of *Dobbs*, even more Americans in polls stated that they wanted abortion mostly if not entirely legal nationwide, according to Pew Research Center.[36] An April 2024 NPR/PBS NewsHour/Marist poll found 84 percent of Americans said women who have abortions should not face penalties like fines or jail time; that response included four in five Republicans.[37] And pollster Perry-Undem in June 2024 reported that, when people were asked if abortion should be regulated by the government or a decision between a "doctor and patient," more than 80 percent of Americans said the latter.[38] Except even that question assumed abortions must be between a "doctor and patient," ignoring SMA. To be clear: without pills and creative ways to get people pills, experts believe that even more pregnant people would almost certainly be dying in the US post-*Dobbs*. That was why, in the summer of 2023, Dr. Linda Prine exhaled a brief sigh of relief when some telehealth shield laws went into effect.

By that summer, in an increasingly scrambled post-*Dobbs* era, 17 states and DC had shield laws better protecting people who traveled for abortions there from a ban or severely restricted state. The telehealth-inclusive shield laws Prine advocated for, which would support people under bans who could not or did not want to travel, passed in just six states: Washington, Massachusetts, New York, Vermont, Colorado, and California.[39] Already, those laws sparked disagreements within the reproductive rights and justice movement.

Drexel University law professor David S. Cohen, who helped outline shield law strategies, knew these laws were not perfect. For one, he would have wanted all the telehealth shield laws that passed to recognize the patient's location of care as the same as the provider's location of care in that shield law state, which would have somewhat better protected abortion-seekers in ban states. "That's not what they do," he told me. "What they do is they say we are going to protect providers and helpers and patients while they're in the state of [say] New York in all these different ways: protection from extradition, from civil and criminal witness requirements, licensure, etcetera, etcetera. And we're going to do so regardless of where the patient is located." At the end of the day, a person ordering pills in a ban state from Aid Access through Prine, who was now better protected under New York's telehealth shield law, would still be physically located in that ban state. "There's nothing New York, Vermont, Colorado, Washington, Massachusetts, or California can do about that," Cohen told me in late 2023. "And so, that is a vulnerability."

And while he did not at all wish to minimize pregnancy-criminalization concerns, concerns that he repeatedly stressed when we spoke, he noted the risk of someone being criminalized under a ban after taking pills was nonetheless remarkably low. A 2023 report from If/When/How: Lawyering for Reproductive Justice found that, from 2000 to 2020, at least 61 people in the US had been criminally investigated or arrested for allegedly ending their own pregnancies or helping someone else do so.[40] Cohen estimated that, over those two decades, there were maybe 100 million instances of people in the country being pregnant. These were 61 people among roughly 100 million. "It is much more likely that you are struck by lightning twice than you get investigated for pregnancy-related crimes," he told me. "Compare that super low risk to all the harms that come from people who are not able to get an abortion when they want one in life. . . . It's not my anatomy. It's not my risk. But I would take those odds if I were in that situation."

As of October 2024, nearly two dozen states banned or severely restricted abortion, 13 of those states banning abortion almost entirely.[41] Millions of pregnant-capable people live in these states. At least 66 clinics that once provided abortions closed after *Dobbs*.[42] Many clinicians fled ban states like Alabama given criminalization risks, leaving maternal-care deserts.[43] There will be reams of research for years to come about post-*Dobbs* ramifications. But from what is known in 2024, *Dobbs* has wrought harms deeply unequally. *KFF* found people of color in states with bans or severe restrictions faced disproportionately greater abortion-access challenges due to "longstanding underlying social and economic inequities, which could exacerbate existing disparities in maternal and infant health."[44]

In the first full year telehealth shield laws were in effect, tens of thousands of people in ban or severely restricted states who could not or did not want to travel were receiving pills from telehealth shield law provision. There were only three such services as of October 2024: Aid Access; the Massachusetts Medication Abortion Access Project (the MAP); and Abuzz.[45] This book introduced many of the people behind them: Dr. Linda Prine and Dr. Rebecca Gomperts (Aid Access); Dr. Angel Foster and Susan Yanow (the MAP); and Dr. Suzanne Poppema (formerly Aid Access, then Abuzz).

All three services provided pills for $150, $250, or on a sliding scale based on what a person said they could afford, including if they could not pay anything. Earlier research showed that half of the women seeking abortion care in the US live below 100 percent of the federal poverty level (which, in 2024 for a single person, meant earning $15,060 a year), and three-quarters reported not having enough money to cover housing, transportation, and food.[46] As stated prior, most abortion-seekers in the US already have children.[47] Every single cent that they had counted. Aid Access's US-based providers in early 2024 were sending about 7,000 doses of pills a month, almost 90 percent of them to people in ban or severely restricted states.[48] Thousands of people could not pay full price for these services. That meant telehealth shield law providers were absorbing costs, struggling to stay afloat, while many within their own movement were not financially supporting them.[49]

In the roughly two years post-*Dobbs*, *Rewire News Group* estimated that more than $100 million in donations paid for people's abortion care, including out-of-state travel.[50] Very little of those millions reportedly went to paying for people using telehealth shield law services in ban states. The high volume of people that telehealth shield law providers served and the movement money available to them to subsidize that care dramatically differed from the volume of people clinics served and the movement money spent on bringing people across state lines to in-person care.[51] Some movement actors saw this equation as woefully unsustainable. It was not that in-person care at a clinic should not be an option. To them, it was that the bulk of movement resources were largely ignoring supporting those who could not or did not want to travel for in-clinic care.

Other movement actors argued that paying for telehealth shield law provision may make big institutions already with targets on their backs—like Planned Parenthood—vulnerable to lawsuits that could tank them, and then where would abortion care be? Telehealth shield laws were also untested in court at this time, and though the anti-abortion movement as of October 2024 had not challenged these laws in court yet, that could change if Trump won the presidency in November 2024 (and he did indeed win). Even prior to the election results, there were criminalization worries. Yes, only 61 people over two decades were known to be criminalized in the US for trying to end their pregnancies or helping someone do so. But that If/When/How report stopped after 2020, excluding post-*Dobbs* realities. Besides, isn't one person criminalized too many?

Then there was an unfortunate truth of America's privatized health care system, where providers competed in a market and where telehealth abortion offered cheaper care than clinics. "And the reality is that abortion clinics are businesses," Cohen told me. In 2024, the *San Francisco Chronicle* reported that, in the first months after *Dobbs*, Planned Parenthood staffers privately lobbied politicians in New York, California, and Massachusetts to *not* pass telehealth shield laws, arguing legal risks were too great.[52] This deeply disappointed several reproductive rights and justice activists who believed that Planned Parenthood acted largely out of financial self-interest.[53] (Planned Parenthood did not respond to my interview requests for this book.)

In Aid Access provision research, the top reason people gave for using that service pre-*Dobbs* was that they could not afford in-clinic care.[54] Some also shared that they had a previous negative experience at a clinic or negative perceptions of clinic-based care.[55] Many people who used Aid Access said they felt scared when ordering pills yet were surprised at their positive experiences with the service, finding it to be trusted and compassionate.[56] After *Dobbs*, a more common reason people have given for using Aid Access is that they don't know how else to get an abortion.[57]

To Cohen, as the country moves further into a post-*Dobbs* era, more abortion-seekers in ban and severely restricted states will be unable or not want to travel for their care. Will more movement resources go to telehealth shield law services? Will there be enough legal support for people who use those services and who provide them? Or will much of the movement look the other way, as if to say, "'We're just going to let that happen and pretend it's not happening,'" Cohen told me in late 2023. "Which is kind of where we are now, right? . . . They are providing care for the people who I think the movement says we want to center in this post-*Dobbs* reality. But they are not being centered."

A more nuanced story on abortion pills post-*Dobbs* seemed to exist among independent abortion clinics, which did not include Planned Parenthood. According to a 2023 Abortion Care Network report, independent abortion clinics represented 61 percent of all US clinics providing abortion care to people at and after 16 weeks of pregnancy, a sweeping 86 percent of all US clinics providing care at or after 22 weeks, and 100 percent of all US clinics providing care after 26 weeks of pregnancy.[58] Yet keeping these clinics open to make this care available proved a delicate balance with competition from telehealth abortion services.

In Washington State just before Dr. Deborah Oyer retired from the independent clinic network Cedar River Clinics in late 2022, an

OBGYN in the state called her. This doctor had a pregnant patient with a "16-week fetal demise" who needed a procedure, as Oyer recalled. But this doctor worked at a Catholic-affiliated hospital, so could not "do abortions," as they explained to her, then asked if Oyer could provide an abortion instead. "This is not an abortion," she replied. "You have a dead fetus. You are not ending a pregnancy. There's no reason that can't be done in a Catholic hospital." The doctor persisted, saying the red tape would be too much to try to perform a procedure. Besides, they did not know how to do this procedure. No one had ever trained them. Oyer's clinic took that patient.

About 40 percent of Washington's hospital beds in 2020 were in Catholic-affiliated hospitals with restrictive abortion policies that acted like de facto abortion bans.[59] *KFF Health News* found in early 2024 that, in Washington, half of all babies were born at Catholic-run hospitals, the highest share in the country.[60] If clinics like Cedar River closed as hospitals like these expanded even in a state like Washington with abortion-protective laws, what would happen to the patients left behind? "We second trimester providers can offer something even the most highly trained OBGYNs often cannot offer," Oyer told me. "And we're losing that skill, and we don't want to lose it more." Post-*Dobbs*, 14 percent of US OBGYN residency programs lost in-state abortion training—and, in states with legal abortion, 46 percent of programs lacked even just routine abortion training.[61] As access worsens and delays for in-clinic care lengthen, more people may need this later abortion care, that skills gap becoming more critical.

Cedar River as of 2023, when Oyer and I spoke, remained one of the nation's high-volume, second-trimester abortion clinics. But they could not stay open only on revenue from later abortion care. If everyone with early pregnancies turned to pills without clinics, Oyer worried independent clinics like Cedar River would fold. Any business tension in abortion could be anti-abortion fodder to demonize providers, Oyer was keenly aware. "But first of all, every business wants to stay in business regardless," she told me. "At the same time, I don't want to take away patients' ability to do the abortion the way they want to do it."

If someone wanted to take these pills, which were safer than Tylenol, without a clinic and licensed provider, who was she to stand in their way? Still, when Cedar River launched their own telehealth abortion service in the pandemic, Oyer noticed some patients wanted "the full meal deal," as she phrased it with a gentle smile. Some wanted an ultrasound, to come in person, to have their hand held. "We can make it as medical as you want, or we can make it as non-medical as you want," Oyer told me. "But please do it with someone knowing. And if not with someone knowing, then make sure that you feel comfortable getting help."

That was why she liked the accompaniment model; you were not alone in your abortion process but supported by an acompañante. "They're sort of like an abortion doula, and I don't really think—this is going to sound sacrilegious—but I don't think you need an abortion trained doula," Oyer told me. "I think what you need is someone in your life who's aware that today is the day." American culture turned abortion into a private experience due to stigma, she believed, but abortion did not need to be that way. "And given how many people have abortions, if everyone who had one said, 'I had one,' that would in fact put an end to the stigma. But that's not going to happen in my lifetime, unfortunately."

For people taking pills alone, especially under bans, it can be scary and legally risky to ask for help or find someone to talk to. For free, confidential peer support during an SMA or anything abortion-related, people can call a resource Socorristas and Las Libres inspired: Reprocare Healthline. I spoke in 2024 to co-directors 26-year-old Phoebe Abramowitz and 32-year-old Lupita Sanchez, both in California. Abramowitz co-founded Reprocare as a "digital-first abortion fund" in 2019. When I asked them both why they thought the American reproductive rights movement did not talk publicly about SMA sooner, they looked at each other. "I think now that it's affecting white people in the US, there is more of a reason to talk about it," Sanchez told me. Abramowitz gently added that the movement pre-*Dobbs* emphasized the US Constitution, which based a right to abortion on a right to privacy between a woman and her doctor. Yet people who took abortion pills on their own did not technically need the consent of a doctor or the state. The movement did not seem to know what to do with that.

In early 2024, the American reproductive rights movement still did not seem to know what to do with people taking pills beyond or in between the law as questions grew over whose abortions now counted.

As Dr. Beverly Winikoff told me, no one in truth really knew how many people in the US were having abortions anymore. Nor did anyone know exactly how many people who wanted abortions post-*Dobbs* were not accessing them. And no one will likely ever know how many people would have had abortions with pills if, more than twenty years ago, the medications had lived up to their full promise.

But despite *Dobbs*, the Guttmacher Institute estimated that the number of abortions in the "US formal healthcare system" increased in 2023 to more than one million.[62] Pills made up 63 percent of those abortions, a major jump from 39 percent in 2017, continuing an upward trend since the pandemic.[63] Guttmacher stated, however, that their 2023 estimate was "almost certainly an undercount."[64] Indeed, it did not include people in ban or severely restrictive states who got pills via telehealth shield law providers, which Guttmacher considered outside the "US formal healthcare system." Guttmacher's estimate also did not include people who got pills via community networks or vendors, groups who were admittedly harder to count given the criminalization they and their pill sources risked.

The Society of Family Planning's #WeCount survey published more expansive data on the number of abortions in 2023, data that included people in ban and restricted states who received pills from telehealth shield law providers.[65] #WeCount found that, in the last few months of 2023 after most telehealth shield laws went into effect, nearly one in five abortions in the US, or about 17,000 each month, were with pills via telehealth.[66] The researchers predicted this number would go up. But like Guttmacher, #WeCount did not include people who got pills through networks or vendors without a licensed provider.

Many of Dr. Heather Skanes's patients in Alabama post-*Dobbs* told her confidentially where they were finding pills, so when she read that #WeCount only included abortions from a licensed provider, she told me frankly, "That's not necessarily where everybody's getting their abortion pills from. I would say it's probably a gross underestimate of the number of abortions."

One study came closer to counting the scope of these alternate pill sources. A March 2024 paper co-authored by Dr. Abigail Aiken, Elisa Wells, and Dr. Rebecca Gomperts counted doses of pills sent "outside the US formal health care setting" during the first six months post-*Dobbs*, before telehealth shield laws went into effect.[67] This included pills through community networks, vendors, and Aid Access (at this time, Aid Access sent pills from India to people in ban states). Compared to just before *Dobbs*, the study found an increase of almost 28,000 doses of pills sent in those first six months from these sources.[68] About 32,000 fewer abortions were reported in the US formal health care system in this same time.[69] These paths to pills beyond or in between the law made up some of that loss. "Without these other routes of access, many, many more people would be forced to give birth when they're not wanting to," Wells told me in early 2024. "But even if you've got one person who's forced to give birth against their will, that's too many."

Jenice Fountain, director of Alabama's abortion fund and reproductive justice nonprofit Yellowhammer Fund, felt disillusioned with #WeCount and Guttmacher surveys missing exactly those people. "Because when I keep seeing those stats, I'm just like, 'Well, who are y'all talking to?'" she told me in May 2024. "Were y'all sure to get folks that weren't already online, super engaged, know where to look? Because y'all are gonna fully forget about Black folks."

Two years after *Dobbs*, abortions in the US did become simpler and cheaper to access than ever before for many people thanks to telehealth abortion. But for other people, namely low-income and rural communities under bans, access became much harder and, given travel costs if seeking in-clinic care, more expensive. Telehealth abortion emerged in the US in the pandemic on top of structural inequities.[70] For years, global feminist SMA movement activists have been asking similar questions as Fountain has: What about the people without internet access? Or who don't know where to look?

When Fountain and I spoke in May 2024, she believed the reproductive rights and justice movement was bracing for a Trump

White House and national abortion ban. Fountain thought if Trump came to power and a national ban happened, Alabama's organizing under a ban for two years may become a blueprint for states that were once safe havens. As a Black birthing person in Alabama, she was terrified by the "really deadly" path that her state hurtled down. "It feels like something that's only going to be survivable if you have the means to survive it," Fountain told me. "And the way the abortion movement has gone so far, looking at the numbers that are reported or the celebrations of the lack of decline in abortion access, it just tells me that people are only paying attention to certain groups of people."

To her, the reproductive rights movement's siloing of abortion as a single issue was "our biggest downfall," a warning harkening back to 1990s reproductive justice actors. "Because what red states or Republican people do well is get on the same page to fuck us over," Fountain told me. "If it's going to take five years of policy change, how do we keep people alive during those five years so they can see the win, too?"

In late March 2024, a Supreme Court mired in ethical scandals heard arguments in that AHM case on mifepristone.[71] Even the most conservative justices expressed a scolding skepticism of the plaintiffs' standing to sue. They poked holes in their argument that the FDA, in approving mifepristone, somehow directly caused anti-abortion doctors current or future harm by somehow forcing these doctors to perform abortions against their conscience.

But then conservative Justice Clarence Thomas asked Danco's lawyer, Jessica Ellsworth, if the company, in distributing mifepristone, had violated the Comstock Act.[72] Ellsworth firmly explained that the FDA's decisions granted Danco the legal authority to distribute mifepristone for medication abortions, adding that the court "should think hard about the mischief it would invite" if it ruled the FDA now responsible for enforcing a statute dormant for nearly a century.[73]

As discussed prior in this book, an anti-abortion White House could very well use the Comstock Act to nationally ban mailing abortion pills and any "instrument" used in an abortion procedure, vague wording that could dangerously extend to obstetrics and gynecological care generally.[74] Project 2025, the roughly 920-page playbook for a second Trump term written by the far-right think tank the Heritage Foundation, proposed wielding the Comstock Act "against providers and distributers of abortion pills that use the mail," stating "abortion pills pose the single greatest threat to unborn children in a post-*Roe* world."[75] If this ban became real, more pregnant people across the country would indeed die, and more people would be forced to give birth.

Whether these justices thought hard about "the mischief it would invite" or, given the approaching November 2024 election, the court's Trump appointees laid low to lull American voters into believing Trump was not responsible for harming and killing women, the court in June 2024 unanimously dismissed this AHM case.[76] Mifepristone and telehealth abortion were safe, temporarily.

Yet the court did not toss out this case on its merits, only its standing. Trump appointee Justice Brett Kavanaugh in his majority opinion left unresolved if the FDA's decisions on mifepristone were legal, his opinion suggesting other ways the plaintiffs could try to ban mifepristone: "The plaintiffs may present their concerns and objections to the President and FDA in the regulatory process, or to Congress and the President in the legislative process. And they may also express their views about abortion and mifepristone to fellow citizens, including in the political and electoral processes."[77] He did not mention the Comstock Act.

In April 2024, the court heard another joined abortion case, *Idaho v. United States* and *Moyle v. United States*, on the Emergency Medical Treatment and Labor Act (EMTALA).[78] Alliance Defending Freedom (ADF) lawyers argued in this case too. EMTALA, a federal law, required hospitals receiving federal funding to provide all patients, including pregnant people, stabilizing, lifesaving treatment in emergencies.[79] The federal government argued Idaho's near-total abortion ban perilously conflicted with EMTALA, forcing providers to delay or deny pregnant people urgent care in the state. While their organs failed, sick pregnant people were reportedly being airlifted from Idaho hospitals for care in another state where no ban existed.[80] The court in June 2024 dismissed that case, too, in an unsigned, one-sentence statement merely punting the case to a lower court decision, without clarifying that EMTALA took precedence over Idaho's ban, that pregnant people's lives did matter.[81] Justice Ketanji Brown Jackson wrote in dissent, "The Court had a chance to bring clarity and certainty to this tragic situation, and we have squandered it."[82]

The court's shrugging of responsibility for the tragedies it wrought with *Dobbs* came four days after *Dobbs*'s two-year mark and the day of the first presidential debate in the 2024 race. The debate was such a disaster for then President Biden that he dropped out of the race soon after.[83] Vice President Kamala Harris suddenly became the Democratic candidate, the first Black and South Asian woman ever to be on the ticket.[84]

But the EMTALA and AHM decisions continued to appear to be part of a Republican strategy to seem moderate on abortion to bring swing voters to Trump—despite national outrage at *Dobbs*.[85] The court in that same term, as if preparing for a Trump White House, eviscerated the authority of federal regulatory agencies (like the FDA) and granted Trump as well as any sitting or former president broad immunity from prosecution.[86] These moves gave the executive branch unprecedented power. The White House could now get away with murder. Of course, it already had.

CHAPTER 17

KNOW THE RIGHT PEOPLE

From her Washington home, Elisa Wells at Plan C in early 2024 continued to be flooded with messages from prescription-less vendors of abortion pills asking to be listed on the Plan C website. "There's nothing really they can do about that," she told me of anti-abortion attempts to stop all supplies of pills. "So, they just create confusion and fear and criminalization and all these other strategies to prevent people from doing it. They're smart. They're doing what they think they need to do. And we're smart, too. We're doing the opposite."

According to Plan C's early 2024 data, the top four states that people searched for in their guide to pills by mail were Texas, Florida, Louisiana, and California. Wells expected that more people would search Plan C for options in Florida since, at the time we spoke, the state had just passed an abortion ban in pregnancies later than six weeks.[1] Louisiana, though not a big state, had a big need under a near-total ban, Wells explained to me. California was a huge state without a ban and with comparatively good access. But people there still wanted to know how to get pills by mail. A *KFF* survey published in August 2024 also found that, while two-thirds of women of reproductive age (18–49) in the US had heard of abortion pills (when just one-third reported knowing about these medications before the pandemic struck), still only 19 percent of women two years after *Dobbs* knew that they could order pills online.[2]

Wells in early 2024 routinely updated Plan C's site with language on legal risks people faced per state when ordering and using pills under bans or severe restrictions. To her, there was a fine line between sharing this information directly and not creating a chilling effect in which people may become too scared to seek help. Wells used with me a 1980s AIDS activist slogan: Silence = Death. To her, this meant quality information saved lives.

She often spoke to If/When/How: Lawyering for Reproductive Justice about how those few people who have been known to be criminalized for ending their pregnancies got in trouble, If/When/ How helping Plan C translate this information clearly to site visitors. Core to those criminalization cases was usually a betrayal: you told someone you trusted, such as a friend or provider, that you took pills, and that person reported you or told someone who reported you. Another risk, according to If/When/How's findings, was if you took pills further along in your pregnancy, then needed to dispose of fetal tissue, which could be difficult to do discreetly to keep yourself safe. How do you lower such risks? "First, you have to know about them," Wells told me in early 2024. "You have to know that people are getting criminalized. Not a lot of people. But now that there's a higher volume and more people are using mailed pills, there are more cases."

According to a 2023 If/When/How report on such cases from 2000 to 2020, people who have been criminalized tended to be among the most surveilled groups: disproportionately people of color and immigrants, almost universally low-income, and, in the moment that led to their criminalization, disproportionately survivors of intimate partner violence.[3] While that report stopped at 2020, If/When/How's chief legal and policy director Sara Ainsworth told me in May 2024 that their organization's post-*Dobbs* clients have predominantly been intimate-partner-violence survivors. And on the If/When/How's Repro Legal Helpline, "very significant numbers of people indicate to us that they are experiencing abuse," Ainsworth told me. "And that they don't want their abuser to know that they need an abortion."

If callers lived in a ban state, they often told the helpline they wanted to order pills online because they did not know how to hide their abortion from their abuser if they traveled for care, then they anxiously asked the hotline if ordering pills was legal.[4] "What that indicates to us is that states stopping access to pills is going to hurt survivors," Ainsworth told me. "States punishing people for obtaining pills hurts survivors of intimate partner violence. And abusers know this. And therefore are really emboldened by state abortion bans to engage in what we call reproductive coercion."

That coercion may mean forcing someone to maintain a pregnancy or forcing a termination, such as by beating a pregnant person to cause a miscarriage.[5] Dr. Diana Greene Foster's *The Turnaway Study* found that if people were in a violent relationship when trying to get an abortion but did not access one, they were more likely than those who did access an abortion to still be in contact with a violent partner two years later—and to be raising a child on their own while experiencing abuse, with that violent partner not helping to raise the child.[6] Research on Aid Access found one reason people often gave for ordering pills was to hide their abortion from their abuser.[7]

Ainsworth told me SMA can be a way for survivors, particularly those in states under bans and unable to travel, to have a discrete abortion if they can get mifepristone and misoprostol or misoprostol alone soon enough in pregnancy. But according to Ainsworth, when survivors have been criminalized, the abuser has known about their abortion and often has used that against them, even calling the police on them.[8] If survivors in a ban state could not safely travel to an abortion-protective state without their abuser knowing, and if the survivor wanted to order pills, Ainsworth advised they first call the Repro Legal Helpline to understand their legal risks and resources. "I think that when we center survivors of intimate partner violence, we understand that only they know when they can get safely out of the relationship," she told me. "And they know that."

Given the expansive and punitive US criminal justice system, community networks in this country appear to have been embedding more legal support than similar models did in countries like Argentina (Socorristas) and Mexico (Las Libres). Since *Dobbs*, some states like Washington have updated their laws to better protect from prosecution community-based providers within such states helping someone access abortions.[9] These may not be licensed or regulated providers, more like acompañantes. Yet those protections did not exist for helpers living in ban states that target providers and, as in Texas, so-called aiders and abettors. Prosecutions of helpers acting in states under bans had not yet happened as of May 2024 when Ainsworth and I spoke, only threats of such prosecutions. If the worst did happen, however, and police were called on a helper or abortion-seeker under a ban, Ainsworth was clear: "There is legal defense for every person in this scenario that is free." This was largely thanks to the Abortion Defense Network of allied nonprofits, private law firms, and government officials.[10]

In early 2023, I spoke to one activist involved in community networks who could not be named for security. It was frustratingly clear to them that mainstream reproductive rights organizations after *Dobbs* would not do the high-risk work of pill distribution to those people with nowhere else to go. Some big groups were even too scared to talk publicly about SMA. The activists willing to take on those risks were deciding if they were safer leaving pill distribution to those in the movement or branching out for help in allied movements. This initially prompted tense debates around risk and trust. But a year later, that changed.

Because by the time I spoke to that activist again in mid-2024, more states had banned abortion, more people needed help, more clinics were backed up, more orders for pills were coming to telehealth shield law providers, and abortion funds, nearly half of which remained all-volunteer operations, were running out of money.[11] The daily grind of people trying to access abortions seemed to be in the headlines less, as if normalized, while Trump's presidential campaign projected confidence and anti-abortion Senator J. D. Vance of Ohio, who supported a national abortion ban, became Trump's running mate.[12] So, when I asked that same activist about earlier tensions among networks a year ago, questions about whether to expand or stay small, they told me, "I think people kind of have less time for that shit right now, you know?" SMA had become a pillar of abortion care, with community networks as one source of pills and support that needed all the help they could get.

There is admitted murkiness when I write about these networks because of what I cannot share and do not know. One activist told me that, if cops showed up at their door for giving free pills to people in a ban state, they would know our interview had tipped them off since they had told hardly anyone else. This was why community networks were and are secretive. Despite such grim risks, networks appeared to run astonishingly safely, Socorristas-like shields up around the abortion-seeker. As I write in early November 2024 with a second Trump term looming, there have been no public reports of people criminalized after receiving pills through community networks, not to my knowledge or according to my sources in these networks. What activists I spoke to worried about acutely were those who did not take pills at all but who miscarried in an abortion-hostile state, then sought medical care only to be criminalized by those who were suspicious they took pills. These scenarios would be like what happened to Brittany Watts in Ohio in 2023 and to several women in Guanajuato, Mexico, late in the first decade of the 2000s. "I think we are entering a new age of criminalization," activist Nancy Cárdenas Peña, director of Abortion on Our Own Terms, told me in March 2024.

Fundamentalist Christian extremists who called themselves "abortion abolitionists" were demanding that women who have abortions should be put in prison for murder.[13] Those voices, predominantly white men fashioning themselves as Operation Rescue's next generation, seemed to be growing louder in an anti-abortion movement furious at a failure to stop all abortions. Yet to be paralyzed with fear was not the answer to Cárdenas Peña. She has found inspiration from SMA activists in Mexico and globally who have been here before, who teach her providers can be anyone. They can be community members. They can be abortion-seekers. They can be you. She saw a "blank canvas" for what future access could look like, allied with other movements. The American reproductive rights, health, and justice movement did play defense on criminalization in this new era, she told me. But it was time to play offense too.

Susan Yanow thought there was at least one thing anyone playing offense could do. Talk about abortion. Talk about pills. In 2023, a reporter asked Yanow if she worried that the federal government would stop all pills flowing into the country. She replied, "Like they stopped fentanyl?" Kinga Jelinska at Women Help Women (WHW) thought the next decade would see SMA activists make their own misoprostol and mifepristone.

As I write in late 2024, these are also just the two abortion pills the world knows right now. A former FDA official told me that American pharmaceutical companies were notorious for having libraries of rejected compounds that, for one reason or another, never went through an FDA approval process.[14] "And so many of these drugs failed early trials because they were accidental abortifacients," they told me. They recalled consulting for one such company after their time at the FDA and being tasked with seeing if any of those rejected drugs could be salvaged. "And I said at one point, 'Well, how about thinking about marketing abortifacients?' It didn't go over well. . . . But an effect of a drug as being an abortifacient is not unusual. And if we, as a society, looked more mindfully for such things, my guess is we could find them."

As I finished this book, Trump won the White House, again. I cannot predict what will happen, but I know it will be devastating. There are nonetheless strategies to try to keep each other safe. In Green Wave countries like Argentina, accompaniment activists understood pills were a tool under bans not just for abortions but also to help bring people's abortion experiences out of isolation and to honor all feelings. They did this—and still do—with hope that love will win. This is not to romanticize networks. The specter of criminalization alone can hurt people. And strategies molded around one context will never take the same shape in another. With a caveat that I will miss nuances, I end this book by introducing voices in three places—Mexico, Brazil, and Texas—who share how they navigated their own or others' abortions with pills under bans. Some can use their real names; others cannot. All do as Yanow encouraged: talk.

We first visit Hidalgo, Mexico, around 2016, when 24-year-old Daniela (Dani) Tellez and two friends had an idea: create a three-person volunteer collective about sexual and reproductive health. They called their collective Di Ramona.

Tellez that same year went to an abortion-access training in Mexico City. At the time, Mexico City had an abortion ban on pregnancies later than 12 weeks, which was the most protective abortion law in

Mexico then. Hidalgo and almost every other state in the country had a near-total abortion ban.[15] At this training, Tellez learned all about abortion pills and stigma. She shared everything she learned there with her friends at Di Ramona, including fellow 24-year-old Mirelle (Miri) Rosales, who had never heard of pills until then. "Wow, is this possible? You don't even have to go to the hospital," Rosales told me in 2023 through an interpreter. "It's not the way it's portrayed in Mexican education, right? Abortion as something extremely horrible and all that. It's something that you can actually do at home. Wow, I do remember that feeling of, maybe, powerful. I don't know if that's the right word, but [powerful] to say: 'I have the information, and I can share it with many more women.'"

In Hidalgo, Di Ramona began accompanying people through their abortions with misoprostol or misoprostol and mifepristone (if they could find mifepristone). The friends kept their accompaniment a secret known through word of mouth. While it was not illegal in Hidalgo in 2016 to accompany someone having an abortion, it was almost entirely illegal for the person they accompanied to have an abortion. Months after Rosales heard about pills, she discovered she was pregnant and turned to Tellez for help. She wanted an abortion but was scared. "My friend, you have the information," Tellez assured her. "You know how to do it, but I am here for you." Tellez stayed on the phone with Rosales as she took pills, gently saying, "If it hurts, rest a little bit. Just take a nap. Have a cup of tea. Anything else, let me know." Rosales shared with Tellez whenever she cramped, threw up, everything. "Instead of making me feel bad, she just received the information and gave me words of support: 'We know that this is normal, but it's going to happen,'" Rosales told me. After Rosales's abortion, she accompanied more and more people.

Accompaniment was not either of their jobs at the time. Rosales worked as a psychologist, and Tellez, who realized how much abortion access meant to her, worked for a Global North–based NGO sending mifepristone and misoprostol to people in countries banning abortion. There were only a few ban countries this NGO did not touch, Brazil among them. Tellez sat on the NGO's help desk, responding to people's emailed questions that did not need a doctor, as Kinga

Jelinska and many others had done. But Tellez quickly realized her prior Mexico City training left some people out.

She had been told at that training that people needed an ultrasound before taking pills, for example. But for people in difficult circumstances, whether living in remote areas or experiencing intimate partner violence, those rules were too impractical and, as Tellez read more medication abortion research, not always necessary. At this NGO, she emailed abortion-seekers in a "very intimate way," careful of the person's possible stigmas. Many confided to her that their partner did not support them. Tellez shared strategies to make their abortion less visible, assuring them an abortion with pills looked like a miscarriage, and that miscarriages were common.[16] That they would be okay.

Tellez supported around 50 people a day at that NGO, much more than the three or five people a day that Di Ramona as a collective accompanied. Tellez began to build at Di Ramona "the best of both worlds" between accompaniment and this NGO's model. When that NGO closed its unit in Mexico, Tellez worked on Aid Access's help desk as it launched, where she provided the same kind of support to people living in the US. She left Aid Access in 2019 to dedicate herself to Di Ramona as the Green Wave surged. Di Ramona went public that year about their accompaniment. "That was our strategy: instead of going more clandestine and secretive, we decided to go all out," Tellez told me. "And also, it was because we were very naive."

Di Ramona was convinced Hidalgo would decriminalize abortion in 2019, so the collective loudly called for abortion to be legal throughout pregnancy as well as for access for nonbinary and trans people. While some activists told people to go to Mexico City for legal care, Tellez publicly challenged that: "Yes, you can go to Mexico City if you want, but a lot of people are having their abortions here in Hidalgo." The state, however, did not decriminalize abortion that year. But when the pandemic struck, Di Ramona's openness meant that people who needed help more easily found them. Tellez noticed that more people later in pregnancies were now seeking abortions, some having wanted their pregnancies until they lost their jobs in the pandemic and could no longer afford a child. Di Ramona drew on regional SMA networks' knowledge of later abortion care with pills to support people. They also needed more help themselves.

The pandemic saw a stream of young people in Hidalgo asking Di Ramona how to be acompañantes. Tellez ran virtual trainings on accompaniment basics until she realized that attendees assumed all they needed to know was how abortion pills worked. She believed their enthusiasm for accompaniment was not enough. "Because you're not knowing the legal context," she told me. "You're not knowing what the medication is doing to your body. You're not knowing how to support alarm signs. You're not knowing what to do if someone in crisis comes to you, and they are very nervous, very anxious, or very depressed. How are you able to contain them in these kinds of situations?"

Di Ramona started what the collective called Escuelita with 12 training sessions over 12 weeks detailing accompaniment. The first session unpacked abortion stigma. The second session was on pills, answering questions Tellez whipped through with me: "What is misoprostol? What does it cause to your body? Why are we using this medication? What's the history of this? Where does it come from? Who decided that abortion can be done with misoprostol and mifepristone?"

They even ran simulations. What to do if a person needed hospital care. How to connect to an allied doctor. Escuelita had a session on the law as well. "Right now, here in 2023, nobody in Mexico can go to jail for having an abortion," Tellez told me. "That's a change that happened in 2021, but it was not happening in 2020 when Escuelita started." When Hidalgo in 2021 did decriminalize abortion, the state put in place a 12-week ban with exceptions for later care.[17] Di Ramona still wanted total legalization of abortion and partnered with Hidalgo's Ministry of Health to improve the quality of legal abortion care. People as of 2023 could call Di Ramona to learn how to access legal abortion, like what abortion funds in the US have done for decades, only legal abortion in Mexico was (and is) free. And someone in Mexico could still often find misoprostol over the counter while mifepristone required a prescription.[18]

When Tellez and I spoke in 2023, an allied provider was prescribing and sending Di Ramona combi-packs costing about $45, and Di

Ramona kept a stock of pills, especially misoprostol. If pills neared their expiration date, then Di Ramona donated those unused pills to other collectives. Di Ramona was continuing to accompany people through their later abortions with pills, if that was what the person said they needed and wanted. Weeks before we spoke, Tellez and another acompañante safely supported a person around 32 weeks pregnant through their abortion with pills over several days, with an allied doctor on call. "If you come to Di Ramona, and you decide to have an abortion, you are going to have an abortion," Tellez told me. "We are going to find a way."

Tellez believed accompaniment should come from the "willingness to do something different for people who are having an abortion," she told me, continuing:

> If I am seeing or feeling that my accompaniment comes from sacrifice, from pain, from heroism, then you are not doing good work because you are putting yourself at the center because "I'm so heroic doing all of this." No, the person who is having the abortion is the person that should be at the center of all this situation. . . . You are not like someone graceful that doesn't make mistakes and is completely perfect because we are doing activism. No, we are people who are doing this because it needs to be done. Because it's important. Because I needed it one time or maybe I will need it someday. Or someone that I love is needing it or will need it. We are all the same.

She believed accompaniment models in Latin America were "radically different" from telehealth-abortion models like Aid Access. Some people may want the latter model, others not. "In these Latin American models, what I have seen is that we are so close to people," Tellez told me. "Not only so you know how to have an abortion and you have access to medication. That's the most superficial part of the accompaniment. We go deep."

Yet to Rosales, being an acompañante was not for everyone. "You can have all the desire to accompany, but you may lack that something to not get caught up in the cases," she told me. "That something that allows you to accompany with love." Rosales referred as well to ancestral knowledge about abortion from Mexican parteras, or midwives. Recall that scientists in the 1960s extracted prostaglandins from corals found in the Gulf of Mexico before misoprostol, a prostaglandin in pill-form, existed. Some seaweeds in the Gulf also contained prostaglandins, with a few parteras rumored to have given seaweeds to women to try to bring back their periods (though it remains unknown just how successful that was). So, when I asked Rosales what she thought about *Dobbs*, she simply said, "Women don't need permission to have abortions."

If an accompaniment network in Mexico had a medical question, one trusted contact was Dr. Suzanne Veldhuis, an abortion provider in the Mexican state of Chiapas. Acompañantes shook up almost everything she thought she knew about abortion. Her medical training taught her that patients needed ultrasounds and blood tests before taking abortion pills, for instance. But once she listened to acompañantes, she realized how much more they understood about supporting people using abortion pills. "They're doing a much better job at this than we are," she told me, referring to doctors. "Especially in this context, where the stigmatization is horrible and people are afraid."

Veldhuis believed even empathetic doctors could fall into a power dynamic that acompañantes, who saw themselves as peers, resisted. But the American anti-abortion movement post-*Dobbs* seemed to Veldhuis in 2023 to grasp the mechanics of accompaniment models better than the American reproductive rights and justice movement did, which worried her. Bans in states like Texas specifically targeted those who helped with another person's abortion; such bans did not exist in Mexico even when abortion was almost entirely illegal there. "I think that is really scary," she told me. "In Mexico, yes, there are people who have been in jail for abortions. But there are accompaniment groups that have been doing this openly for over 20 years and never faced any legal issues. Because the state doesn't have the interest [or] the possibility to really prosecute people for this."

A context closer to ban states in a post-*Dobbs* US may be Brazil, which is one of the most dangerous countries for people to access or spread misoprostol beyond the law. Activists there still have been finding a way. As mentioned in an earlier chapter, Brazil's FDA equivalent, the National Health Surveillance Agency (ANVISA), classified misoprostol as a controlled substance in the 1990s, then, early in the first decade of the 2000s, restricted simply sharing information about misoprostol online or on social media.[19] A person could be imprisoned for breaking through that censorship. When American reproductive justice activist Renee Bracey Sherman testified to Congress in July 2022 and shared SMA protocols, she warned in her testimony that some US states were already trying to make it illegal for people to spread information about abortion pills. This was the reality in Brazil.

Even WOW did not mail pills into Brazil because it was too dangerous; state surveillance there had grown too sophisticated.[20] There were nonetheless two main ways people in Brazil could get misoprostol and, if lucky, mifepristone beyond the law: from street vendors who sold prescription-less pills or from feminist networks giving pills for free and providing accompaniment. Those feminist networks operated within Brazil and would almost certainly be imprisoned if caught, like the community networks carefully operating in ban states in the US. I spoke to several of these feminist activists in Brazil, one of whom was Mana, a pseudonym she picked.

Mana, who was around my age, had not had an abortion yet, but many in her collective had and then became activists. She noticed that sometimes vendors claiming to sell misoprostol did not give women enough pills or shared the wrong instructions. *Swallow all pills, lie on your back, lift your legs up.* "Stupid things," Mana told me. She began accompanying people and moving pills around very slowly when her friend got pregnant in 2016 and needed an abortion. That friend knew well-connected feminists, who found her misoprostol pills. Yet this friend never used those pills because, before she could, she miscarried. "Lucky her," Mana told me sarcastically. Her friend held onto those pills and gave them to another friend in need. When a different friend of Mana's sought pills for an abortion, Mana asked that first friend for help. A tiny network formed. They had no social media presence and saw themselves as a collective only in recent years with the Green Wave. Mana has since been surprised to meet more collectives in Brazil: "We have been finding one another, other groups, other collectives that are doing the same."

When Mana's collective began, a Global North–based NGO in the global feminist SMA movement supplied them pills. Their collective later spread out their pill sources across Latin America, which felt "more equal" to Mana because of shared, on-the-ground risks. The most dangerous part of Mana's activism has been the pill distribution and transportation, not when pills were with the abortion-seeker and Mana accompanied them. Brazil, like the US, is massive. To move pills discreetly was complex and extremely tense. Mana hated that stress. Sometimes the collective only had misoprostol pills since that medication was more accessible in the region. No one in her collective, including Mana, knew everything about how pills traveled. The less a person knew, the less likely information leaked that may harm someone—all for pills safer than Tylenol.

Mana checked her phone often as we spoke, just as Socorrista Lucía Baez in Argentina did. She, too, accompanied someone over text while we talked. Many people Mana accompanied grappled with guilt or guilt about *not* feeling guilt. Mana sensed people wanted her to validate them, but she never asked why a person wanted an abortion. Often the only people in that person's life who knew about their abortion were Mana and one of that person's friends. "They are the ones who are always doing this work of supporting women," she told me of friends. "Always, always, always." Accompanying teens and preteens have been "the most delicate cases" for Mana. These young people were usually too scared to tell their parents. Sometimes Mana would be on the phone with a girl as young as twelve having her abortion at home with her unaware parents in the next room.

Abortion-seekers found Mana through word of mouth. Whenever someone asked for help, activists could rarely be completely certain the person was not the police or an extremist trying to entrap them. They had strategies to try to vet the person and developed collective-wide security protocols (which they voted on). These included the use of pseudonyms, encrypted messaging apps, and virtual private networks to hide locations. Most members were volunteers, but this meant their collective tended to be middle-class and white, people who could afford to do time-intensive, high-risk activism for free. While some activists believed it was politically important that their accompaniment not be a paid job, others disagreed. There were also ongoing debates about how public their collective should be.

Mana's collective entered more dangerous waters in 2019 after Brazil elected president the far-right, anti-abortion politician Jair Bolsonaro, a Trump ally.[21] Bolsonaro acted like the dictators of South America's recent past, even describing Brazil's military dictatorship from 1964 to 1985 as a "very good" period.[22] Attacks on democracy and abortion under Bolsonaro in Brazil and Trump in the US soon mimicked each other. Months after *Dobbs* and three years after the January 6th riots of Trump extremists in DC, Bolsonaro extremists mobbed federal buildings in Brazil's capital to overthrow the newly elected president, Luis Inácio Lula da Silva (known as Lula).[23] Bolsonaro lied that he, not Lula, won the election, as Trump lied that he, not Biden, won the 2020 election. Mana and I spoke around when a Brazilian court banned Bolsonaro from running for president until 2030.[24] No US court successfully banned Trump from running as the 2024 Republican presidential candidate. Mana worried what the rising far-right in the US meant for Brazil and abortion-seekers. She hoped Bolsonaro's successor, Lula, would be different.

Except in early 2024, a year after Mana and I spoke, Dr. Carmen Barroso, longtime Brazilian activist for global reproductive and sexual rights, told me that Lula had been a "grave disappointment" on abortion. Barroso now lived in Oregon and believed anti-abortion tactics were spreading between the US and Brazil.[25] About to turn 80 when we spoke, she remembered RU-486 and misoprostol surfacing in Brazil three decades ago. When I asked her why an anti-rights campaign, with abortion as one target, was gaining ground in Brazil and the US, she sighed: "The easiest answer is that this world is very unequal and becoming more and more unequal."

Wealth and income inequality have worsened in many countries over the past four decades.[26] Women have experienced that inequality acutely. According to the United Nations, of the less than two-thirds of women in the paid labor force worldwide, more than half work in the "informal economy," earning low wages without a social safety net.[27] This figure did not include unpaid labor like parenting and domestic work, which women around the world continue to disproportionately do, largely invisibly and woefully unsupported.[28]

The millions globally who do not benefit from these stark inequalities, "the underdogs," Barroso told me, become "prey of demagogues, who can manipulate what is most precious to individuals: their bodies, their families, their relationships." What better way to manipulate that which is most precious than to ban abortion? Barroso warned me it was not hard for demagogues to win elections, having witnessed it happen in Brazil before, only the tools of these demagogues have changed. "In my youth, we were fighting the military because they were the ones taking power with weapons, destroying democracy with weapons," she told me. "Now, the weapon is in the minds of people, who are so fragilized, not fragile. There's an educational system that hides the capacity to think. And there is this religious fanaticism that is easy to manipulate. We are in a very dangerous situation."

I end this book back in the US, where this country is indeed in a very dangerous situation. And where an abortion-seeker I spoke to wanted you to hear her story.

Alauni, who lived in Texas when we spoke in 2023, was a 24-year-old Black single parent and intimate-partner-violence survivor. She chose her pseudonym. Alauni has had two abortions with pills: one at a New Mexico clinic pre-*Dobbs*, one at her Texas home under a ban post-*Dobbs*. She has three daughters, aged six, four, and two, and worked gig jobs that paid barely above the minimum wage and did not offer benefits. When Alauni needed an abortion in January 2023 with Texas's abortion funds still closed, she was around six weeks pregnant. "I guess you have to go underground to find the pills," she told me. "Or just know people. Know the *right* people." She took a chance and asked a trusted person for help. That person luckily was tied to a community network.

When Alauni got mifepristone and misoprostol, she knew how to take them because of her prior medication abortion. She told me that her SMA felt no different physically from her earlier abortion at a clinic, only she could now better plan when to take the pills at home, with her three kids around her and with her abuser no longer in her life. "And it was just on my time." One of her daughters, her four-year-old, had disabilities and needed much of Alauni's attention. Alauni learned sign language for her daughter (she was nonverbal). "People always ask me, 'How do you do it?'" she told me. "And I'm just like, 'I'm her mom.'"

Alauni did not know what their lives would have looked like if she did not find pills, if she would have been forced to give birth to a fourth child, knowing she "could not care for them like they should be cared for." For a while, Alauni thought that if she had another daughter, she would name her Alauni. But when she realized she no longer wanted another child, at least not now, she turned "Alauni" into her pseudonym to safely share her post-*Dobbs* story with you.

This book began with voices of abortion-seekers like Alauni unnamed in research papers. It ends with her, still unnamed, yet talking when others cannot or do not want to, knowing that preciousness of her body, her family, and her relationships of which Barroso spoke. But a decades-long, transnational movement to control these pills as a way to control the people who need them reveals the threatening power in women, pregnant people, and allies who continue to help each other, not necessarily the power in these pills alone. Some post-*Dobbs* stories hailed these pills as "saving" abortion in the US, echoing a 1990s fantasy of pills ending America's "abortion wars." What that misses is people: We cannot make sense of where we have been and where we go without Alauni and Barroso on one side of a border, Tellez and Mana on another.

Trump in 2024 beat for the second time a woman running for president, for the first time a Black and South Asian woman running for president. His appointees dominated the Supreme Court and, in 2024, gave the presidency unprecedented power. Not only that but Trump entered the White House with a Republican-controlled Congress filled with more Trump loyalists than when he first came to office in 2016.[29] That trifecta stood prepared to aggressively pursue a far-right agenda, including sweeping conservative appointments to the federal judiciary and a merciless gutting of federal regulatory authority.[30] Project 2025 made explicit that abortion pills and those who provide them will be one of this agenda's biggest targets.

I wish I could write that Trump's reelection shocked me. It did not. This book felt to me for a while like we were hurtling toward a country that would not believe, understand, or care that Trump, if elected president again, could ban abortion. According to *CNN* exit polling in November 2024, nearly half of voters who said that abortion should be legal in most cases also supported Trump.[31]

But the many voices in this book, including Alauni's, also hurtled me personally toward hope in some people, more than I may realize, who resist how they can, no matter how small, and who will not stop.

Pills are not enough. They never will be. Pills do not expand Medicaid. Do not subsidize childcare. Do not close the gender pay gap. Not everyone who needs an abortion will want to or can use pills, nor should they have to, if all were equal. And abortion access under Trump will very likely become more unequal.[32] But as Dr. Beverly Winikoff told me, pills have a habit of finding their way to people, if not nearly enough. Knowledge of and access to pills have been rising in the US. We would almost certainly be in a worse maternal mortality crisis if these medications never existed and if the many people in this history gave up on these pills when they had ample opportunity to. This may offer little comfort in these dangerous times. Yet I, for one, will take it.

The lives of these pills and the support networks around them seem to be only just beginning, particularly in this country. It took five decades to demolish *Roe*, which was flawed from its start. It may take another five decades to enshrine expansive abortion protections, to make mifepristone and misoprostol available over the counter and affordable (even free), to reach broad reproductive justice goals beyond abortion. That may not happen in my lifetime. But I will hold onto what Socorristas, currently in a far-right backlash of their own, have taught me: do not underestimate love, and do not forget each other. We are all we have.

EPILOGUE

When I was twelve, my Catholic school required I volunteer at a charity each week. I was not thrilled. A neighbor asked me for help at her small nonprofit for "new moms and babies," as she told me. I begrudgingly volunteered to stick stamps on envelopes at their office space after school. One day, a young woman with a baby on her hip came into their office and hurriedly asked me for free diapers. Her eyes did not meet mine. My neighbor stepped in and addressed the woman with a saccharine voice I had not heard from her before, handing a few diapers over while trying to convince this woman to stay. The woman grabbed the diapers and vanished. She looked scared. Something felt wrong.

When she left, I took out a letter in one of those envelopes that I had been stamping. I read it closely for the first time. I saw "life" and "babies" written over and over, the pregnant person mentioned nowhere, and I realized what had been staring at me that whole time but that I could not or did not want to see before. I was inside of an anti-abortion crisis pregnancy center that, in tacit exchange for providing low-income parents a measly couple of free diapers, shamed or scared women into giving birth rather than listening to what may have been really going on in each of their lives. I stopped volunteering there. I avoided that neighbor. I tried not to think about that place. But I believe what frightened my younger self most in that moment was imagining what might have happened to me had I never paid attention, never left. Would I have become that neighbor?

I have not had an abortion but may one day. All of us, including me, know and deeply love someone in our lives who has had an abortion, even if that person never told you. Women of my generation and younger in the US today now have fewer rights than those of my mother's generation, with a gender pay gap that has barely moved in two decades.[1] When I started this book, abortion in the US was legal, if marginally and highly unequally. When I finished this book, abortion was (and is) illegal in about half the country—and, in my last days of writing, a known racist, misogynist responsible for the US Supreme Court ushering in state abortion bans was elected president by this nation for the second time.

But this book is about slivers of hope even amid crushing despair. These tiny abortion pills terrified the American far-right enough that a federal judge briefly, nationally banned mifepristone, that case winding its way through courts as I interviewed those who first studied the medication and, today in their nineties, wanted their memories recorded to fight back with the truth. It was too late to stop all abortion pills everywhere, they argued to me. It was not too late to help one another under what, as I write, look like very bleak years ahead. The parallel history in this book of vibrant activism under abortion bans across mainly Latin America, maneuvering around that other abortion pill, misoprostol, has been even more integral to our knowledge of both medications, our reimagining and revolutionizing of abortion care, and our rebuilding of communities that, despite the odds, protect and empower each other. And their next chapters, now in this country, are just beginning.

ACKNOWLEDGMENTS

This book would never have existed without the nearly 200 people who generously spoke with me for my reporting and research. Each person's perspective made this project all the richer. You squeezed in interviews between a fervent commitment to help abortion-seekers, patients, and each other. I am in awe. Those whom I do not name know who you are: thank you. I especially must thank Dr. Beverly Winikoff, Kinga Jelinska, Dr. Carole Joffe, Dr. Caitlin Gerdts, Dr. Tracy Weitz, Dr. Rebecca Gomperts, Francine Coeytaux, Dr. Paul Blumenthal, Dr. Sara Larrea, Renee Bracey Sherman, Lucía Baez, Amelia Bonow, and Ruth Zurbriggen.

This book would also never have existed without Samuel Freedman, my Columbia Journalism School professor, who took a chance on me and this project based on an email that I wrote to him in pandemic-era lockdowns. My Columbia classmates—particularly Josie Cox, Julia Love, and the late Blake Schmidt—were nothing but encouraging as I workshopped very early versions of this book before any of us knew what would unfold in the US. You took my words seriously. Thank you to Jessica Papin, my supremely poised and sharp agent. Thank you to my thoughtful and, above all, kind editor Haley Lynch and to all the dedicated, patient folks at Beacon Press. It would have been much harder for me to write this emotionally (and physically) exhausting book if I did not trust these words and stories would be safe in your hands.

Thank you to my gracious interpreter Adrián Espinoza Staines, whose warmth and sincerity immediately put interviewees at ease. We were a team. Thank you to the librarians at Harvard University's Schlesinger Library, Columbia University's Rare Book & Manuscript

Library, Barnard College, and Smith College's Sophia Smith Collection of Women's History. Thank you to the Pulitzer Center on Crisis Reporting as well as to my Columbia Journalism School professors, who taught me more about grit and rigor than they may realize: Joanne Faryon, Christopher Weaver, Daniel Alarcón, and Heba Elorbany. And to Jamal Watson, officially my first editor and one of my biggest, early champions.

There are too many people to name and dearly thank who listened to me talk about this book for four years—or, before a book existed, helped me own and trust my words. Here are a few. To my wonderfully talented teachers Karen Randall, Theresa Padden, Sunnie Evers, Pam Cobrin, Wendy Schor-Haim, Margaret Vandenburg, Cecelia Brun Lie-Spahn, Mary Gordon, Peter Platt, Abigail Lewis, and many others. How grateful I am to you. To my writing group colleagues Jean Lee, Cleo Levin, Anna Jordan, and Shira Schindel. To my beloved friends Eleonora, Masha, Ankhi, Briar, Callie, Rosie, Amanda, Elisa, Elizabeth, Megan, Nora, Elissa, and Aliza. Our talks buoyed and grounded me all at once. To my parents, Madeleine and Jack, and my brother, Gerry, and my little sister, Hannah (you are stronger than you know), thank you for supporting me and my grand dreams in your own ways. To my late aunt Marian, who gave me history books when I was a child, knowing I would one day write one.

To the person who read every sentence before anyone else did, who listened to me talk about this book idea on a long walk in the pandemic while you were dazed from starting rounds of chemotherapy, with strands of your hair falling out, strands you tried to hide under your hat so as not to worry me. You did not want to talk about cancer. You wanted to talk about this book. I questioned aloud to you if I could or even should write such a wildly ambitious book, if this might all be a mistake. You then gently held my hand and told me life is precious, so why not try? Thank you, Carter, my partner in life and love.

And to Maureen, my aunt who cannot speak but has much to say, always. This book is dedicated to you.

NOTES

CHAPTER 1: THE PILL THAT MAKES YOUR PERIOD COME BACK

1. Regina Maria Barbosa and Margareth Arilha, "The Brazilian Experience with Cytotec," *Studies in Family Planning* 24, no. 4 (1993): 236–40, https://doi.org/10.2307/2939191.
2. Aníbal Faúndes et al., "Post-Abortion Complications After Interruption of Pregnancy With Misoprostol," *Advances in Contraception: The Official Journal of the Society for the Advancement of Contraception* 12, no. 1 (1996): 1–9, doi:10.1007/BF01849540, https://pubmed.ncbi.nlm.nih.gov/8739511/.
3. Barbosa and Arilha, "The Brazilian Experience with Cytotec."
4. S. H. Costa and M. P. Vessey, "Misoprostol and Illegal Abortion in Rio de Janeiro, Brazil," *The Lancet* 341, no. 8855 (May 1993): 1258–61, https://doi.org/10.1016/0140-6736(93)91156-g.
5. Costa and Vessey, "Misoprostol and Illegal Abortion in Rio de Janeiro, Brazil."
6. Marion Lipschutz and Rosa Rosenblatt, *The Abortion Pill*, First Run/Icarus Films, 1997, 56 min.
7. Paul W. Collins, "Misoprostol: Discovery, Development, and Clinical Applications," *Medicinal Research Reviews* 10, no. 2 (Apr. 1990): 149–72, https://doi.org/10.1002/med.2610100202.
8. Cleveland Clinic, "Prostaglandins," Nov. 4, 2022, https://my.clevelandclinic.org/health/articles/24411-prostaglandins.
9. Lawarence Galton, "The New Mystery—Maybe," *New York Times*, Dec. 5, 1971, https://www.nytimes.com/1971/12/05/archives/the-new-mystery-maybe-miracle-drug-the-new-mystery-maybe-miracle.html.
10. Gina Kolata, "US May Allow Anti-Ulcer Drug Tied to Abortion," *New York Times*, Oct. 29, 1988, https://www.nytimes.com/1988/10/29/world/us-may-allow-anti-ulcer-drug-tied-to-abortion.html.
11. Barbosa and Arilha, "The Brazilian Experience with Cytotec."
12. Citeline, Pink Sheet: "Searle Cytotec Concomitant. . . . ," *Citeline*, https://insights.citeline.com/PS010737/SEARLE-CYTOTEC-CONCOMITANT-USE-WITH-ASPIRIN-STUDIES/. Also see Mariana Prandini Assis, 2023 interview with author.
13. Citeline, Pink Sheet: "Searle Cytotec Concomitant. . . . ," *Citeline*, https://insights.citeline.com/PS010737/SEARLE-CYTOTEC-CONCOMITANT-USE-WITH-ASPIRIN-STUDIES/. Also see Mariana Prandini Assis, 2023 interview with author.
14. Human Rights Watch, "History of Brazil's Law on Abortion," *Human Rights Watch*, https://www.hrw.org/legacy/women/abortion/brazil.html#:~:text=History%20of%20Brazil's%20Law%20on,woman's%20life%20is%20in%20danger.
15. Jan E. Dickinson, "Confusion, Inequity and Inconsistency: Abortion in Australia," *Australian and New Zealand Journal of Obstetrics and Gynaecology* 55, no. 2 (Apr. 2015): 103–4, https://doi.org/10.1111/ajo.12332.

16. Marge Berer, "Abortion Law and Policy Around the World: In Search of Decriminalization," *Health and Human Rights* 19, no. 1 (2017): 13–27, https://pmc.ncbi.nlm.nih.gov/articles/PMC5473035/pdf/hhr-19-013.pdf.

17. Human Rights Watch, "History of Brazil's Law on Abortion."

18. Human Rights Watch, "History of Brazil's Law on Abortion."

19. James Brooke, "Ulcer Drug Tied to Numerous Abortions in Brazil," *New York Times*, May 19, 1993, https://www.nytimes.com/1993/05/19/health/ulcer-drug-tied-to-numerous-abortions-in-brazil.html.

20. For a glossary of abortion terms, see World Health Organization, Abortion Care Guidelines, 2022, https://srhr.org/abortioncare/key-terms/glossary/. For a dilation and curettage definition, see Mayo Clinic, "Dilation and Curettage (D&C)," https://www.mayoclinic.org/tests-procedures/dilation-and-curettage/about/pac-20384910.

21. Barbosa and Arilha, "The Brazilian Experience with Cytotec."

22. Barbosa and Arilha, "The Brazilian Experience with Cytotec."

23. H. L. L. Coêlho et al., "Misoprostol and Illegal Abortion in Fortaleza, Brazil." *The Lancet* 341, no. 8855 (May 1993): 1261–63, https://doi.org/10.1016/0140-6736(93)91157-h. https://www.contraceptionjournal.org/article/0010-7824(94)90084-1/abstract.

24. Costa and Vessey, "Misoprostol and Illegal Abortion in Rio de Janeiro, Brazil."

25. Cristiane da Silva Cabral et al., "Direito Ao Aborto: Caminhos Traçados No Brasil—Entrevista Com Margareth Arilha," *Cadernos de Saúde Pública* 36, no. suppl. 1 (2020), https://doi.org/10.1590/0102-311x00118319.

26. da Silva Cabral et al., "Direito Ao Aborto: Caminhos Traçados No Brasil—Entrevista Com Margareth Arilha."

27. da Silva Cabral et al., "Direito Ao Aborto: Caminhos Traçados No Brasil—Entrevista Com Margareth Arilha."

28. da Silva Cabral et al., "Direito Ao Aborto: Caminhos Traçados No Brasil—Entrevista Com Margareth Arilha."

29. da Silva Cabral et al., "Direito Ao Aborto: Caminhos Traçados No Brasil—Entrevista Com Margareth Arilha."

30. Lipschutz and Rosenblatt, *The Abortion Pill.*

31. Kolata, "US May Allow Anti-Ulcer Drug Tied to Abortion."

32. Kolata, "US May Allow Anti-Ulcer Drug Tied to Abortion." Also see Assis, 2023 interview with author.

33. Kolata, "US May Allow Anti-Ulcer Drug Tied to Abortion."

34. Kolata, "US May Allow Anti-Ulcer Drug Tied to Abortion."

35. Kolata, "US May Allow Anti-Ulcer Drug Tied to Abortion."

36. Kolata, "US May Allow Anti-Ulcer Drug Tied to Abortion."

37. CNN, "The Catholic Church Once Allowed for Abortions. Everything Changed in 1873," CNN, July 3, 2022, https://www.cnn.com/videos/politics/2022/07/03/abortion-law-roe-v-wade-history-orig-dp-kj.cnn.

38. Barbosa and Arilha, "The Brazilian Experience with Cytotec."

39. Helena Lutéscia Coêlho et al., "Misoprostol: The Experience of Women in Fortaleza, Brazil," *Contraception* 49, no. 2 (Feb. 1994): 101–10, https://doi.org/10.1016/0010-7824(94)90084-1.

40. Coêlho et al., "Misoprostol: The Experience of Women in Fortaleza, Brazil."

41. Helena L. L. Coêlho et al., "Selling Abortifacients over the Counter in Pharmacies in Fortaleza, Brazil," *The Lancet* 338, no. 8761 (1991): 247, ISSN 0140–6736, https://doi.org/10.1016/0140-6736(91)90379-4, https://www.sciencedirect.com/science/article/pii/0140673691903794.

42. W. Wilson Downie, "Misuse of Misoprostol," *The Lancet* 338, no. 8761 (July 1991): 247, https://doi.org/10.1016/0140-6736(91)90378-3.

43. Walter Fonseca et al., "Misoprostol and Congenital Malformations," *The Lancet* 338, no. 8758 (July 1991): 56, https://doi.org/10.1016/0140-6736(91)90046-r.

44. Fonseca et al., "Misoprostol and Congenital Malformations."
45. Downie, "Misuse of Misoprostol."
46. Barbosa and Arilha, "The Brazilian Experience with Cytotec."
47. Ana Cristina de Lima Pimentel et al., "A Breve Vida Do Norplant® No Brasil: Controvérsias E Reagregações Entre Ciência, Sociedade e Estado," *Ciência & Saúde Coletiva* 22, no. 1 (Jan. 2017): 43–52, https://doi.org/10.1590/1413-81232017221.05932016.
48. Pimentel et al., "A Breve Vida Do Norplant® No Brasil: Controvérsias E Reagregações Entre Ciência, Sociedade e Estado."
49. Dorothy E. Roberts, "From Norplant to the Contraceptive Vaccine: The New Frontier of Population Control," *Killing the Black Body: Race, Reproduction, and the Meaning of Liberty* (New York, NY: Vintage, 1999), 104–49.
50. For a detailed history of the population-control movement, see Matthew James Connelly, *Fatal Misconception: The Struggle to Control World Population* (Cambridge, MA: Belknap Press of Harvard University, 2008).
51. Connelly, *Fatal Misconception.*
52. Connelly, *Fatal Misconception.*
53. Loretta J. Ross and Rickie Solinger, "A Reproductive Justice History," in *Reproductive Justice: An Introduction* (Oakland: University of California Press, 2017), 9–57.
54. Pimentel et al., "A Breve Vida Do Norplant® No Brasil: Controvérsias E Reagregações Entre Ciência, Sociedade e Estado."
55. Morgani Guzzo, "Brasil: As Regras Que Puseram o Misoprostol 'Na Cadeia,'" *Portal Catarinas*, Sept. 15, 2021, https://catarinas.info/as-regras-que-puseram-o-misoprostol-na-cadeia/.
56. Barbosa and Arilha, "The Brazilian Experience with Cytotec."
57. Barbosa and Arilha, "The Brazilian Experience with Cytotec."
58. Barbosa and Arilha, "The Brazilian Experience with Cytotec."
59. Barbosa and Arilha, "The Brazilian Experience with Cytotec."
60. Barbosa and Arilha, "The Brazilian Experience with Cytotec."
61. Barbosa and Arilha, "The Brazilian Experience with Cytotec."
62. Barbosa and Arilha, "The Brazilian Experience with Cytotec."
63. Barbosa and Arilha, "The Brazilian Experience with Cytotec."
64. Barbosa and Arilha, "The Brazilian Experience with Cytotec."
65. Barbosa and Arilha, "The Brazilian Experience with Cytotec."
66. Barbosa and Arilha, "The Brazilian Experience with Cytotec."
67. Barbosa and Arilha, "The Brazilian Experience with Cytotec."
68. Barbosa and Arilha, "The Brazilian Experience with Cytotec."
69. Barbosa and Arilha, "The Brazilian Experience with Cytotec."
70. Barbosa and Arilha, "The Brazilian Experience with Cytotec."
71. Barbosa and Arilha, "The Brazilian Experience with Cytotec."
72. Barbosa and Arilha, "The Brazilian Experience with Cytotec."
73. Barbosa and Arilha, "The Brazilian Experience with Cytotec."
74. Barbosa and Arilha, "The Brazilian Experience with Cytotec."
75. Barbosa and Arilha, "The Brazilian Experience with Cytotec."
76. Barbosa and Arilha, "The Brazilian Experience with Cytotec."
77. Barbosa and Arilha, "The Brazilian Experience with Cytotec."
78. Barbosa and Arilha, "The Brazilian Experience with Cytotec."
79. Barbosa and Arilha, "The Brazilian Experience with Cytotec."
80. Barbosa and Arilha, "The Brazilian Experience with Cytotec."
81. Barbosa and Arilha, "The Brazilian Experience with Cytotec."
82. Barbosa and Arilha, "The Brazilian Experience with Cytotec."
83. Barbosa and Arilha, "The Brazilian Experience with Cytotec."
84. Barbosa and Arilha, "The Brazilian Experience with Cytotec."

85. World Health Organization Human Reproduction Programme, *Abortion Care Guideline* (Geneva, Switzerland: World Health Organization, 2022), 68–72, https://www.who.int/publications/i/item/9789240039483.

86. World Health Organization Human Reproduction Programme, *Abortion Care Guideline*.

87. World Health Organization Human Reproduction Programme, *Abortion Care Guideline*.

88. World Health Organization Human Reproduction Programme, *Abortion Care Guideline*.

89. World Health Organization Human Reproduction Programme, *Abortion Care Guideline*.

90. Mariana Prandini Assis and Joanna N. Erdman, "In the Name of Public Health: Misoprostol and the New Criminalization of Abortion in Brazil," *Journal of Law and the Biosciences* 8, no. 1 (Jan. 2021), https://doi.org/10.1093/jlb/lsab009.

91. Assis and Erdman, "In the Name of Public Health: Misoprostol and the New Criminalization of Abortion in Brazil."

92. Guzzo, "Brasil: As Regras Que Puseram o Misoprostol 'Na Cadeia.'"

93. Mariana Prandini Assis, "Liberating Abortion Pills in Legally Restricted Settings: Activism as Public Criminology," in *The Routledge International Handbook of Public Criminologies*, ed. Kathryn E. Henne and Rita Shah (New York: Routledge, Taylor & Francis Group, 2020), 120–30; Assis, 2023 interview with the author.

94. da Silva Cabral et al., "Direito Ao Aborto: Caminhos Traçados No Brasil—Entrevista Com Margareth Arilha."

CHAPTER 2: A PARENTHETICAL

1. Ronald Bentley, *Biographical Memoirs: Volume 82* (Washington, DC: National Academies Press, 2003), 221–41, https://doi.org/10.17226/10683.

2. National Human Genome Research Institute, "Eugenics: Its Origin and Development (1883–Present)," National Institutes of Health, updated Nov. 30, 2021, https://www.genome.gov/about-genomics/educational-resources/timelines/eugenics.

3. *Buck v. Bell*, 274 U.S. 200 (1927).

4. R. Kurzrok and C. C. Lieb, "Biochemical Studies of Human Semen. II. The Action of Semen on the Human Uterus," *Experimental Biology and Medicine* 28, no. 3 (Dec. 1, 1930): 268–72, https://doi.org/10.3181/00379727-28-5265.

5. Bentley, *Biographical Memoirs: Volume 80*, 221–41.

6. Bentley, *Biographical Memoirs: Volume 80*.

7. U. S. von Euler, "On the Specific Vaso-dilating and Plain Muscle Stimulating Substances from Accessory Genital Glands in Man and Certain Animals (Prostaglandin and Vesiglandin)," *Journal of Physiology* 88, no. 2 (Nov. 6, 1936): 213–34, https://doi.org/10.1113/jphysiol.1936.sp003433.

8. Audre Lorde, "The Master's Tools Will Never Dismantle the Master's House," in *Sister Outsider: Essays and Speeches* (Berkeley, CA: Crossing Press, 2007), 110–14.

9. Sune Bergström, "The Prostaglandins: From the Laboratory to the Clinic (Nobel Lecture)," *Angewandte Chemie International Edition in English* 22, no. 11 (Nov. 1983): 858–66, https://doi.org/10.1002/anie.198308581.

10. Bergström, "The Prostaglandins: From the Laboratory to the Clinic (Nobel Lecture)."

11. Sarah McCammon, "How the Approval of the Birth Control Pill 60 Years Ago Helped Change Lives," NPR, May 9, 2020, https://www.npr.org/2020/05/09/852807455/how-the-approval-of-the-birth-control-pill-60-years-ago-helped-change-lives#:~:text=How%20The%20Approval%20Of%20The,Ago%20Helped%20Change%20Lives%20:%20%20NPR&text=Weekend%20Edition%20Saturday-,How%20The%20Approval%20Of%20The%20Birth%20Control%20Pill%2060%20Years,lives%20of%20millions%20of%20Americans.

12. Marc Bygdeman, 2023 interview with the author; Kristina Gemzell Danielsson, 2023 interview with the author.

13. Per Gunnar Cassel, "Induced Legal Abortion in Sweden During 1939–1974: Change in Practice and Legal Reform," Stockholm University Demography Unit, 2009, https://www.su.se/polopoly_fs/1.18721.1320939636!/WP_2009_1.pdf.

14. Cassel, "Induced Legal Abortion in Sweden During 1939–1974."

15. Dan Balz, "Sweden Sterilized Thousands of 'Useless' Citizens for Decades," *Washington Post*, Aug. 29, 1997, https://www.washingtonpost.com/archive/politics/1997/08/29/sweden-sterilized-thousands-of-useless-citizens-for-decades/3b9abaac-c2a6-4be9-9b77-a147f5dc841b/.

16. U. Roth-Brandel et al., "Prostaglandins for Induction of Therapeutic Abortion," *The Lancet* 295, no. 7639 (Jan. 1970): 190–91, https://doi.org/10.1016/s0140-6736(70)90427-7.

17. Roth-Brandel et al., "Prostaglandins for Induction of Therapeutic Abortion."

18. S. M. M. Karim and G. M. Filshie, "Therapeutic Abortion Using Prostaglandin F2A," *The Lancet* 295, no. 7639 (Jan. 1970): 157–59, https://doi.org/10.1016/S0140-6736(70)90402-2; S. M. M. Karim et al., "Induction of Labour with Prostaglandin F2A," *BJOG: An International Journal of Obstetrics & Gynaecology* 76, no. 9 (Sept. 1969): 769–82, https://doi.org/10.1111/j.1471-0528.1969.tb06177.x.

19. Lawarence Galton, "The New Mystery—Maybe," *New York Times*, Dec. 5, 1971, https://www.nytimes.com/1971/12/05/archives/the-new-mystery-maybe-miracle-drug-the-new-mystery-maybe-miracle.html.

20. Paul F. Van Look and Jane Cottingham, "The World Health Organization's Safe Abortion Guidance Document," *American Journal of Public Health* 103, no. 4 (Apr. 2013): 593–96, https://doi.org/10.2105/ajph.2012.301204.

21. Van Look and Cottingham, "The World Health Organization's Safe Abortion Guidance Document."

22. World Health Organization and Halfdan Mahler, *The Work of WHO, 1976–1977: Biennial Report of the Director-General to the World Health Assembly and to the United Nations*, 1978, https://iris.who.int/handle/10665/86039.

23. World Health Organization and Mahler, *The Work of WHO, 1976–1977.*

24. World Health Organization, *Proposed Regular Programme and Budget Estimates for the Financial Year 1 January—31 December 1972. . . .* , Dec. 1970, https://iris.who.int/handle/10665/85827.

25. Étienne-Émile Baulieu and Mort Rosenblum, *The "Abortion Pill": RU-486, A Woman's Choice* (New York, NY: Simon & Schuster, 1991), 29.

26. Paul F. A. Van Look, formerly of the WHO, 2023 interview with the author; United States, Department of Treasury, Internal Revenue Service, Return of Organization Exempt from Income Tax (Form 990): The Susan Thompson Buffett Foundation.

27. Bergström, "The Prostaglandins: From the Laboratory to the Clinic (Nobel Lecture)."

28. M. Bygdeman et al., "Self-Administration of Prostaglandin for Termination of Early Pregnancy," *Contraception* 24, no. 1 (July 1981): 45–52, https://doi.org/10.1016/0010-7824(81)90067-6.

29. Bygdeman et al., "Self-Administration of Prostaglandin for Termination of Early Pregnancy."

30. Bygdeman et al., "Self-Administration of Prostaglandin for Termination of Early Pregnancy."

31. Bygdeman et al., "Self-Administration of Prostaglandin for Termination of Early Pregnancy."

CHAPTER 3: THE DAWN OF RU-486

1. Jeremy Cherfas, "Dispute Surfaces over Paternity of RU 486," *Science* 246, no. 4933 (Nov. 24, 1989): 994, https://doi.org/10.1126/science.2587988; and Steven

Greenhouse, "A New Pill, a Fierce Battle," *New York Times Magazine*, Feb. 12, 1989, https://www.nytimes.com/1989/02/12/magazine/a-new-pill-a-fierce-battle.html.

2. Cherfas, "Dispute Surfaces over Paternity of RU 486," 994.

3. Mayo Clinic, "Cushing Syndrome," June 7, 2023, accessed Nov. 11, 2024, https://www.mayoclinic.org/diseases-conditions/cushing-syndrome/symptoms-causes/syc-20351310.

4. Cherfas, "Dispute Surfaces over Paternity of RU 486," 994.

5. Cherfas, "Dispute Surfaces over Paternity of RU 486."

6. Étienne-Émile Baulieu and Mort Rosenblum, *The "Abortion Pill": RU-486, A Woman's Choice* (New York: Simon & Schuster, 1991), 55.

7. Baulieu and Rosenblum, *The "Abortion Pill,"* 56.

8. Baulieu and Rosenblum, *The "Abortion Pill,"* 57–62.

9. Suzanne White Junod, "FDA's Approval of the First Oral Contraceptive, Enovid," *Update*, July–Aug. 1998, https://www.fda.gov/media/110456/download.

10. Audiey Kao, "History of Oral Contraception," *Virtual Mentor* 2, no. 6 (2000): 55–56, doi: 10.1001/virtualmentor.2000.2.6.dykn1–0006, https://journalofethics.ama-assn.org/article/history-oral-contraception/2000-06.

11. PBS *American Experience*, "A Timeline of Contraception," https://www.pbs.org/wgbh/americanexperience/features/pill-timeline/.

12. Martha J. Bailey, "More Power to the Pill: The Impact of Contraceptive Freedom on Women's Life Cycle Labor Supply," *Quarterly Journal of Economics* 121, no. 1 (Feb. 1, 2006): 289–320, https://doi.org/10.1162/003355306776083491.

13. PBS *American Experience*, "A Timeline of Contraception."

14. Baulieu and Rosenblum, *The "Abortion Pill,"* 57.

15. Erin Blakemore, "The First Birth Control Pill Used Puerto Rican Women as Guinea Pigs," *History.com*, Aug. 24, 2023, https://www.history.com/news/birth-control-pill-history-puerto-rico-enovid.

16. Blakemore, "The First Birth Control Pill Used Puerto Rican Women as Guinea Pigs."

17. Blakemore, "The First Birth Control Pill Used Puerto Rican Women as Guinea Pigs."

18. Blakemore, "The First Birth Control Pill Used Puerto Rican Women as Guinea Pigs."

19. Blakemore, "The First Birth Control Pill Used Puerto Rican Women as Guinea Pigs."

20. PBS *American Experience*, "A Timeline of Contraception."

21. Jamie Ducharme, "Hormonal Birth Control Doesn't Deserve Its Bad Reputation," *TIME*, Apr. 3, 2024, https://time.com/6962771/is-hormonal-birth-control-safe-health-risks/.

22. Baulieu and Rosenblum, *The "Abortion Pill,"* 72–75.

23. Baulieu and Rosenblum, *The "Abortion Pill,"* 13.

24. Baulieu and Rosenblum, *The "Abortion Pill,"* 83–85.

25. Baulieu and Rosenblum, *The "Abortion Pill,"* 83–85.

26. Cherfas, "Dispute Surfaces over Paternity of RU 486," 994.

27. Baulieu and Rosenblum, *The "Abortion Pill,"* 18, 26–29.

28. Baulieu and Rosenblum, *The "Abortion Pill,"* 85–86.

29. Baulieu and Rosenblum, *The "Abortion Pill,"* 87.

30. Baulieu and Rosenblum, *The "Abortion Pill,"* 16.

31. United Press International, "Legal-Abortion Bill Advances in France After Heated Debate," *New York Times*, Nov. 29, 1974, https://www.nytimes.com/1974/11/29/archives/legalabortion-bill-advances-in-france-after-heater-debate.html?timespast Highlight=Simone,Veil,and,abortion.

32. Jess McHugh, "How 343 Women Made French History by Talking About Their Abortions," *TIME*, Nov. 26, 2018, https://time.com/5459995/manifesto-343-abortion-france/.

33. McHugh, "How 343 Women Made French History by Talking About Their Abortions."

34. Baulieu and Rosenblum, *The "Abortion Pill,"* 36.

35. Solène Cordier, "Access to Abortion in France Remains Fraught with Obstacles," *Le Monde*, Mar. 19, 2024, https://www.lemonde.fr/en/opinion/article/2024/03/19/access-to-abortion-in-france-remains-fraught-with-obstacles_6635616_23.html.
36. Elisabeth Aubény, 2023 interview with author.
37. Aubény, 2023 interview with author.
38. Greenhouse, "A New Pill, a Fierce Battle."
39. Baulieu and Rosenblum, *The "Abortion Pill,"* 84–85.
40. Baulieu and Rosenblum, *The "Abortion Pill,"* 85–86.
41. W. Herrmann et al., "Effet d'un stéroide anti-progestérone chez la femme: Interruption du cycle menstruel et de la grossesse au début," *Comptes rendus de l'Académie des Sciences III* (1982): 933–38.
42. Paul F. A. Van Look, 2023 interview with the author; Marc Bygdeman, 2023 interview with the author.
43. Baulieu and Rosenblum, *The "Abortion Pill,"* 22.
44. Académie des Sciences Institut de France, "History of the French Académie des sciences," 2016, https://www.academie-sciences.fr/en/Histoire-de-l-Academie-des-sciences/history-of-the-french-academie-des-sciences.html.
45. Howard Markel, "The Day Marie Curie Got Snubbed by the French Science World," PBS, Jan. 23, 2021, https://www.pbs.org/newshour/science/the-day-marie-curie-got-snubbed-by-the-french-science-world.
46. Ioana Fechete, "Accomplishments of Yvonne Choquet-Bruhat: The First Woman Member of the French Academy of Sciences," *Comptes Rendus. Chimie* 19, no. 11–12 (Oct. 13, 2016): 1382–87, https://doi.org/10.1016/j.crci.2016.09.005.
47. Baulieu and Rosenblum, *The "Abortion Pill,"* 22.
48. Baulieu and Rosenblum, *The "Abortion Pill."*
49. Baulieu and Rosenblum, *The "Abortion Pill."*
50. Richard Eder, "Birth Control: 4-Day Pill Is Promising in Early Test," *New York Times*, Apr. 20, 1982, https://www.nytimes.com/1982/04/20/science/birth-control-4-day-pill-is-promising-in-early-test.html.
51. Baulieu and Rosenblum, *The "Abortion Pill,"* 27.
52. Pam Belluck, "The Father of the Abortion Pill," *New York Times*, Jan. 17, 2023, https://www.nytimes.com/2023/01/17/health/abortion-pill-inventor.html.
53. World Health Organization, Prevention of Maternal Mortality: Report of a WHO Interregional Meeting (Geneva, Switzerland, 1985), 11–15.
54. Baulieu and Rosenblum, *The "Abortion Pill,"* 81.
55. Baulieu and Rosenblum, *The "Abortion Pill."*
56. Baulieu and Rosenblum, *The "Abortion Pill."*
57. Baulieu and Rosenblum, *The "Abortion Pill,"* 30.
58. Bygdeman, 2023 interview with the author. Also see Christian Fiala and Kristina Gemzell-Danielsson, "Review of Medical Abortion Using Mifepristone in Combination with a Prostaglandin Analogue," *Contraception* 74, no. 1 (July 2006): 66–86, https://doi.org/10.1016/j.contraception.2006.03.018.
59. L. Kovacs et al., "Termination of Very Early Pregnancy by RU 486—an Antiprogestational Compound," *Contraception* 29, no. 5 (May 1984): 399–410, https://doi.org/10.1016/0010-7824(84)90014-3.
60. Bygdeman, 2023 interview with the author.
61. Baulieu and Rosenblum, *The "Abortion Pill,"* 35.
62. M. Bygdeman and P. F. A. Van Look, "7 Anti-Progesterones for the Interruption of Pregnancy," *Baillière's Clinical Obstetrics and Gynaecology* 2, no. 3 (Sept. 1988): 617–29, https://doi.org/10.1016/s0950-3552(88)80048-8.

CHAPTER 4: THE MORAL PROPERTY OF WOMEN

1. The Rockefeller Foundation, https://www.rockefellerfoundation.org/report/bellagio-center-villa-serbelloni-a-brief-history/.

2. Étienne-Émile Baulieu and Mort Rosenblum. *The "Abortion Pill": RU-486, A Woman's Choice* (New York: Simon & Schuster, 1991), 35.

3. B. Couzinet et al., "Termination of Early Pregnancy by the Progesterone Antagonist RU 486 (Mifepristone)," *New England Journal of Medicine* 315, no. 25 (1986): 1565–70, doi:10.1056/NEJM198612183152501.

4. Mary W. Rodger and David T. Baird, "Induction of Therapeutic Abortion in Early Pregnancy with Mifepristone in Combination with Prostaglandin Pessary," *The Lancet* 330, no. 8573 (Dec. 1987): 1415–18, https://doi.org/10.1016/s0140-6736(87)91126-3.

5. Christian Fiala and Kristina Gemzell-Danielsson, "Review of Medical Abortion Using Mifepristone in Combination with a Prostaglandin Analogue," *Contraception* 74, no. 1 (July 2006): 66–86, https://doi.org/10.1016/j.contraception.2006.03.018.

6. A. Ulmann, "The Development of Mifepristone: A Pharmaceutical Drama in Three Acts," *Journal of the American Medical Women's Association* 55 (1972), no. 3, suppl. (2000): 117–20, https://pubmed.ncbi.nlm.nih.gov/10846319/.

7. E. Aubény et al., "Etude clinique de 353 cas d'IVG de moins de 49 jours d'amenorrhee realisee par. . . ." [Clinical trial of pregnancy terminations in 353 patients where amenorrhea was present for less than 49 days. . . .], *Fertilité, Contraception, Sexualité* 17, no. 4 (1989): 307–14, https://pubmed.ncbi.nlm.nih.gov/12282175/.

8. Baulieu and Rosenblum, *The "Abortion Pill,"* 91.

9. Oceane Duboust and Natalie Huet, "France Fears Abortion Pill Shortage as US States Stockpile Misoprostol amid Supreme Court Battle," *Euro News*, Apr. 20, 2023, https://www.euronews.com/health/2023/04/20/france-fears-abortion-pill-shortage-as-us-states-stockpile-misoprostol-amid-supreme-court-.

10. Aria Bendix, "What the Supreme Court's Decision in the Legal Fight over Abortion Pills Means for Access to Mifepristone," NBC News, Apr. 12, 2023, https://www.nbcnews.com/health/womens-health/abortion-pill-lawsuit-mifepristone-questions-future-access-rcna79455.

11. Randall Balmer, "The Real Origins of the Religious Right," *Politico Magazine*, May 27, 2014, https://www.politico.com/magazine/story/2014/05/religious-right-real-origins-107133/.

12. Kristen Hwang, "How California Created the Nation's Easiest Abortion Access—and Then Went Further," *CalMatters*, Apr. 21, 2022, updated Mar. 26, 2024, https://calmatters.org/explainers/abortion-in-california-laws/.

13. For a rigorous legal history of abortion in the US after *Roe*, see Mary Ziegler, *Abortion and the Law in America: Roe v. Wade to the Present* (Cambridge, UK: Cambridge University Press, 2020), 73–87.

14. R. Alta Charo, "A Political History of RU-486," in *Biomedical Politics*, ed. Kathi E. Hanna (Washington, DC: National Academies Press, 1991), https://www.ncbi.nlm.nih.gov/books/NBK234199/.

15. Emma Wallenbrok, "Inside the *Handbook on Abortion*," *Slate*, June 8, 2022, https://slate.com/news-and-politics/2022/06/fetal-photos-jack-barbara-willke-handbook-on-abortion.html.

16. Wallenbrok, "Inside the *Handbook on Abortion*."

17. Charo, "A Political History of RU-486."

18. Baulieu and Rosenblum, *The "Abortion Pill,"* 37.

19. Baulieu and Rosenblum, *The "Abortion Pill,"* 36.

20. Gina Kolata, "Boycott Threat Blocking Sale of Abortion-Inducing Drug," *New York Times*, Feb. 22, 1988, https://www.nytimes.com/1988/02/22/us/boycott-threat-blocking-sale-of-abortion-inducing-drug.html.

21. Steven Greenhouse, "A New Pill, a Fierce Battle," *New York Times Magazine*, Feb. 12, 1989, https://www.nytimes.com/1989/02/12/magazine/a-new-pill-a-fierce-battle.html.

22. Baulieu and Rosenblum, *The "Abortion Pill,"* 38–39; United States Holocaust Memorial Museum, "At the Killing Centers," Holocaust Encyclopedia, Mar. 3, 2023, https://encyclopedia.ushmm.org/content/en/article/at-the-killing-centers.

23. Baulieu and Rosenblum, The "Abortion Pill," 48.
24. Gina Kolata, "France and China Allow Sale of a Drug for Early Abortion," New York Times, Sept. 24, 1988, https://www.nytimes.com/1988/09/24/us/france-and-china-allow-sale-of-a-drug-for-early-abortion.html.
25. Baulieu and Rosenblum, The "Abortion Pill," 104–7.
26. Tessa Berenson Rogers, "Here's How China's One-Child Policy Started in the First Place," TIME, Oct. 29, 2015, https://time.com/4092689/china-one-child-policy-history/.
27. Baulieu and Rosenblum, The "Abortion Pill," 104–7.
28. Baulieu and Rosenblum, The "Abortion Pill," 43–44.
29. Greenhouse, "A New Pill, a Fierce Battle."
30. Baulieu and Rosenblum, The "Abortion Pill," 43–44.
31. Ulmann, "The Development of Mifepristone," 117–20.
32. Carol Pogash, "Does the Abortion Pill Have a Future in America?" San Francisco Examiner, Apr. 14, 1991, https://sfexaminer.newspapers.com/image/462261395.
33. Baulieu and Rosenblum, The "Abortion Pill," 43–46.
34. Brian Knowlton, "Facing US Boycott, Drugmaker Returns Pill Rights to Creator: Opponents of Abortion Force Shift by Hoechst," International Herald Tribune and New York Times, Apr. 9, 1997, https://www.nytimes.com/1997/04/09/IHT-facing-us-boycott-drugmaker-returns-pill-rights-to-creator-opponents-of.html.
35. Charo, "A Political History of RU-486."
36. Charo, "A Political History of RU-486."
37. Charo, "A Political History of RU-486."
38. Baulieu and Rosenblum, The "Abortion Pill," 48.
39. Baulieu and Rosenblum, The "Abortion Pill," 48.
40. Baulieu and Rosenblum, The "Abortion Pill," 49.
41. Baulieu and Rosenblum, The "Abortion Pill," 49.
42. Steven Greenhouse, "France Ordering Company to Sell Its Abortion Drug," New York Times, Oct. 29, 1988, https://www.nytimes.com/1988/10/29/world/france-ordering-company-to-sell-its-abortion-drug.html.
43. Baulieu and Rosenblum, The "Abortion Pill," 50.
44. Greenhouse, "France Ordering Company to Sell Its Abortion Drug."
45. Gina Kolata, "US May Allow Anti-Ulcer Drug Tied to Abortion," New York Times, Oct. 29, 1988, https://www.nytimes.com/1988/10/29/world/us-may-allow-anti-ulcer-drug-tied-to-abortion.html.
46. James Brooke, "Ulcer Drug Tied to Numerous Abortions in Brazil," New York Times, May 19, 1993, https://www.nytimes.com/1993/05/19/health/ulcer-drug-tied-to-numerous-abortions-in-brazil.html.
47. Rémi Peyron et al., "Early Termination of Pregnancy with Mifepristone (RU 486) and the Orally Active Prostaglandin Misoprostol," New England Journal of Medicine 328, no. 21 (1993): 1509–13, doi:10.1056/NEJM199305273282101, https://www.nejm.org/doi/full/10.1056/NEJM199305273282101.

CHAPTER 5: "OBSCENE, LEWD, OR LASCIVIOUS"

1. Faye Wattleton, "An Abortion Pill: Too Good to Be True," Life on the Line (New York, NY: Ballantine, 1996), 414–16.
2. Marianne Szegedy-Maszak, "Calm, Cool and Beleaguered," New York Times Magazine, Aug. 6, 1989, https://www.nytimes.com/1989/08/06/magazine/calm-cool-and-beleaguered.html.
3. MAKERS, "Faye Wattleton, My Illegal Abortion," YouTube Video, 1:31, July 12, 2018, https://www.youtube.com/watch?v=V9iOJEwrHis.
4. Leslie J. Reagan, When Abortion Was a Crime: Women, Medicine, and Law in the United States, 1867–1973 (Berkeley: University of California Press, 1997), 8–9.
5. Reagan, When Abortion Was a Crime, 8.

6. Reagan, *When Abortion Was a Crime*, 10–11.
7. Rund Abdelfatah et al., "Before Roe: The Physicians' Crusade," NPR, *Throughline*, May 19, 2022, https://www.npr.org/2022/05/18/1099795225/before-roe-the -physicians-crusade.
8. Reagan, *When Abortion Was a Crime*, 10–11.
9. Abdelfatah et al., "Before Roe: The Physicians' Crusade."
10. Reagan, *When Abortion Was a Crime*, 10–11.
11. Horatio Robinson Storer, *Why Not? A Book for Every Woman: The Prize Essay to Which the American Medical Association Awarded the Gold Medal for MDC-CCLXV* (Boston, MA: Lee and Shepard, 1867).
12. Reagan, *When Abortion Was a Crime*, 11–12.
13. Abdelfatah et al., "Before Roe: The Physicians' Crusade."
14. Mabel Felix et al., "The Comstock Act: Implications for Abortion Care Nation-wide," *KFF*, Apr. 15, 2024, https://www.kff.org/womens-health-policy/issue-brief/the -comstock-act-implications-for-abortion-care-nationwide/.
15. Grace Haley, "The Comstock Act," *Abortion, Every Day*, July 30, 2023, https:// jessica.substack.com/p/the-comstock-act?utm_source=publication-search.
16. Reagan, *When Abortion Was a Crime*, 13–14.
17. Reagan, *When Abortion Was a Crime*, 13–14.
18. Maria Vullo, "People v. Sanger and the Birth of Family Planning Clinics in Amer-ica," *Judicial Notice*, Oct. 2021, https://history.nycourts.gov/wp-content/uploads /2021/10/Judicial-Notice-Issue-09_People-v-Sanger.pdf.
19. Linda Gordon, *Woman's Body, Woman's Right: Birth Control in America* (New York, NY: Penguin Books, 1976), 281.
20. Anna Purna Kambhampaty, "Why Planned Parenthood Is Removing Founder Mar-garet Sanger's Name from a New York City Clinic," *TIME*, July 21, 2020, https:// time.com/5869743/planned-parenthood-margaret-sanger/.
21. Doris A. Dirks and Patricia Relf, *To Offer Compassion: A History of the Clergy Consultation Service on Abortion* (Madison: University of Wisconsin Press, 2017).
22. Sandee LaMotte, "These Women Ran an Underground Abortion Network in the 1960s. Here's What They Fear Might Happen Today," CNN, Apr. 23, 2023, https:// www.cnn.com/2023/04/23/health/abortion-lessons-jane-wellness/index.html#:~ :text=What%20started%20as%20referrals%20to,which%20is%20amazing% 2C%20right?%E2%80%9D.
23. For a deep, inside account of the Janes, see Laura Kaplan, *The Story of Jane: The Legendary Underground Feminist Abortion Service* (Chicago, IL: University of Chi-cago Press, 1995).
24. Kaplan, *The Story of Jane*.
25. Kaplan, *The Story of Jane*.
26. *Roe v. Wade*, 410 U.S. 113 (1973), https://supreme.justia.com/cases/federal/us/410 /113/.
27. Julia Longoria et al., "Part 1: The Viability Line," *More Perfect*, WNYC Studios, June 8, 2023, https://www.wnycstudios.org/podcasts/radiolabmoreperfect/episodes /part-1-viability-line.
28. Angela Y. Davis, *Women, Race and Class* (New York, NY: Vintage Books, 1983), 204.
29. Davis, *Women, Race and Class*, 205.
30. Carole E. Joffe, *Doctors of Conscience: The Struggle to Provide Abortion Before and After Roe v. Wade* (Boston, MA: Beacon Press, 1996).
31. Faye Wattleton, "Refusing to Surrender the Poor," *Life on the Line* (New York, NY: Ballantine, 1996), 204–12.
32. Faye Wattleton, "Refusing to Surrender the Poor," *Life on the Line* (New York, NY: Ballantine, 1996), 204–12.
33. Joffe, *Doctors of Conscience*.

34. Marlene Gerber Fried, "The Hyde Amendment: 30 Years of Violating Women's Rights," *Center for American Progress*, Oct. 6, 2006, https://www.americanprogress .org/article/the-hyde-amendment-30-years-of-violating-womens-rights/.

35. Fried, "The Hyde Amendment."

36. Marianne Szegedy-Maszak, "Calm, Cool and Beleaguered," *New York Times Magazine*, Aug. 6, 1989, https://www.nytimes.com/1989/08/06/magazine/calm-cool-and -beleaguered.html.

37. Faye Wattleton, "Roe v. Wade: Completing the Revolution," in *Life on the Line* (New York, NY: Ballantine, 1996), 147–51.

38. *Harris v. McRae*, 448 U.S. 297 (1980), https://supreme.justia.com/cases/federal/us /448/297/.

39. Alina Salganicoff et al., "The Hyde Amendment and Coverage for Abortion Services Under Medicaid in the Post-Roe Era," *KFF*, Mar. 14, 2024, https://www.kff.org /womens-health-policy/issue-brief/the-hyde-amendment-and-coverage-for-abortion -services-under-medicaid-in-the-post-roe-era/.

40. Szegedy-Maszak, "Calm, Cool and Beleaguered."

41. Szegedy-Maszak, "Calm, Cool and Beleaguered."

42. Szegedy-Maszak, "Calm, Cool and Beleaguered."

43. Francis Wilkinson, "The Gospel According to Randall Terry," *Rolling Stone*, Oct. 5, 1989, https://www.rollingstone.com/culture/culture-news/the-gospel-according -to-randall-terry-47951/.

44. Ziegler, *Abortion and the Law in America*, 98–100.

45. Ziegler, *Abortion and the Law in America*.

46. David A. Grimes et al., "An Epidemic of Antiabortion Violence in the United States," *American Journal of Obstetrics and Gynecology* no. 165, 5, part 1 (1991): 1263– 68, doi:10.1016/0002–9378(91)90346-s.

47. Stanley K. Henshaw et al., "Abortion Services in the United States, 1991 and 1992," *Family Planning Perspectives* 26, no. 3 (1994): 100–112, https://doi.org/10.2307 /2136033.

48. Baulieu and Rosenblum, The *"Abortion Pill,"* 93–94.

49. Baulieu and Rosenblum, The *"Abortion Pill."*

50. Baulieu and Rosenblum, The *"Abortion Pill,"* 102–3.

51. Baulieu and Rosenblum, The *"Abortion Pill,"* 103.

52. Baulieu and Rosenblum, The *"Abortion Pill,"* 95–97.

53. Baulieu and Rosenblum, The *"Abortion Pill,"* 98.

54. Baulieu and Rosenblum, The *"Abortion Pill."*

55. Faye Wattleton, "An Abortion Pill: Too Good to Be True," in *Life on the Line* (New York, NY: Ballantine, 1996), 416–17.

56. Five former FDA officials at the agency during the late 1980s and/or 1990s and involved in mifepristone's journey, 2023 and 2024 interviews with author.

57. Wattleton, "An Abortion Pill," 415.

58. R. Alta Charo, "A Political History of RU-486," in *Biomedical Politics*, ed. Kathi E. Hanna (Washington, DC: National Academies Press, 1991), https://www.ncbi.nlm .nih.gov/books/NBK234199/.

59. Charo, "A Political History of RU-486."

60. Charo, "A Political History of RU-486."

61. André Ulmann, 2023 interview with author; Paul Van Look, 2023 interview with author; Beverly Winikoff, 2023 interviews with author; Marc Bygdeman, 2023 interview with author; Kristina Gemzell Danielsson, 2023 interview with author.

62. Rob Stein, "Abortion Pill 'Well-Liked' in US study," *UPI*, Oct. 1, 1990, https://www .upi.com/Archives/1990/09/30/Abortion-pill-well-liked-in-US-study/4808654667200/.

63. Beth Ann Krier, "RU-486: The Abortion Battle's New Frontier. . . . ," *Los Angeles Times*, Apr. 22, 1990, https://www.latimes.com/archives/la-xpm-1990-04-22-vw-373 -story.html.

64. "The Import Ban on RU486," Congressional Hearing, US House of Representatives Small Business Subcommittee on Regulation, Business Opportunity, and Energy, C-SPAN video, Nov. 19, 1990, https://www.c-span.org/video/?15059-1/import-ban -ru486.

65. "The Import Ban on RU486."

66. Ziegler, *Abortion and the Law in America*, 103–9.

67. *Webster v. Reproductive Health Services*, 492 U.S. 490 (1989), https://supreme .justia.com/cases/federal/us/492/490/.

68. Lisa M. Koonin et al., "Abortion Surveillance—United States, 1992," *Morbidity and Mortality Weekly Report*, Centers for Disease Control and Prevention, May 3, 1996, https://www.cdc.gov/mmwr/preview/mmwrhtml/00041486.htm.

69. Marcia Ann Gillespie et al., "We Remember: African American Women Are for Reproductive Freedom," 1989, https://birthequity.org/wp-content/uploads/2022/01 /WeRememberBrochure-1.pdf.

70. Gillespie et al., "We Remember."

71. Natelegé Whaley, "Black Women and the Fight for Abortion Rights: How This Brochure Sparked the Movement for Reproductive Freedom," NBC News, Mar. 25, 2019, https://www.nbcnews.com/news/nbcblk/black-women-fight-abortion-rights -how-brochure-sparked-movement-reproductive-n983216.

72. Wattleton, "An Abortion Pill," 416–17.

73. Wattleton, "An Abortion Pill," 438.

74. Ziegler. *Abortion and the Law in America*, 117–20.

75. Ziegler. *Abortion and the Law in America*, 117–20.

CHAPTER 6: THE BELLY OF THE BEAST

1. Much of this chapter comes from "RU 486 Abortion Pill," Congressional Hearing, US House of Representatives Small Business Subcommittee on Regulation, Business Opportunity, and Energy, C-SPAN video, Dec. 5, 1991, https://www.c-span.org /program/house-committee/ru-486-abortion-pill/16828.

2. Much of this chapter comes from Beverly Winikoff, 2021 and 2023 interviews with author.

3. "RU 486 Abortion Pill."

4. "RU 486 Abortion Pill."

5. US Government Accountability Office, *National Institutes of Health: Problems in Implementing Policy on Women in Study Populations*, GAO (Washington, DC, 1990), https://www.gao.gov/assets/t-hrd-90-50.pdf.

6. Marie Bass, co-founder of Reproductive Health Technologies Project, 2023 interview with author.

7. Reproductive Health Technologies Project archives and 2017 oral history interviews at Schlesinger Library, Radcliffe Institute for Advanced Study at Harvard University, author accessed 2023.

8. Lawrence Lader, *Abortion* (Boston, MA: Beacon Press, 1966).

9. Elaine Woo, "Lawrence Lader, 86; Activist for Abortion Rights Whose Book Was Cited in Roe Case," *Los Angeles Times*, May 14, 2006, https://www.latimes.com /archives/la-xpm-2006-may-14-me-lader14-story.html.

10. Lawrence Lader, "Perilous Years (1975–1990)," in *A Private Matter: RU 486 and the Abortion Crisis* (Amherst, NY: Prometheus, 1995), 104.

11. Lader, "Perilous Years (1975–1990)."

12. Lader, "Perilous Years (1975–1990)," 104–5.

13. Lawrence Lader, *RU 486: The Pill That Could End the Abortion Wars and Why American Women Don't Have It* (Reading, MA: Addison-Wesley, 1991).

14. Lader, *RU 486*, 135.

15. *United States v. One Package*, 13 F. Supp. 334 (S.D.N.Y. 1936), https://law.justia .com/cases/federal/appellate-courts/F2/86/737/1567252/.

16. Lader, *RU 486*, 135.

17. Aaron Zitner, "What Ever Happened to RU-486?" *Boston Globe*, Nov. 23, 1997, https://www.newspapers.com/image/441463829/?match=1.

18. Lawrence Lader, "Abortion and the Population Problem," in *A Private Matter: RU 486 and the Abortion Crisis* (Amherst, NY: Prometheus, 1995), 175.

19. Angela Hume, "Rage Is Your Bitter Fuel," *Deep Care: The Radical Activists Who Provided Abortions, Defied the Law, and Fought to Keep Clinics Open* (Edinburgh, UK: AK Press, 2023), 245–52.

20. Tamar Lewin, "Woman at Center of Debate: Model of an Ardent Feminist," *New York Times*, July 16, 1992, https://www.nytimes.com/1992/07/16/us/woman-at -center-of-debate-model-of-an-ardent-feminist.html.

21. Lawrence Lader, "Challenging the RU 486 Ban," in *A Private Matter: RU 486 and the Abortion Crisis* (Amherst, NY: Prometheus, 1995), 134.

22. Lewin, "Woman at Center of Debate: Model of an Ardent Feminist."

23. *Benten v. Kessler*, 799 F. Supp. 281 (E.D.N.Y. 1992), https://law.justia.com/cases /federal/district-courts/FSupp/799/281/1379485/.

24. *Benten v. Kessler*, 505 U.S. 1084 (1992), https://supreme.justia.com/cases/federal /us/505/1084/.

25. Mark Stencel, "Clinton's Pledges," *Washington Post*, Jan. 20, 1993, https://www .washingtonpost.com/archive/politics/1993/01/20/clintons-pledges/606b7724-a040 -48a8-a406-f6488a35b954/.

26. Hume, "Rage Is Your Bitter Fuel," 251.

27. Lewin, "Woman at Center of Debate: Model of an Ardent Feminist." See also S. J. Diamond, "An Unorthodox 'Everywoman. . . . ,'" *Los Angeles Times*, July 23, 1992, https://www.latimes.com/archives/la-xpm-1992-07-23-vw-4217-story.html.

28. William Clinton, "Remarks on Signing Memorandums on Medical Research and Re- productive Health and an Exchange with Reporters, Jan. 22, 1993," Gerhard Peters and John T. Woolley, The American Presidency Project, https://www.presidency.ucsb .edu/documents/remarks-signing-memorandums-medical-research-and-reproductive -health-and-exchange-with.

29. Lewin, "Woman at Center of Debate: Model of an Ardent Feminist."

30. Hume, "Rage Is Your Bitter Fuel," 245–52, 253, 255.

31. Marion Lipschutz and Rosa Rosenblatt, *The Abortion Pill*, First Run/Icarus Films, 1997, 56 min.

32. William Clinton, Memorandum, "Importation of RU-486," Jan. 22, 1993, Federal Register 58, no. 23 (Feb. 5, 1993), https://archives.federalregister.gov/issue_slice /1993/2/5/7451-7468.pdf.

33. William Clinton, "Remarks on Signing Memorandums."

34. "March for Life" Rally, C-SPAN video, Jan. 22, 1993, https://www.c-span.org/video /?37354-1/march-life-rally.

35. Emily Langer, "Nellie Gray, March for Life Founder, Dead at 88," *Washington Post*, Aug. 14, 2012, https://www.washingtonpost.com/local/obituaries/nellie-gray-march -for-life-founder-dead-at-88/2012/08/14/c496d1ea-e637-11e1-8741-940e3f6dbf48 _story.html.

36. "Defining the Health Agenda," National Rainbow Coalition Panel, C-SPAN video, June 11, 1993, https://www.c-span.org/video/?42828-1/defining-health-agenda.

37. Bela Ganatra, "Coercion, Control or Choice?" *Seminar*, Dec. 2003, https://www .india-seminar.com/2003/532/532%20bela%20ganatra.htm. Also see Byllye Avery, "Empowerment Through Wellness," *Yale Journal of Law and Feminism* 4, no. 147 (1991), 147–54.

38. "Defining the Health Agenda."

39. Jael Miriam Silliman et. al, *Undivided Rights: Women of Color Organize for Repro- ductive Justice* (Chicago, IL: Haymarket Books, 2016), 7–25.

40. Loretta J. Ross and Rickie Solinger, "A Reproductive Justice History," *Reproductive Justice: An Introduction* (Oakland: University of California Press, 2017), 9.

CHAPTER 7: "THE PILL THAT CHANGES EVERYTHING"

1. Larry Rohter, "Doctor Is Slain During Protest over Abortions," *New York Times*, Mar. 11, 1993, https://www.nytimes.com/1993/03/11/us/doctor-is-slain-during-protest-over-abortions.html.

2. Rohter, "Doctor Is Slain During Protest over Abortions."

3. Karissa Haugeberg, *Women Against Abortion: Inside the Largest Moral Reform Movement of the Twentieth Century* (Champaign: University of Illinois Press, 2017), 107.

4. Haugeberg, *Women Against Abortion*, 110–12.

5. Haugeberg, *Women Against Abortion*, 119.

6. Haugeberg, *Women Against Abortion*, 100.

7. Haugeberg, *Women Against Abortion*, 117.

8. Haugeberg, *Women Against Abortion*, 105.

9. Haugeberg, *Women Against Abortion*, 109.

10. Haugeberg, *Women Against Abortion*, 126.

11. Haugeberg, *Women Against Abortion*, 137.

12. Haugeberg, *Women Against Abortion*, 117.

13. "The Pill That Changes Everything," *TIME*, June 14, 1993, https://content.time.com/time/covers/0,16641,19930614,00.html.

14. A. Ulmann, "The Development of Mifepristone: A Pharmaceutical Drama in Three Acts," *Journal of the American Medical Women's Association 55* (1972), no. 3, suppl. (2000): 117–20, https://pubmed.ncbi.nlm.nih.gov/10846319/.

15. Ulmann, "The Development of Mifepristone."

16. Ulmann, "The Development of Mifepristone."

17. Marion Lipschutz and Rosa Rosenblatt, *The Abortion Pill*, First Run/Icarus Films, 1997, 56 min.

18. George Brown, former vice president at the Population Council, 2024 interview with author.

19. For extensive details on Danco's history, see Hannah Levintova, "The Abortion Pill's Secret Money Men," *Mother Jones*, Mar.–Apr. 2023, https://www.motherjones.com/politics/2023/01/abortion-pill-mifepristone-mifeprex-roe-dobbs-private-equity/.

20. Abigail Brone and Lauren Mascarenhas, "The Abortion Pill," *Shoe Leather, Columbia Journalism School*, May 2020, https://shoeleather.podcasts.library.columbia.edu/podcast/the-abortion-pill/.

21. Ronald Smothers, "Abortion Doctor and Bodyguard Slain in Florida; Protestor Is Arrested in Pensacola's 2d Clinic Killing," *New York Times*, July 30, 1994, https://www.nytimes.com/1994/07/30/us/death-doctor-overview-abortion-doctor-bodyguard-slainin-florida-protester.html.

22. John Kifner, "Anti-Abortion Killings: The Overview; Gunman Kills 2 at Abortion Clinics in Boston Suburb," *New York Times*, Dec. 31, 1994, https://www.nytimes.com/1994/12/31/us/anti-abortion-killings-overview-gunman-kills-2-abortion-clinics-boston-suburb.html.

23. Knuvl Sheikh, "Dr. Wayne Bardin, 85, Innovative Researcher on Birth Control, Dies," *New York Times*, Nov. 14, 2019, https://www.nytimes.com/2019/11/14/science/dr-wayne-bardin-dead.html.

24. Beverly Winikoff, 2023 interviews with author; Brown, 2024 interview with author.

25. Ibid.

26. Charlotte Ellertson et al., "Can Women Use Medical Abortion Without Medical Supervision?" *Reproductive Health Matters 5*, no. 9 (Jan. 1997): 149–61, https://doi.org/10.1016/s0968-8080(97)90019-7.

27. Much of this section about the Population Council's medication abortion trials at this Seattle clinic comes from Suzanne T. Poppema and Mike Henderson, "Appendix C," *Why I Am An Abortion Doctor* (Amherst, NY: Prometheus, 1996), 245–53.

28. Poppema and Henderson, "Appendix C," 252.

29. Poppema and Henderson, "Appendix C," 251–52.

30. Poppema and Henderson, *Why I Am An Abortion Doctor*, 89.
31. Suzanne Poppema, 2023 interview with author.
32. LaTasha B. Craig et al., "To the Point: Gender Differences in the Obstetrics and Gynecology Clerkship," *American Journal of Obstetrics and Gynecology* 219, no. 5 (Nov. 2018): 430–35, https://doi.org/10.1016/j.ajog.2018.05.020.
33. Robert D. McFadden, "Kenneth C. Edelin, Doctor at Center of Landmark Abortion Case, Dies at 74," *New York Times*, Dec. 30, 2013, https://www.nytimes.com/2013/12/31/us/kenneth-c-edelin-physician-at-center-of-landmark-abortion-case-dies-at-74.html.
34. US Congress, House of Representatives, *Partial-Birth Abortion Ban Act of 1995*, HR 1833, 104th Congress, introduced in House June 14, 1995, https://www.congress.gov/bill/104th-congress/house-bill/1833.
35. Julie Rovner, "'Partial-Birth Abortion': Separating Fact from Spin," NPR, Feb. 21, 2006, https://www.npr.org/2006/02/21/5168163/partial-birth-abortion-separating-fact-from-spin.
36. Rovner, "'Partial-Birth Abortion.'"
37. Katharine Q. Seelye, "Dole's Switch on Abortion Leads Quickly to Furor on G.O.P. Right," *New York Times*, Dec. 19, 1995, https://www.nytimes.com/1995/12/19/us/dole-s-switch-on-abortion-leads-quickly-to-furor-on-gop-right.html.
38. The details on Mifeprex's approval process come from this report: US Government Accountability Office, *Food and Drug Administration: Approval and Oversight of the Drug Mifeprex*, GAO-08-751 (Washington, DC, 2008), https://www.gao.gov/assets/gao-08-751.pdf.
39. Brone and Mascarenhas, "The Abortion Pill."
40. Gina Kolata, "Panel Advises F.D.A. To Allow Abortion Pill," *New York Times*, July 20, 1996, https://www.nytimes.com/1996/07/20/us/panel-advises-fda-to-allow-abortion-pill.html.
41. US Food and Drug Administration, *New Drug Application for the Use of Mifepristone for Interruption of Early Pregnancy* (Maryland, 1996), Reproductive Health Drugs Advisory Committee, Center for Drug Evaluation and Research, accessed via Freedom of Information Act and transcript on file with author.
42. Elizabeth Pirruccello Newhall, "The Courage to Listen to Your Heart," in *Women of Courage: Inspiring Stories from the Women Who Lived Them*, ed. Katherine Martin (Novato, CA: New World Library, 1999), 131–37.
43. US Food and Drug Administration, *New Drug Application for the Use of Mifepristone for Interruption of Early Pregnancy*.
44. US Government Accountability Office, *Food and Drug Administration: Approval and Oversight of the Drug Mifeprex*.
45. US Food and Drug Administration's Center for Drug Evaluation and Research, *Approval Package for Mifeprex, Application Number 20687 Approvable Letter* (Maryland, 1996), https://www.accessdata.fda.gov/drugsatfda_docs/nda/2000/20687_Mifepristone_approvableltr.pdf.
46. US Food and Drug Administration, *Drug Approval Package, Mifeprex (Mifepristone) Tablet, Application Number 20687*, (Maryland, 2000), https://www.accessdata.fda.gov/drugsatfda_docs/nda/2000/20687_mifepristone.cfm. Mifeprex's FDA approval package includes the medication's detailed medical review, chemistry review, environmental assessment, pharmacology review, statistical review, approval letter, approvable letters, and approved labeling text.
47. Levintova, "The Abortion Pill's Secret Money Men."
48. Beverly Winikoff, 2023 interviews with author; George Brown, 2024 interview with author. Former Population Council member, 2023 interview with author.
49. Caryle Murphy and Kathleen Day, "Abortion Pill's US Debut Snagged by Business Dispute," *Washington Post*, Jan. 12, 1997, https://www.washingtonpost.com/archive/politics/1997/01/12/abortion-pills-us-debut-snagged-by-business-dispute/8e500dd4-3aba-40b7-b3a2-3bff7fcd4850/.

50. Marie Bass, 2023 interview with author; Amy Allina, former Reproductive Health Technologies Project staff member and board member, 2023 interviews with author; Reproductive Health Technologies Project archives and 2017 oral history interviews at Schlesinger Library, Radcliffe Institute for Advanced Study at Harvard University, author accessed 2023.

51. Levintova, "The Abortion Pill's Secret Money Men."

52. Rachel Zimmerman, "Abortion-Pill Venture Keeps to Shadows Awaiting Approval," *Wall Street Journal*, Sept. 5, 2000, https://www.wsj.com/articles/SB968103355754 057093.

53. Levintova, "The Abortion Pill's Secret Money Men."

54. Murphy and Day, "Abortion Pill's US Debut Snagged by Business Dispute."

55. Murphy and Day, "Abortion Pill's US Debut Snagged by Business Dispute."

56. Winikoff, 2023 interviews with author; Brown, 2024 interview with author; former Population Council members, 2023 interviews with author.

57. Aaron Zitner, "What Ever Happened to RU-486?" *Boston Globe*, Nov. 23, 1997, https://www.newspapers.com/image/441463829/?match=1.

58. Lawrence Lader, "Making an American Abortion Pill," in *A Private Matter: RU 486 and the Abortion Crisis* (Amherst, NY: Prometheus, 1995), 146.

59. David Horne, 2023 interview with author.

60. Lawrence Lader, *A Private Matter: RU 486 and the Abortion Crisis* (Amherst, NY: Prometheus, 1995), 141–62.

61. Eric Schaff, 2023 interview with author; Mitchell Creinin, 2023 interviews with author.

62. Eric A. Schaff et al., "Low-Dose Mifepristone 200 mg and Vaginal Misoprostol for Abortion," *Contraception* 59, no. 1 (Jan. 1999): 1–6, https://doi.org/10.1016/s0010 -7824(98)00150-4; Eric A. Schaff et al., "Vaginal Misoprostol Administered 1, 2, or 3 Days After Mifepristone for Early Medical Abortion," *JAMA* 284, no. 15 (Oct. 18, 2000): 1948, https://doi.org/10.1001/jama.284.15.1948; Eric A. Schaff et al., "Vaginal Misoprostol Administered at Home After Mifepristone (RU486) for Abortion," *Journal of Family Practice* 44, no. 4 (Apr. 1997): 353–60, https://pubmed.ncbi.nlm .nih.gov/9108832/.

63. Zitner, "What Ever Happened to RU-486?"

CHAPTER 8: A FANTASY

1. Katharine Q. Seelye, "House Votes to Block F.D.A. on Approval of Abortion Pill," *New York Times*, June 25, 1998, https://www.nytimes.com/1998/06/25/us/house -votes-to-block-fda-on-approval-of-abortion-pill.html.

2. Jim Yardley and David Rohde, "Abortion Doctor in Buffalo Slain; Sniper Attack Fits Violent Pattern," *New York Times*, Oct. 25, 1998, https://www.nytimes.com /1998/10/25/nyregion/abortion-doctor-in-buffalo-slain-sniper-attack-fits-violent -pattern.html.

3. Carole Joffe and Tracy A. Weitz, "Normalizing the Exceptional: Incorporating the 'Abortion Pill' into Mainstream Medicine," *Social Science & Medicine* 56, no. 12 (June 2003): 2353–66, doi:10.1016/s0277–9536(02)00240-x, https://www.science direct.com/science/article/abs/pii/S027795360200240X?via%3Dihub.

4. Margaret Talbot, "The Little White Bombshell," *New York Times Magazine*, July 11, 1999, https://www.nytimes.com/1999/07/11/magazine/the-little-white-bombshell.html.

5. United States Holocaust Memorial Museum, "King Christian X of Denmark," Holocaust Encyclopedia, https://encyclopedia.ushmm.org/content/en/article/king -christian-x-of-denmark.

6. Kaiser Family Foundation, "1995 Survey of Obstetricians/Gynecologists on Contraception and Unplanned Pregnancy: Attitudes and Practices with Regard to Abortion," conducted by Fact Finders, Inc., Albany, NY, Henry J. Kaiser Family Foundation, https://files.kff.org/attachment/chartpack-kaiser-family-foundation-1995-survey-of -obstetriciangynecologists.

7. Mitchell D. Creinin, "Medical Abortion Regimens: Historical Context and Overview," *American Journal of Obstetrics & Gynecology* 183, no. 2 S3-S9 (Aug. 2000), doi:10.1067/mob.2000.107948, https://www.ajog.org/article/S0002-9378(00)84053-3/abstract.

8. Carole Joffe, "'You Need a Community with You': Becoming an Abortion Provider," *Dispatches from the Abortion Wars: The Cost of Fanaticism to Doctors, Patients, and the Rest of Us* (Boston, MA: Beacon Press, 2009), 39–44.

9. Carole Joffe, "Reactions to Medical Abortion Among Providers of Surgical Abortion: An Early Snapshot," *Family Planning Perspectives* 31, no. 1 (Jan./Feb. 1999): 35–38, https://doi.org/10.2307/2991555.

10. Joffe, "Reactions to Medical Abortion Among Providers of Surgical Abortion."

11. Joffe, "Reactions to Medical Abortion Among Providers of Surgical Abortion."

12. Rachel K. Jones et al., "Abortion Incidence and Service Availability in the United States, 2020," *Perspectives on Sexual and Reproductive Health* 54, no. 4 (Nov. 20, 2022): 128–41. https://doi.org/10.1363/psrh.12215.

13. Talbot, "The Little White Bombshell."

14. Rachel Zimmerman, "Abortion-Pill Venture Keeps to Shadows Awaiting Approval," *Wall Street Journal*, Sept. 5, 2000, https://www.wsj.com/articles/SB968103355754057093.

15. Zimmerman, "Abortion-Pill Venture Keeps to Shadows Awaiting Approval."

16. "Bush Backs RU-486 Limits," *ABC News*, Oct. 11, 2000, https://abcnews.go.com/Politics/story?id=122727&page=1.

17. Five former FDA officials involved with mifepristone while at the agency, 2023 and 2024 interviews with author.

18. US Government Accountability Office, *Food and Drug Administration: Approval and Oversight of the Drug Mifeprex*, GAO-08–751 (Washington, DC, 2008), https://www.gao.gov/assets/gao-08-751.pdf.

19. US Government Accountability Office, *Food and Drug Administration.*

20. US Government Accountability Office, *Food and Drug Administration.*

21. "Abortion Drugs," Feminist Majority Foundation Conference, C-SPAN video, Apr. 2, 2000, https://www.c-span.org/video/?156360-1/abortion-drugs.

22. "Abortion Drugs."

23. "Abortion Drugs."

24. "Abortion Drugs."

25. Sheryl Gay Stolberg, "F.D.A. Adds Hurdles in Approval of Abortion Pill," *New York Times*, June 8, 2000, https://www.nytimes.com/2000/06/08/us/fda-adds-hurdles-in-approval-of-abortion-pill.html.

26. Stolberg, "F.D.A. Adds Hurdles in Approval of Abortion Pill."

27. Joffe and Weitz, "Normalizing the Exceptional: Incorporating the 'Abortion Pill.'"

28. US Government Accountability Office, *Food and Drug Administration.*

29. US Government Accountability Office, *Food and Drug Administration.*

30. "Presidential Candidates Debate: Governor George W. Bush and Vice President Al Gore," C-SPAN video, Oct. 3, 2000, https://www.c-span.org/video/?159295-1/presidential-candidates-debate.

31. "Presidential Candidates Debate."

32. Robin Toner, "The 2000 Campaign: Abortion; from Social Security to Environment, the Candidates' Positions," *New York Times*, Nov. 5, 2000, https://www.nytimes.com/2000/11/05/us/2000-campaign-abortion-social-security-environment-candidates-positions.html.

33. Eric A. Schaff et al., "Vaginal Misoprostol Administered 1, 2, or 3 Days After Mifepristone for Early Medical Abortion," *JAMA* 284, no. 15 (Oct. 18, 2000): 1948, https://doi.org/10.1001/jama.284.15.1948.

34. Eric Schaff, 2023 interview with author; Deborah Oyer, 2023 interview with author; Beverly Winikoff, 2023 interviews with author; Mitchell Creinin, 2023 interview with

author; Elizabeth Newhall, 2023 interview with author; Suzanne Poppema, 2023 interview with author; Karen Meckstroth, 2023 interview with author.

35. Sources familiar with Danco, the American abortion-provider community, and the medication abortion researcher community at this time, 2023 and 2024 interviews with author.

36. Christian Sinave et al., "Toxic Shock Syndrome due to *Clostridium Sordellii*: A Dramatic Postpartum and Postabortion Disease," *Clinical Infectious Diseases* 35, no. 11 (Dec. 2002): 1441–43, https://doi.org/10.1086/344464; Abigail Brone and Lauren Mascarenhas, "The Abortion Pill," *Shoe Leather, Columbia Journalism School*, May 2020, https://shoeleather.podcasts.library.columbia.edu/podcast/the-abortion-pill/.

37. "*Clostridium sordellii* Toxic Shock Syndrome After Medical Abortion with Mifepristone and Intravaginal Misoprostol—United States and Canada, 2001–2005," *Morbidity and Mortality Weekly Report*, Centers for Disease Control and Prevention, July 29, 2005, https://www.cdc.gov/mmwr/preview/mmwrhtml/mm5429a3.htm.

38. Christine S. Ho et al., "Undiagnosed Cases of Fatal Clostridium-Associated Toxic Shock in Californian Women of Childbearing Age," *American Journal of Obstetrics & Gynecology* 201, no. 5 (2009): 459.e1–7, doi:10.1016/j.ajog.2009.05.023.

39. US Congress, House of Representatives, Committee on Government Reform, *RU-486: Demonstrating A Low Standard for Women's Health? Hearings before the Subcommittee on Criminal Justice, Drug Policy, and Human Resources,* 109th Congress, 2nd sess., 2006, 109–202.

40. US Government Accountability Office, *Food and Drug Administration.*

41. US Government Accountability Office, *Food and Drug Administration.*

42. Diana Greene Foster, *The Turnaway Study: Ten Years, a Thousand Women, and the Consequences of Having—or Being Denied—an Abortion* (New York, NY: Scribner, 2020).

43. US Food and Drug Administration, *Mifepristone US Post-Marketing Adverse Events Summary through 12/31/2022*, US Food and Drug Administration (Maryland), https://www.fda.gov/media/164331/download.

44. US Food and Drug Administration, *Mifepristone US Post-Marketing Adverse Events Summary through 12/31/2022.*

45. Elizabeth G. Raymond and David A. Grimes, "The Comparative Safety of Legal Induced Abortion and Childbirth in the United States," *Obstetrics and Gynecology* 119, no. 2, part 1 (2012): 215–19, doi:10.1097/AOG.0b013e31823fe923.

46. Linda Prine, 2023 interview with author.

47. Gina Kolata, "Many Doctors Find Array of Obstacles to the Abortion Pill," *New York Times*, Sept. 30, 2000, https://www.nytimes.com/2000/09/30/us/many-doctors-find-array-of-obstacles-to-the-abortion-pill.html.

48. Na'amah Razon et al., "Exploring the Impact of Mifepristone's Risk Evaluation and Mitigation Strategy (REMS). . . . ," *Contraception* 109 (May 2022): 19–24, https://doi.org/10.1016/j.contraception.2022.01.017.

49. Richard Hausknecht, "Physicians for Reproductive Choice and Health: The Reminiscences of Richard Hausknecht," Fly on the Wall Productions, April 2001, Columbia Center for Oral History, Columbia University Libraries, https://oralhistoryportal.library.columbia.edu/document.php?id=ldpd_13794994.

50. R. K. Jones et al., "Abortion in the United States: Incidence and Access to Services, 2005," *Perspectives on Sexual and Reproductive Health* 40, no. 1 (Mar. 2008): 6–16, https://doi.org/10.1363/4000608.

51. Lawrence B. Finer and Junhow Wei, "Effect of Mifepristone on Abortion Access in the United States," *Obstetrics & Gynecology* 114, no. 3 (2009): 623–30, doi: 10.1097/AOG.0b013e3181b2a74d, https://journals.lww.com/greenjournal/Abstract/2009/09000/Effect_of_Mifepristone_on_Abortion_Access_in_the.21.aspx.

52. Mary Ziegler, *Abortion and the Law in America: Roe v. Wade to the Present* (Cambridge, UK: Cambridge University Press, 2020), 191–201.

53. Nicole Dube, *States Allowing Non-Physicians to Provide Abortion Services*, Office of Legislative Research, Connecticut General Assembly, July 29, 2022, https://www.cga.ct.gov/2022/rpt/pdf/2022-R-0167.pdf.

54. Charlotte Ellertson et al., "Can Women Use Medical Abortion Without Medical Supervision?" *Reproductive Health Matters* 5, no. 9 (Jan. 1997): 149–61, https://doi.org/10.1016/s0968-8080(97)90019-7.

55. Paul Blumenthal, 2023 interview with author; Beverly Winikoff, 2023 interviews with author; Daniel Grossman, 2021 interview with author; Ushma Upadhyay, 2021 interview with author; Mitchell Creinin, 2023 interviews with author; Tracy Weitz, 2023 interview with author.

CHAPTER 9: "THE MOST NORMAL THING TO DO"

1. Verónica Cruz Sánchez, 2023 interview with author through an English-Spanish interpreter.

2. Elizabeth Navarro, "An Abortion Network That Works," *Lux Magazine*, Issue 5, 2022, https://lux-magazine.com/article/an-abortion-network-that-works-las-libres/.

3. "Abortion Surfaces as Key Issue in Mexican Politics," *Guttmacher Policy Review* 3, no. 5 (Oct. 1, 2000), Guttmacher Institute, https://www.guttmacher.org/gpr/2000/10/abortion-surfaces-key-issue-mexican-politics.

4. Human Rights Watch, "Abortion: Mexico," *Human Rights Watch*, 2006, https://www.hrw.org/legacy/women/abortion/mexico.html.

5. Consejo Nacional de Evaluación de la Política de Desarrollo Social, *Distribution of People by Poverty Condition in Guanajuato*, Data México (2020), https://www.economia.gob.mx/datamexico/en/profile/geo/guanajuato?redirect=true#population-and-housing.

6. For a thoughtful book on feminist abortion activism with pills in Mexico, including the role some parteras in the State of Chiapas have played, see Georgina Sánchez-Ramírez and Suzanne Veldhuis, *Realidades y retos del aborto con medicamentos en México* (Chetumal, Quintana Roo: ECOSUR: Ipas México, 2022).

7. Deborah Billings, 2023 interviews with author.

8. Madeleine Belfrage, 2023 interview with author. Also see Madeleine Belfrage "Revolutionary Pills? Feminist Abortion, Pharmaceuticalization, and Reproductive Governance," *International Feminist Journal of Politics* 25, no. 1 (Jan. 2023): 6–29, doi:10.1080/14616742.2022.2154688. And see Madeleine Belfrage, "Reclaiming Autonomy: The Changing Landscape of Mexican Abortion Activism," *Signs: Journal of Women in Culture and Society* 49, no. 3 (Mar. 2024): 535–56, https://doi.org/10.1086/727986.

9. Feminist doctors and activists active in Mexico in the 1990s, 2023 interviews with author.

10. For a detailed tracing of transnational mifepristone and misoprostol supply routes, as well as post-2000 cross-border activism on abortion pills in primarily the Global North, see Sydney Calkin, *Abortion Pills Go Global: Reproductive Freedom Across Borders* (Oakland: University of California Press, 2023).

11. Deborah L. Billings et al., "Pharmacy Worker Practices Related to Use of Misoprostol for Abortion in One Mexican State," *Contraception* 79, no. 6 (2009): 445–51, doi:10.1016/j.contraception.2008.12.011.

12. Deborah L. Billings, "Misoprostol Alone for Early Medical Abortion in a Latin American Clinic Setting," *Reproductive Health Matters* 12, no. 24, suppl. (2004): 57–64, doi:10.1016/s0968–8080(04)24010–1.

13. There were and are acompañantes across Latin America who do not identify as women. I use "women" here because Verónica Cruz Sánchez referred to acompañantes at Las Libres as women early in the first decade of the 2000s.

14. Billings, "Misoprostol Alone for Early Medical Abortion in a Latin American Clinic Setting," 57–64.

15. Ipas, "About Us," *Ipas*, accessed 2023, https://www.ipas.org/about-us/.
16. Anu Kumar, president and CEO of Ipas, and Traci Baird, former Ipas employee, joint 2023 interview with author; Ann Leonard, former Ipas executive, 2023 interview with author; Virginia Chambers, former Ipas employee, 2023 interview with author; Paul Blumenthal, former advisor to Ipas, 2023 interviews with author.
17. Jeffrey Collins, "Judge Says South Carolina Can Enforce 6-Week Abortion Ban amid Dispute over When a Heartbeat Begins," *Associated Press*, May 17, 2024, https://apnews.com/article/abortion-south-carolina-fetal-heartbeat-fa742d40c8e15df41c8545d8a33a1838.
18. "Human Rights Watch Honors Mexican Activist: Honoree Secures Access to Legal Abortion for Rape Victims," *Human Rights Watch*, Oct. 30, 2006, https://www.hrw.org/news/2006/10/30/human-rights-watch-honors-mexican-activist.
19. Navarro, "An Abortion Network That Works."
20. For an excellent book on this larger, global feminist movement for self-managed abortion, see Naomi Braine, *Abortion Beyond the Law: Building a Global Feminist Movement for Self-Managed Abortion* (London: Verso, 2023).
21. Verónica Cruz Sánchez, 2023 interview with author through an interpreter.
22. Ann Friedman, "Mail-Order Abortions: Pfizer's Little Secret," *Mother Jones*, Nov./Dec. 2006, https://www.motherjones.com/politics/2006/11/mail-order-abortions-cytotec/.
23. Andrea Rowan, "Prosecuting Women for Self-Inducing Abortion: Counterproductive and Lacking Compassion," *Guttmacher Policy Review* 18, no. 3 (2015), https://www.guttmacher.org/sites/default/files/article_files/gpr1807015.pdf; Tovia Smith, "Teenager's Home Abortion May Spur Charges," NPR, Mar. 29, 2007, https://www.npr.org/2007/03/29/9213707/teenagers-home-abortion-may-spur-charges.
24. For an excruciating and thorough book on this pregnancy criminalization trend in the US, see Michele Goodwin, *Policing the Womb: Invisible Women and the Criminalization of Motherhood* (Cambridge, UK: Cambridge University Press, 2020).
25. The term "self-managed abortion" remains a subject of debate within the American reproductive rights, health, and justice movements as I write in late 2024. Some argue the term "self-sourced abortion" is clearer. But the movements in the first decade of the 2000s and in the early 2010s did not yet often use "self-managed abortion," and the term "self-induced abortion" sometimes appeared instead, as in this instance. See also Susan Yanow, *The Best Defense Is a Good Offense: Misoprostol, Abortion, and the Law: Conference Summary and Strategic Recommendations*, Gynuity Health Projects and the Reproductive Health Technologies Project, Aug. 2009, https://gynuity.org/assets/resources/Goldman_best_defense_web.pdf.
26. Friedman, "Mail-Order Abortions: Pfizer's Little Secret."
27. Friedman, "Mail-Order Abortions: Pfizer's Little Secret."
28. Susan Yanow, *The Best Defense Is a Good Offense.*
29. Bob Herbert, "In America; Stillborn Justice," *New York Times*, May 24, 2001, https://www.nytimes.com/2001/05/24/opinion/in-america-stillborn-justice.html.
30. Michele Goodwin, "Pregnancy and State Power," *Policing the Womb: Invisible Women and the Criminalization of Motherhood* (Cambridge, UK: Cambridge University Press, 2020), 16–23.
31. James C. McKinley Jr., "Mexico City Legalizes Abortion Early in Term," *New York Times*, Apr. 25, 2007, https://www.nytimes.com/2007/04/25/world/americas/25mexico.html; Mary Cuddehe, "Mexico's Abortion Wars," *The Atlantic*, Oct. 2009, https://www.theatlantic.com/magazine/archive/2009/10/mexicos-abortion-wars/307768/.
32. United Nations, Human Rights Committee, *Red Nacional de Organismos Civiles de Derechos Humans "Todos los Derechos para Todas y Todas," Mexico Report*, New York, NY, 2010, https://www2.ohchr.org/english/bodies/hrc/docs/ngos/RNOCDH_mexico98.pdf.

33. Elisabeth Malkin, "Many States in Mexico Crack Down on Abortion," *New York Times*, Sept. 22, 2010, https://www.nytimes.com/2010/09/23/world/americas /23mexico.html.

34. Ana Labandera et al., "Implementation of the Risk and Harm Reduction Strategy Against Unsafe Abortion in Uruguay: From a University Hospital to the Entire Country," *International Journal of Gynaecology and Obstetrics: The Official Organ of the International Federation of Gynaecology and Obstetrics* 134, S1 (2016): S7–S11, doi:10.1016/j.ijgo.2016.06.007.

35. Patrick Adams, "From Uruguay, a Model for Making Abortion Safer," *New York Times*, June 28, 2016, https://www.nytimes.com/2016/06/28/opinion/from-uruguay -a-model-for-making-abortion-safer.html.

36. Leonel Briozzo, 2023 interview with author through English-Spanish interpreter.

37. Giselle Carino, CEO of Fòs Feminista (a funder of Iniciativas Sanitarias), 2023 interview with author.

38. Labandera et al., "Implementation of the Risk and Harm Reduction Strategy Against Unsafe Abortion in Uruguay," S7–S11.

39. Shelly Makleff et al., "Experience Obtaining Legal Abortion in Uruguay: Knowledge, Attitudes, and Stigma Among Abortion Clients," *BMC Women's Health* 19, no. 155 (2019), https://doi.org/10.1186/s12905-019-0855-6.

40. Makleff et al., "Experience Obtaining Legal Abortion in Uruguay."

41. Lucía Berro Pizzarossa and Patty Skuster, "Toward Human Rights and Evidence-Based Legal Frameworks for (Self-Managed) Abortion: A Review of the Last Decade of Legal Reform," *Health and Human Rights* 23, no. 1 (2021): 199–212. https://pmc.ncbi.nlm.nih.gov/articles/PMC8233026/.

42. Paul F. A. Van Look and Jane Cottingham, "The World Health Organization's Safe Abortion Guidance Document," *American Journal of Public Health* 103, no. 4 (2013): 593–96, doi:10.2105/AJPH.2012.301204, https://pmc.ncbi.nlm.nih.gov /articles/PMC3673261/#bib9.

43. World Health Organization, *Safe Abortion: Technical and Policy Guidance for Health Systems* (Geneva, Switzerland: World Health Organization, 2003), https:// iris.who.int/bitstream/handle/10665/42586/9241590343-eng.pdf?sequence=1&is Allowed=y.

44. Socorristas en Red, "Sistematización," *Socorristas en Red*, https://socorristasenred .org/category/sistematizaciones/.

CHAPTER 10: LOOPHOLES

1. Sara Corbett, "The Pro-Choice Extremist," *New York Times Magazine*, Aug. 26, 2001, https://www.nytimes.com/2001/08/26/magazine/the-pro-choice-extremist.html.

2. Anita Hardon, "Reproductive Health Care in the Netherlands: Would Integration Improve It?" *Reproductive Health Matters* 11, no. 21 (2003), 59–73, doi:10.1016 /S0968–8080(03)02165–7.

3. B. Becker, "78,000 Women Die Each Year from Unsafe Abortions Worldwide. It Is Estimated That There Are 20 Million Unsafe Abortions Per Year on a Global Basis," *Reproductive Freedom News* 8, no. 3 (1999): 1, 5. https://pubmed.ncbi.nlm.nih.gov /12294838/.

4. Rebecca Gomperts, 2020, 2021, 2022 interviews with author.

5. For extensive details on Women on Waves's first abortion boat campaign, see "Book About the Abortionship Campaign in Ireland," *Women on Waves*, 2001, https:// www.womenonwaves.org/en/page/7056/book-about-the-abortionship-campaign -in-ireland.

6. Marijke Alblas, 2021 interview with author.

7. Feminist Majority Foundation, "FMF Assists Launch of Women on Waves," *Feminist Majority Foundation Blog*, June 15, 2001, https://feminist.org/news/fmf-assists -launch-of-women-on-waves/.

8. Gunilla Kleiverda, 2021 interview with author.
9. Rebecca Gomperts, "Women on Waves: Where Next for the Abortion Boat?," *Reproductive Health Matters* 10, 19 (2002): 180–3, doi:10.1016/s0968–8080(02) 00004–6, https://pubmed.ncbi.nlm.nih.gov/12369324/.
10. Corbett, "The Pro-Choice Extremist."
11. Feminist Majority Foundation, "Mifepristone Approved in Europe," *Feminist Majority Foundation Blog*, July 6, 1999, https://feminist.org/news/mifepristone-approved -in-europe/.
12. Mary Muldowney, formerly of Irish Women on Waves, 2021 interview with author. Also see "Book about the Abortionship Campaign in Ireland," *Women on Waves*, 2001, https://www.womenonwaves.org/en/page/7056/book-about-the-abortionship -campaign-in-ireland.
13. David Stout, "Man Accused of Killing New York Obstetrician Is Arrested," *New York Times*, Mar. 29, 2001, https://www.nytimes.com/2001/03/29/nyregion/man -accused-of-killing-new-york-obstetrician-is-arrested.html.
14. Muldowney, 2021 interview with author.
15. Marlise Simons, "Dutch Ship Offers Abortions; to Make Ireland Its First Call," *New York Times*, June 11, 2001, https://www.nytimes.com/2001/06/11/world/dutch-ship -offers-abortions-to-make-ireland-its-first-call.html.
16. Mark Brennock, "Decision on Rape Girl Likely to Be Left to Supreme Court," *Irish Times*, Nov. 24, 1997, https://www.irishtimes.com/news/decision-on-rape-girl-likely -to-be-left-to-supreme-court-1.129742.
17. Women on Waves, "Book About the Abortionship Campaign in Ireland."
18. Brian Lavery, "Ship Planning to Offer Abortions Makes Waves, but Hits Shoal at Irish Port," *New York Times*, June 17, 2001, https://www.nytimes.com/2001/06/17 /world/ship-planning-to-offer-abortions-makes-waves-but-hits-shoal-at-irish-port .html.
19. Diana Whitten, *Vessel*, Sovereignty Productions, 2014, 86 min., https://vesselthefilm .com/.
20. Whitten, *Vessel*.
21. Corbett, "The Pro-Choice Extremist."
22. Whitten, *Vessel*.
23. Whitten, *Vessel*.
24. Corbett, "The Pro-Choice Extremist."
25. Sydney Calkin, *Abortion Pills Go Global: Reproductive Freedom Across Borders* (Oakland: University of California Press, 2023), 127–45.
26. Henry McDonald, Emma Graham-Harrison, and Sinead Baker, "Ireland Votes by Landslide to Legalise Abortion," *The Guardian*, May 26, 2018, https://www.the guardian.com/world/2018/may/26/ireland-votes-by-landslide-to-legalise-abortion.
27. Ireland, Oireachtas, *Health (Regulation of Termination of Pregnancy) Act 2018*, commenced Jan. 1 2019, https://data.oireachtas.ie/ie/oireachtas/act/2018/31/eng /enacted/a3118.pdf.
28. Women on Waves, "Abortion Ship Portugal 2004," *Women on Waves*, 2004, https:// www.womenonwaves.org/en/page/483/abortion-ship-portugal-2004.
29. Susan Davies and Rebecca Gomperts, "On Deck for Abortion Rights: Women on Waves Sails to Portugal," *Thresholds* 34 (2007): 26–28, doi: https://doi.org/10.1162 /thld_a_00223.
30. World Health Organization, *Safe Abortion*.
31. Women on Waves, "Talkshow Teachings: How to Induce Abortion," 2004, https:// www.womenonwaves.org/en/page/797/talkshow-teachings-how-to-induce-abortion.
32. Whitten, *Vessel*.
33. Women on Waves, "Live on Television: Explaining How to Do an Abortion on Television," 2004, https://www.womenonwaves.org/en/page/608/live-on-television.
34. Gomperts, 2022 interview with author.

35. Sydney Calkin, "How Indian Abortion Pills Travel the Globe," *Abortion Pills Go Global: Reproductive Freedom Across Borders* (Oakland: University of California Press, 2023), 25–45.

36. Women on Web, "Who We Are," *Women on Web*, https://www.womenonweb.org/en/page/521/who-we-are.

37. Rebecca Gomperts et al., "Using Telemedicine for Termination of Pregnancy With Mifepristone and Misoprostol in Settings Where There Is No Access to Safe Services," *BJOG: An International Journal of Obstetrics & Gynaecology* 115, no. 9 (July 14, 2008): 1171–78, https://doi.org/10.1111/j.1471-0528.2008.01787.x.

38. Juliette Jowit, "From Nagpur to Northern Ireland: Pill Pipeline Helping Women Get Round Abortion Laws," *The Guardian*, Jan. 6, 2016, https://www.theguardian.com/world/2016/jan/06/nagpur-to-northern-ireland-pill-pipeline-helping-women-get-round-abortion-ban.

39. Emily Bazelon, "The Dawn of the Post-Clinic Abortion," *New York Times*, Aug. 28, 2014, https://www.nytimes.com/2014/08/31/magazine/the-dawn-of-the-post-clinic-abortion.html.

40. Kinga Jelinska, former Women on Web manager, 2023 interviews with author; Susan Yanow, former Women on Web employee, 2023 interview with author; Sara Larrea, former Women on Web employee, 2023 interview with author; Gomperts, 2022 interview with author.

41. Bazelon, "The Dawn of the Post-Clinic Abortion."

42. Louise Finer and Johanna B. Fine, "Abortion Law Around the World: Progress and Pushback," *American Journal of Public Health* 103, no. 4 (2013): 585–89, doi:10.2105/AJPH.2012.301197, https://pmc.ncbi.nlm.nih.gov/articles/PMC3673257/pdf/AJPH.2012.301197.pdf.

43. Gomperts, 2022 interview with author.

44. Jessica Griffin, "Does Facebook Have an Anti-Choice Agenda? Censorship of Information on Misoprostol Raises Questions," *Rewire News Group*, Jan. 2, 2012, https://rewirenewsgroup.com/2012/01/02/facebook-censors-information-on-misoprostol/.

45. Angel M. Foster et al., "Evidence of Global Demand for Medication Abortion Information: An Analysis of www.medicationabortion.com," *Contraception* 89, no. 3 (2014): 174–80, doi:10.1016/j.contraception.2013.05.005.

46. Angel Foster, 2023 interview with author.

47. Angel M. Foster et al., "Community-Based Distribution of Misoprostol for Early Abortion: Evaluation of a Program Along the Thailand-Burma Border," *Contraception* 96, no. 4 (2017): 242–47, doi:10.1016/j.contraception.2017.06.006.

48. Ellen Tousaw et al., "'It Is Just Like Having a Period With Back Pain': Exploring Women's Experiences with Community-Based Distribution of Misoprostol for Early Abortion on the Thailand-Burma Border," *Contraception* 97, no. 2 (2018): 122–29, doi:10.1016/j.contraception.2017.06.015.

49. Larrea, 2023 interviews with author.

50. Ximena Casas, "'Why Do They Want to Make Me Suffer Again?' The Impact of Abortion Prosecutions in Ecuador," *Human Rights Watch*, July 14, 2021, https://www.hrw.org/report/2021/07/14/why-do-they-want-make-me-suffer-again/impact-abortion-prosecutions-ecuador.

51. Women on Waves, "From the Virgin: The Call for Safe Abortion," *Women on Waves*, 2008, https://www.womenonwaves.org/en/page/1886/from-the-virgin-the-call-for-safe-abortion.

52. Raquel Irene Drovetta, "Safe Abortion Information Hotlines: An Effective Strategy for Increasing Women's Access to Safe Abortions in Latin America," *Reproductive Health Matters* 23, no. 45 (2015): 47–57, doi:10.1016/j.rhm.2015.06.004.

53. Drovetta, "Safe Abortion Information Hotlines."

54. Drovetta, "Safe Abortion Information Hotlines."

55. Women on Waves, "Late Night Action to Publicize Hotline," *Women on* Waves, 2009, https://www.womenonwaves.org/en/page/2359/late-night-action-to-publicize-hotline.
56. Raquel Drovetta, 2023 interview with author; Human Rights Watch, "Abortion: Argentina," *Human Rights Watch*, 2004, https://www.hrw.org/legacy/women/abortion /argentina.html#:~:text=History%20of%20Argentina's%20Law%20on%20Abortion &text=In%201922%2C%20the%20penal%20code,pregnant%20woman%20was %20mentally%20disabled.
57. Women on Waves, "Safe Abortion Hotline Launched in Buenos Aires," *Women on Waves*, 2009, https://www.womenonwaves.org/en/page/2360/safe-abortion-hotline -launched-in-buenos-aires.
58. Jelinska, 2023 interviews with author; Yanow, 2023 interview with author; Inna Hudaya, head of Samsara abortion hotline in Indonesia and former Women on Waves partner (current Women Help Women partner as of 2024), 2023 interview with author; 2023 interviews with Women Help Women partners running abortion-pills hotlines in Nigeria and Kenya.
59. Larrea, 2023 interview with author; Stephanie (Stefy) Altamirano, 2023 interview with author through English-Spanish interpreter.
60. Casas, "'Why Do They Want to Make Me Suffer Again?'"
61. Mariana Prandini Assis, "Misoprostol on Trial: A Descriptive Study of the Criminalization of an Essential Medicine in Brazil," *Cadernos de Saude Publica* 37, no. 10 (2021), doi:10.1590/0102–311X00272520, https://www.scielo.br/j/csp/a/fJK7WG zJQrd9NCbyRztLxjR/?lang=en.
62. Stephanie Nolen, "When Brazil Banned Abortion Pills, Women Turned to Drug Traffickers," *New York Times*, June 28, 2022, https://www.nytimes.com/2022/06 /28/health/brazil-abortion-pills.html.
63. Zoë Carpenter, "Las Comadres Is Fighting to Make Abortion Safe in Ecuador— Even While It's Illegal," *The Nation*, May 7, 2019, https://www.thenation.com /article/world/abortion-activism-prosecutions-ecuador/.
64. Altamirano, 2023 interview with author through English-Spanish interpreter.
65. Women Help Women, "Our Teams," *Women Help Women*, https://womenhelp.org /en/page/428/our-teams.
66. Center for Reproductive Rights, *Self-Managed Abortion: Legal Analysis by Country*, Center for Reproductive Rights, 2024, https://reproductiverights.org/wp-content /uploads/2024/09/Self-managed-abortion-Legal-Analysis-by-Country.pdf.
67. World Health Organization Human Reproduction Programme, *Abortion Care Guideline*.

CHAPTER 11: QUESTIONING EVERYTHING, COMPLETELY

1. Uki Goñi, "Argentina Senate Rejects Bill to Legalise Abortion," *The Guardian*, Aug. 9, 2018, https://www.theguardian.com/world/2018/aug/09/argentina-senate-rejects -bill-legalise-abortion.
2. Human Rights Watch, "Abortion: Argentina," *Human Rights Watch*, https://www.hrw .org/legacy/women/abortion/argentina.html#:~:text=History%20of%20Argentina's %20Law%20on,pregnant%20woman%20was%20mentally%20disabled.
3. Human Rights Watch, "Abortion: Argentina."
4. Daniel Politti and Ernesto Londoño, "Argentina's Senate Narrowly Rejects Legalizing Abortion," *New York Times*, Aug. 9, 2018, https://www.nytimes.com/2018/08 /09/world/americas/argentina-abortion-vote.html.
5. Lucía Baez, Socorristas en Red member, 2023 interviews with author.
6. Ruth Zurbriggen, co-founder of Socorristas en Red, 2023 interview with author through English-Spanish interpreter.
7. Victoria Rodriguez Rey, "'Cooking Is an Act of Humanity and Element of Resistance and Power,'" *Río Negro*, Aug. 3, 2022, https://www.rionegro.com.ar/gastronomia /8m-cocinar-es-un-acto-de-humanidad-y-un-elemento-de-resistencia-y-poder -2189800/.

8. Alejandro Rebossio, "What Drives . . . Ruth Zurbriggen. 'We Ensure That Violent and Abusive People End Up in Jail,'" *El País*, Oct. 1, 2014, https://elpais.com/elpais /2014/09/24/planeta_futuro/1411581598_142614.html; Reuters, "Chronology: Argentina's Turbulent History of Economic Crises," *Reuters*, July 30, 2014, https:// www.reuters.com/article/business/chronology-argentinas-turbulent-history-of -economic-crises-idUSKBN0FZ23N/.

9. María Alicia Gutiérrez, "Politics of Recognition: The National Campaign for the Right to Legal, Safe, and Free Abortion in Argentina," *South Atlantic Quarterly* 122, no. 2 (2023): 386–96, https://doi.org/10.1215/00382876-10405147.

10. "Las Madres de Plaza de Mayo—1992, Argentina," Sakharov Prize, European Parliament, https://www.europarl.europa.eu/sakharovprize/en/las-madres-de-plaza-de -mayo-1992-argenti/products-details/20200330CAN54167#:~:text=The%20'Mothers %20of%20the%20Plaza,and%20torture%20of%20political%20opponents.

11. "Las Madres de Plaza de Mayo—1992, Argentina."

12. Gutiérrez, "Politics of Recognition," 386–96.

13. Belén Grosso et al., "Políticas *de y con* los cuerpos. . . . ," in *La diferencia desquiciada. Géneros y diversidades sexuales*, ed. Ana María Fernández and Wiliam Sigueira Peres (Buenos Aires: Biblos, 2013), https://larevuelta.com.ar/wp-content/uploads /2017/09/2012-Texto-Socorro-Rosa-Las-Revueltas-Agosto.pdf.

14. Belén Grosso et al., "Políticas *de y con* los cuerpos."

15. Belén Grosso et al., "Políticas *de y con* los cuerpos."

16. Belén Grosso et al., "Políticas *de y con* los cuerpos."

17. Rebossio, "What Drives . . . Ruth Zurbriggen."

18. Ruth Zurbriggen et al., *El Aborto con Medicamentos en el Segundo Trimestre de Embarazo: Una Investigación Socorrista Feminista* (Buenos Aires: Ediciones La Parte Maldita, 2018).

19. Emilié Suarez, 2023 interview with author through English-Spanish interpreter.

20. Tom Phillips, Amy Booth, and Uki Goñi, "Argentina Legalises Abortion in Landmark Moment for Women's Rights," *The Guardian*, Dec. 30, 2020, https://www .theguardian.com/world/2020/dec/30/argentina-legalises-abortion-in-landmark -moment-for-womens-rights.

21. Harriet Barber, "'The Stigma Has Returned': Abortion Access in Turmoil in Javier Milei's Argentina," *The Guardian*, Mar. 18, 2024, https://www.theguardian.com /global-development/2024/mar/18/argentina-abortion-javier-milei.

22. Sonia Santoro, "Persecuted for Complying with the Law," *Página 12*, Dec. 28, 2022, https://www.pagina12.com.ar/511455-perseguidas-por-cumplir-la-ley.

CHAPTER 12: UNAPOLOGETIC LOVE

1. Ruth Zurbriggen et al., "Accompaniment of Second-Trimester Abortions: The Model of the Feminist Socorrista Network of Argentina," *Contraception* 97, no. 2 (2018): 108–15, doi:10.1016/j.contraception.2017.07.170.

2. Caitlin Gerdts and Inna Hudaya, "Quality of Care in a Safe-Abortion Hotline in Indonesia: Beyond Harm Reduction," *American Journal of Public Health* 106, no. 11 (2016): 2071–75, doi:10.2105/AJPH.2016.303446.

3. World Health Organization, *Safe Abortion: Technical and Policy Guidance for Health Systems*, (Geneva, Switzerland: World Health Organization, 2003) https://iris.who.int /bitstream/handle/10665/42586/9241590343-eng.pdf?sequence=1&isAllowed=y.

4. Inna Hudaya, 2023 interview with author.

5. Ruth Zurbriggen, 2023 interview with author; Caitlin Gerdts, 2023 interview with author; Hudaya, 2023 interview with author; Sybil Nmezi, 2023 interview with author; Kinga Jelinska, 2023 interview with author.

6. Caitlin Gerdts et al., "Second-Trimester Medication Abortion Outside The Clinic Setting: An Analysis of Electronic Client Records from a Safe Abortion Hotline in Indonesia," *BMJ Sexual & Reproductive Health* 44 (2018): 286–91, https://srh.bmj .com/content/familyplanning/44/4/286.full.pdf.

7. Ika Ayu Kristianingrum et al., "Overcoming Challenges in Research on Self-Managed Medical Abortion: Lessons from a Collaborative Activist-Researcher Partnership," *Sexual and Reproductive Health Matters* 30, no. 1 (2022): 2077282, doi:10.1080/26410397.2022.2077282.

8. Sophia Chae et al., "Reasons Why Women Have Induced Abortions: A Synthesis of Findings from 14 Countries," *Contraception* 96, no. 4 (2017): 233–41, doi:10.1016/j.contraception.2017.06.014.

9. Heidi Moseson et al., "Effectiveness of Self-Managed Medication Abortion with Accompaniment Support in Argentina and Nigeria (SAFE). . . . ," *The Lancet Global Health* 10, no. 1 (2022): e105–e113, doi:10.1016/S2214–109X(21)00461–7.

10. World Health Organization Human Reproduction Programme, *Abortion Care Guideline* (Geneva, Switzerland: World Health Organization, 2022), https://www.who.int/publications/i/item/9789240039483.

11. Moseson et al., "Effectiveness of Self-Managed Medication Abortion with Accompaniment Support in Argentina and Nigeria (SAFE)," e105–e113; Elizabeth G. Raymond et al., "Clinical Outcomes of Medication Abortion Using Misoprostol -Only: A Retrospective Chart Review at an Abortion Provider Organization in the United States," *Contraception* 126 (2023): 110109, doi:10.1016/j.contraception.2023.110109.

12. Gerdts, 2023 interview with author.

13. Kristianingrum et al., "Overcoming Challenges in Research on Self-Managed Medical Abortion," 2077282.

14. Emily Widra, "States of Incarceration: The Global Context 2024," Prison Policy Initiative, June 2024, https://www.prisonpolicy.org/global/2024.html.

15. Elizabeth Kai Hinton et al., "An Unjust Burden: The Disparate Treatment of Black Americans in the Criminal Justice System," *Vera Institute of Justice*, May 2018, https://www.vera.org/publications/for-the-record-unjust-burden.

16. Center for Reproductive Rights, *Self-Managed Abortion: Legal Analysis by Country*, Center for Reproductive Rights, 2024, https://reproductiverights.org/wp-content/uploads/2024/09/Self-managed-abortion-Legal-Analysis-by-Country.pdf.

17. Bela Ganatra, head of the Prevention of Unsafe Abortion unit in the Sexual and Reproductive Health and Research division of the Human Reproduction Programme at the World Health Organization, 2023 interview with author.

18. Center for Reproductive Rights, *European Abortion Laws: A Comparative Overview*, Center for Reproductive Rights, Sept. 2023, https://reproductiverights.org/wp-content/uploads/2023/09/European-Abortion-Laws-A-Comparative-Overview-new-9-13-23.pdf.

19. Carter Sherman, "US Supreme Court Unanimously Upholds Access to Abortion Pill Mifepristone," *The Guardian*, June 13, 2024, https://www.theguardian.com/us-news/ng-interactive/2024/jun/13/supreme-court-abortion-pill-access.

CHAPTER 13: "REALLY, REALLY, *REALLY* THIS MAKES NO SENSE"

1. Julie Rovner, "Clash over Abortion Stalls Health Bill, Again," NPR and *KFF Health News*, Mar. 21, 2018, https://www.npr.org/sections/health-shots/2018/03/21/595191785/clash-over-abortion-hobbles-a-health-bill-again-here-s-how.

2. Erin Matson, co-founder and president of Reproaction, a US reproductive justice advocacy group, 2023 interview with author.

3. Gardiner Harris, "Plan to Widen Availability of Morning-After Pill Is Rejected," *New York Times*, Dec. 7, 2011, https://www.nytimes.com/2011/12/08/health/policy/sebelius-overrules-fda-on-freer-sale-of-emergency-contraceptives.html.

4. Jackie Calmes and Gardiner Harris, "Obama Endorses Decision to Limit Morning-After Pill," *New York Times*, Dec. 8, 2011, https://www.nytimes.com/2011/12/09/us/obama-backs-aides-stance-on-morning-after-pill.html.

5. Mary Ziegler, *Dollars for Life: The Anti-Abortion Movement and the Fall of the Republican Establishment* (New Haven: Yale University Press, 2022).

6. Anna North, "The Downfall of Roe v. Wade Started in 2010," *Vox*, Dec. 23, 2019, https://www.vox.com/2019/12/23/21024312/abortion-laws-2019-ohio-georgia-roe-wade.

7. Kathryn Kolbert and Julie F. Kay, "A Wolf at the Door: New Supreme Court Majority Puts Procreative and Sexual Freedoms at Risk," in *Controlling Women: What We Must Do Now to Save Reproductive Freedom* (New York: Hachette Books, 2021), 131–37.

8. Tom Dart, "Wendy Davis's Remarkable Filibuster to Deny Passage of Abortion Bill," *The Guardian*, June 26, 2013, https://www.theguardian.com/world/2013/jun/26/texas-senator-wendy-davis-abortion-bill-speech.

9. Dart, "Wendy Davis's Remarkable Filibuster to Deny Passage of Abortion Bill."

10. Alana Rocha et al., "Running Out the Clock: The Wendy Davis Abortion Filibuster, 5 Years Later," *Texas Tribune*, June 25, 2018, https://www.texastribune.org/2018/06/25/wendy-davis-abortion-filibuster-five-year-anniversary/.

11. Amy Littlefield, "Where the Pro-Choice Movement Went Wrong," *New York Times*, Dec. 1, 2021, https://www.nytimes.com/2021/12/01/opinion/abortion-planned-parenthood-naral-roe-v-wade.html.

12. Francine Coeytaux, 2023 interview with author. Also see Francine Coeytaux oral history interview in 2017 in the Reproductive Health Technologies Project archives at Schlesinger Library, Radcliffe Institute for Advanced Study at Harvard University, author accessed in 2023.

13. Francine Coeytaux, Leila Hessini, and Amy Allina, "Bold Action to Meet Women's Needs: Putting Abortion Pills in US Women's Hands," *Women's Health Issues: Official Publication of the Jacobs Institute of Women's Health* 25, no. 6 (2015): 608–11, doi:10.1016/j.whi.2015.08.004.

14. Molly Redden, "Purvi Patel Has 20-Year Sentence for Inducing Own Abortion Reduced," *The Guardian*, July 22, 2016, https://www.theguardian.com/us-news/2016/jul/22/purvi-patel-abortion-sentence-reduced.

15. Emily Bazelon, "A Mother in Jail for Helping Her Daughter Have an Abortion," *New York Times Magazine*, Sept. 22, 2014, https://www.nytimes.com/2014/09/22/magazine/a-mother-in-jail-for-helping-her-daughter-have-an-abortion.html.

16. Public Health Institute, Ipas, National Women's Health Network, Reproductive Health Technologies Project, *Abortion Pills in US Women's Hands: Bold Action to Meet Women's Needs—Report on Meeting Held 12/4/13 in Washington, DC* (Washington, DC, Dec. 2013), courtesy of Francine Coeytaux, on file with author.

17. Public Health Institute, Ipas, National Women's Health Network, Reproductive Health Technologies Project, *Abortion Pills in US Women's Hands*.

18. Carrie N. Baker, "History and Politics of Medication Abortion in the United States and the Rise of Telemedicine and Self-Managed Abortion," *Journal of Health Politics, Policy and Law* 48, no. 4 (2023): 485–510, doi:10.1215/03616878-10449941.

19. Amy Allina, 2023 interview with author.

20. Coeytaux, Hessini, and Allina, "Bold Action to Meet Women's Needs," 608–11.

21. Monica Simpson, "Reproductive Justice and 'Choice': An Open Letter to Planned Parenthood," *Rewire News Group*, Aug. 5, 2014, https://rewirenewsgroup.com/2014/08/05/reproductive-justice-choice-open-letter-planned-parenthood/.

22. Jackie Calmes, "Advocates Shun 'Pro-Choice' to Expand Message," *New York Times*, July 28, 2014, https://www.nytimes.com/2014/07/29/us/politics/advocates-shun-pro-choice-to-expand-message.html?_r=0.

23. Loretta Ross, "Defeating Personhood: A Critical but Incomplete Victory for Reproductive Justice," *Rewire News Group*, Nov. 9, 2011, https://rewirenewsgroup.com/2011/11/09/personhood-defeated-in-mississippi/.

24. Elisa Wells et al., "Evaluation of Different Models of Access to Misoprostol at the Community Level to Improve Maternal Health Outcomes in Ethiopia, Ghana, and

Nigeria," *International Journal of Gynaecology and Obstetrics: The Official Organ of the International Federation of Gynaecology and Obstetrics* 133, no. 3 (2016): 261–65, doi:10.1016/j.ijgo.2016.04.002.

25. Banchiamlack Dessalegn, "What Ethiopia Can Teach the US About Abortion Rights," *Al Jazeera*, Sept. 28, 2022, https://www.aljazeera.com/opinions/2022/9/28/what-ethiopia-can-teach-america-about-abortion-rights#:~:text=Ethiopia%20%E2%80%93%20like%20other%20countries%20in,choice%20groups%20could%20not%20ignore.

26. Nancy Cárdenas Peña, 2024 interview with author.

27. Daniel Grossman et al., "Effectiveness and Acceptability of Medical Abortion Provided Through Telemedicine," *Obstetrics and Gynecology* 118, no. 2, part 1 (2011): 296–303, doi:10.1097/AOG.0b013e318224d110.

28. Elizabeth Raymond et al., "TelAbortion: Evaluation of a Direct to Patient Telemedicine Abortion Service in the United States," *Contraception* 100, no. 3 (2019): 173–77, doi:10.1016/j.contraception.2019.05.013.

29. US Government Accountability Office, *Food and Drug Administration: Information on Mifeprex Labeling Changes and Ongoing Monitoring Efforts*, GAO-18–292 (Washington, DC, 2018), https://www.gao.gov/assets/gao-18-292.pdf.

30. Sources familiar with Danco, the FDA's 2016 approval of revisions to Mifeprex's label, and the reproductive health, rights, and justice advocacy communities at that time, 2023 and 2024 interviews with author.

31. Plan C, "About Us," *Plan C Pills*, https://www.plancpills.org/about#:~:text=Plan%20C%20is%20a%20public,of%20abortion%20pills%20by%20mail, accessed 2024.

32. Amy Merrill, 2023 interview with author.

33. Coeytaux, 2023 interview with author; Elisa Wells, 2023 interview with author.

34. Sources in the American reproductive health, rights, and justice movement familiar with these dynamics, 2023 and 2024 interviews with author.

35. Susan Yanow, 2023 interview with author.

36. Chloe Murtagh et al., "Exploring the Feasibility of Obtaining Mifepristone and Misoprostol from the Internet," *Contraception* 97, no. 4 (2018): 287–91, doi:10.1016/j.contraception.2017.09.016.

37. Chelsea Conaboy, "She Started Selling Abortion Pills Online. Then the Feds Showed Up," *Mother Jones*, Mar./Apr. 2019, https://www.motherjones.com/politics/2019/02/she-started-selling-abortion-pills-online-then-the-feds-showed-up/.

38. Karen Madden, "Grand Rapids Man Pleads Not Guilty to Trying to Poison Wausau Woman to Kill Her Unborn Baby," *Wausau Daily Herald*, June 12, 2018, https://www.wausaudailyherald.com/story/news/2018/06/12/jeffrey-s-smith-pleads-not-guilty-trying-poison-pregnant-woman/693821002/.

39. United States Attorney's Office, Western District of Wisconsin, 2020, "New York Woman Sentenced for Selling Abortion-Inducing Pills Illegally Smuggled Into US," July 10, 2020, https://www.justice.gov/usao-wdwi/pr/new-york-woman-sentenced-selling-abortion-inducing-pills-illegally-smuggled-us.

40. Conaboy, "She Started Selling Abortion Pills Online."

41. Abigail R. A. Aiken, Jennifer E. Starling, and Rebecca Gomperts, "Factors Associated with Use of an Online Telemedicine Service to Access Self-managed Medical Abortion in the US," *JAMA Network Open* 4, no. 5 (2021): e2111852, doi:10.1001/jamanetworkopen.2021.11852.

42. Linda Prine, 2023 interview with author.

43. US Food and Drug Administration, 2019, "Warning Letter: Aidaccess.org," https://www.fda.gov/inspections-compliance-enforcement-and-criminal-investigations/warning-letters/aidaccessorg-575658-03082019.

44. Sarah McCammon, "European Doctor Who Prescribes Abortion Pills to US Women Online Sues FDA," NPR, Sept. 9, 2019, https://www.npr.org/2019/09/09/758871490/european-doctor-who-prescribes-abortion-pills-to-u-s-women-online-sues-fda.

45. *Gomperts v. Azar*, Case No. 1:19-cv-00345-DCN (D. Idaho Jul. 13, 2020), https://casetext.com/case/gomperts-v-azar.

46. US Food and Drug Administration, *Policy for Certain REMS Requirements During the COVID-19 Public Health Emergency: Guidance for Industry and Health Care Professionals*, US Food and Drug Administration, Mar. 2020, https://www.supremecourt.gov/opinions/URLs_Cited/OT2020/20A34/20A34-5.pdf.

47. *American College of Obstetricians and Gynecologists v. FDA*, Case No. 8:20-cv-01320-TDC (D. Maryland, May 27, 2020), https://www.acog.org/-/media/project/acog/acogorg/files/advocacy/acog-v-fda-complaint-mifepristone-covid19.pdf?rev=45c9d9540fb94f90a4c0e5d2ef88531b&hash=C3293DFE0EF86FFF1304D0C5280D3EE7.

48. Laurie Sobel et al., "State Action to Limit Abortion Access During the COVID-19 Pandemic," *KFF*, Aug. 10, 2020, https://www.kff.org/coronavirus-covid-19/issue-brief/state-action-to-limit-abortion-access-during-the-covid-19-pandemic/.

49. *American College of Obstetricians and Gynecologists v. FDA*.

50. Aamna Mohdin, "Relaxation of UK Abortion Rules Welcomed by Experts," *The Guardian*, Mar. 30, 2020, https://www.theguardian.com/world/2020/mar/30/relaxation-of-uk-abortion-rules-welcomed-by-experts-coronavirus.

51. Jordan A. Parsons and Elizabeth Chloe Romanis, "2020 Developments in the Provision of Early Medical Abortion by Telemedicine in the UK," *Health Policy* 125, no. 1 (2021): 17–21, doi:10.1016/j.healthpol.2020.11.006.

52. Abigail Aiken et al., "Effectiveness, Safety and Acceptability of No-Test Medical Abortion (Termination of Pregnancy) Provided via Telemedicine: A National Cohort Study," *BJOG: An International Journal of Obstetrics and Gynaecology* 128, no. 9 (2021): 1464–74, doi:10.1111/1471–0528.16668; Patricia Lohr of British Pregnancy Advisory Service, 2023 interview with author; Abigail Aiken, 2023 interview with author.

53. Aiken et al., "Effectiveness, Safety and Acceptability of No-Test Medical Abortion (Termination of Pregnancy) Provided Via Telemedicine," 1464–74.

54. *American College of Obstetricians and Gynecologists v. FDA*.

55. Jessica Nouhavandi, co-founder and lead pharmacist of Honeybee Health, early 2024 interview with author.

56. Baker, "History and Politics of Medication Abortion in the United States and the Rise of Telemedicine and Self-Managed Abortion," 485–510.

57. Deborah Oyer, former director of Cedar River Clinics, 2023 interview with author; Wells, 2023 and 2024 interviews with author; Coeytaux, 2023 and 2024 interview with author.

58. *FDA v. American College of Obstetricians and Gynecologists (ACOG)*, 592 U.S. (2021), https://www.supremecourt.gov/opinions/20pdf/20a34_3f14.pdf.

59. Will Feuer and Nate Rattner, "US Reports Record Number of Covid Deaths in January as New Strains Threaten Progress," *CNBC*, Jan. 27, 2021, https://www.cnbc.com/2021/01/27/us-reports-record-number-of-covid-deaths-in-january.html.

60. Erica Chong et al., "Expansion of a Direct-to-Patient Telemedicine Abortion Service in the United States and Experience During the COVID-19 Pandemic," *Contraception* 104, no. 1 (2021): 43–48, doi:10.1016/j.contraception.2021.03.019.

61. Laurie Sobel, Alina Salganicoff, and Mabel Felix, "Legal Challenges to the FDA Approval of Medication Abortion Pills," *KFF*, Mar. 13, 2023, https://www.kff.org/womens-health-policy/issue-brief/legal-challenges-to-the-fda-approval-of-medication-abortion-pills/.

62. R. K. Jones, M. Kirstein, and J. Philbin, "Abortion Incidence and Service Availability in the United States, 2020," *Perspectives on Sexual and Reproductive Health* 54, no. 4 (2022): 128–41, doi:10.1363/psrh.12215, https://onlinelibrary.wiley.com/doi/epdf/10.1363/psrh.12215.

63. Ashley Kirzinger et al., "Abortion Knowledge and Attitudes: KFF Polling and Policy Insights," *KFF*, Jan. 22, 2020, https://www.kff.org/womens-health-policy/poll -finding/abortion-knowledge-and-attitudes-kff-polling-and-policy-insights/.
64. Kirzinger et al., "Abortion Knowledge and Attitudes."

CHAPTER 14: "WE ARE GOING TO LOSE OUR RIGHT TO ABORTION ACCESS TOMORROW"

1. Cathy Torres, 2024 interview with author.
2. Manny Fernandez, "Abortion Law Pushes Texas Clinics to Close Doors," *New York Times*, Mar. 6, 2014, https://www.nytimes.com/2014/03/07/us/citing-new-texas -rules-abortion-provider-is-shutting-last-clinics-in-2-regions.html.
3. Attorney General of Texas, "Health Care Professionals and Facilities, Including Abortion Providers, Must Immediately Stop All Medically Unnecessary Surgeries and Procedures to Preserve Resources to Fight COVID-19 Pandemic," Press Release, Mar. 23, 2020, https://www.texasattorneygeneral.gov/news/releases/health-care -professionals-and-facilities-including-abortion-providers-must-immediately-stop -all#.XnkW2CKrfO8.twitter.
4. Shannon Najmabadi, "Federal Appeals Court Allows Medication Abortions in Texas During Coronavirus Pandemic," *Texas Tribune*, Apr. 13, 2020, https://www .texastribune.org/2020/04/13/texas-abortion-ban-medication-abortions-allowed -during-coronavirus/.
5. S.B. 8, 87th Leg § 171.205 (Tex. 2021), https://capitol.texas.gov/tlodocs/87R/billtext /pdf/SB00008F.pdf.
6. "Civil Liability for Violation or Aiding or Abetting Violation," *Texas Health and Safety Code* § 171.208, accessed 2024, https://statutes.capitol.texas.gov/Docs/HS /htm/HS.171.htm#171.208. Also see Texas State Law Library, "Legal FAQs: What Does Senate Bill 8 Say About Abortions?" accessed 2024, https://www.sll.texas.gov /faqs/abortion-senate-bill-8/#:~:text=Senate%20Bill%208%20is%20also,inducing %20an%20abortion%20a%20crime.
7. Selena Simmons-Duffin and Carrie Feibel, "The Texas Abortion Ban Hinges on 'Fetal Heartbeat.' Doctors Call That Misleading," NPR, originally Sept. 2, 2021, updated May 3, 2022, https://www.npr.org/sections/health-shots/2021/09/02/1033727679 /fetal-heartbeat-isnt-a-medical-term-but-its-still-used-in-laws-on-abortion.
8. Shannon Najmabadi, "Gov. Greg Abbott Signs into Law One of Nation's Strictest Abortion Measures, Banning Procedure as Early as Six Weeks into a Pregnancy," *Texas Tribune*, May 19, 2021, https://www.texastribune.org/2021/05/18/texas -heartbeat-bill-abortions-law/.
9. "Civil Liability for Violation or Aiding or Abetting Violation."
10. Tracy Droz Tragos, *Plan C*, Dinky Pictures, 2023, 99 min., https://plancmovie.com/.
11. US Census Bureau, "Total Population—Texas," *2020 Decennial Census*, Data.census .gov, https://data.census.gov/profile/Texas?g=040XX00US48.
12. Carrie Baker, "Texas Law Prohibiting Mailing Abortion Pills Won't Stop Texans Seeking Pills Online," *Ms. Magazine*, Oct. 11, 2021, https://msmagazine.com/2021 /10/11/texas-mail-abortion-pills-online-plan-c-sb4/.
13. Torres, 2024 interview with author.
14. Torres, 2024 interview with author; Nancy Cárdenas Peña, 2024 interview with author; sources familiar with these dynamics, 2023 and 2024 interviews with author.
15. Ariane de Vogue, "Texas 6-Week Abortion Ban Takes Effect After Supreme Court Inaction," CNN, Sept. 1, 2021, https://www.cnn.com/2021/09/01/politics/texas -abortion-supreme-court-sb8-roe-wade/index.html.
16. *Whole Woman's Health v. Austin Reeve Jackson, Judge,* 594 U.S. (2021), https://www .supremecourt.gov/opinions/20pdf/21a24_8759.pdf.
17. *Whole Woman's Health v. Austin Reeve Jackson, Judge,* 594 U.S. (2021).

18. Torres, 2024 interview with author.
19. Mandi Cai, "Before Roe v. Wade Was Overturned, at Least 50,000 Texans Received Abortions in the State Each Year. Here's a Look Behind the Numbers," *Texas Tribune*, originally May 9, 2022, updated June 24, 2022, https://www.texastribune.org /2022/05/09/texas-abortions-by-the-numbers/.
20. Eleanor Klibanoff, "Five Abortions a Month: How Dobbs Changed Texas," *Texas Tribune*, June 24, 2022, https://www.texastribune.org/2024/06/24/abortion-dobbs -anniversary-pregnancy-complications/; Christopher Adams, "Number of Texans Receiving Abortions Out of State Quadrupled Between 2021 and 2023," *KXAN News*, originally Sept. 3, 2024, updated Nov. 1, 2024, https://www.kxan.com/news /texas-abortion/texas-abortion-data/#:~:text=Still%2C%20the%20total%20number %20of,according%20to%20the%20HHSC%20data.
21. Abigail R. A. Aiken et al., "Association of Texas Senate Bill 8 With Requests for Self-Managed Medication Abortion." *JAMA Network Open* 5, no. 2 (2022): e221122, doi:10.1001/jamanetworkopen.2022.1122.
22. Sarah McCammon, "Threats to Abortion Access Drive Demand for Abortion Pills, Analysis Suggests," NPR, Jan. 2, 2024, https://www.npr.org/2024/01/02/1220733428 /medication-abortion-advance-provision.
23. Abby Vesoulis, "How Texas' Abortion Ban Will Lead to More At-Home Abortions," *TIME*, Sept. 21, 2021, https://time.com/6099921/texas-self-managed-abortions/.
24. Vanessa Romo, "Mexico's Supreme Court Has Voted to Decriminalize Abortion," NPR, Sept. 7, 2021, https://www.npr.org/2021/09/07/1034925270/mexico-abortion -decriminalized-supreme-court.
25. Natalie Kitroeff, "A Plan Forms in Mexico: Help Americans Get Abortions," *New York Times*, Dec. 20, 2021, https://www.nytimes.com/2021/12/20/world/americas /mexico-abortion-pill-activists.html.
26. Kebé, Elizabeth Ling, and Kylee Sunderlin, *A Repro Legal Helpline Report: State Violence and the Far-Reaching Impact of Dobbs*, If/When/How: Lawyering for Reproductive Justice, 2024, https://ifwhenhow.org/wp-content/uploads/2024/06 /Repro-Legal-Helpline-Report-June-24.pdf.
27. Linda Prine, 2023 interview with author.
28. Tom Philpott, "A Texas Woman Has Been Charged with Murder for an Alleged Self-Induced Abortion," *Mother Jones*, Apr. 9, 2022, https://www.motherjones.com /politics/2022/04/lizelle-herrera-texas-greg-abbott-sb-8/.
29. "Criminal Homicide: Applicability to Certain Conduct," *Texas Penal Code* § 19.06, https://statutes.capitol.texas.gov/Docs/PE/htm/PE.19.htm; S.B. 8, 87th Leg § 171.205 (Tex. 2021), https://capitol.texas.gov/tlodocs/87R/billtext/pdf/SB00008F.pdf.
30. Eleanor Klibanoff, "Texas Woman Charged With Murder for Self-Induced Abortion Sues Starr County District Attorney," *Texas Tribune*, Mar. 30, 2024, https://www .texastribune.org/2024/03/30/texas-woman-sues-abortion-arrest-starr-county/.
31. Mary Ziegler, "Lizelle Herrera's Texas Arrest Is a Warning," *NBC News*, Apr. 16, 2022, https://www.nbcnews.com/think/opinion/lizelle-herreras-texas-abortion-arrest -warning-rcna24639.
32. Julianne McShane, "Texas District Attorney Drops Case Against Woman Charged With Murder for Self-Induced Abortion," *NBC News*, Apr. 10, 2022, https://www .nbcnews.com/news/texas-district-attorney-says-indictment-woman-charged-murder -self-indu-rcna23782.
33. Ziegler, "Lizelle Herrera's Texas Arrest Is a Warning."
34. Josh Gerstein and Alexander Ward, "Supreme Court Has Voted to Overturn Abortion Rights, Draft Opinion Shows," *Politico*, originally May 2, 2022, updated May 3, 2022, https://www.politico.com/news/2022/05/02/supreme-court-abortion -draft-opinion-00029473.
35. Politico Staff, "Read Justice Alito's Initial Draft Abortion Opinion Which Would Overturn Roe v. Wade," *Politico*, May 2, 2022, https://www.politico.com/news

/2022/05/02/read-justice-alito-initial-abortion-opinion-overturn-roe-v-wade-pdf
-00029504.

36. US Constitution, amend. XIV, https://www.archives.gov/milestone-documents/14th
-amendment; US Constitution, amend. XIX, https://www.archives.gov/milestone
-documents/19th-amendment.

37. Politico Staff, "Read Justice Alito's Initial Draft Abortion Opinion Which Would
Overturn Roe v. Wade."

38. Pew Research Center, "Public Opinion on Abortion: Views on Abortion, 1995–
2024," May 13, 2024, https://www.pewresearch.org/religion/fact-sheet/public
-opinion-on-abortion/.

39. Politico Staff, "Read Justice Alito's Initial Draft Abortion Opinion Which Would
Overturn Roe v. Wade."

40. Carole Joffe, 2023 interview with author.

41. Mississippi State Department of Health, *Mississippi Maternal Mortality Report
2016–2020*, Dec. 2023, https://msdh.ms.gov/page/resources/20200.pdf.

42. Mississippi State Department of Health, *Mississippi Maternal Mortality Report
2016–2020*.

43. Eleanor Klibanoff, "New Texas Law Increasing Penalties for Abortion Providers
Goes into Effect Aug. 25," *Texas Tribune*, originally July 26, 2022, updated July 27,
2022, https://www.texastribune.org/2022/07/26/texas-abortion-ban-dobbs/.

44. Eleanor Klibanoff, "Texans Who Perform Abortions Now Face up to Life in Prison,
$100,000 Fine," *Texas Tribune*, Aug. 25, 2022, https://www.texastribune.org/2022
/08/25/texas-trigger-law-abortion/.

45. Torres, 2024 interview with author; sources familiar with these dynamics, 2023 and
2024 interviews with author.

46. Klibanoff, "Texans Who Perform Abortions Now Face up to Life in Prison,
$100,000 Fine."

47. Attorney General of Texas, "Advisory on Texas Law Upon Reversal of *Roe v. Wade*,"
June 21, 2022, Advisory, https://www.texasattorneygeneral.gov/sites/default/files
/images/executive-management/Post-Roe%20Advisory.pdf.

48. Nina Totenberg and Sarah McCammon, "Supreme Court Overturns Roe v. Wade,
Ending Right to Abortion Upheld for Decades," NPR, June 24, 2022, https://www
.npr.org/2022/06/24/1102305878/supreme-court-abortion-roe-v-wade-decision
-overturn.

49. Lawrence Hurley, "Trump's Justices Decisive in Long Campaign to Overturn Roe v.
Wade," *Reuters*, June 24, 2022, https://www.reuters.com/legal/government/trumps
-justices-decisive-long-campaign-overturn-roe-v-wade-2022-06-24/.

50. *Dobbs v. Jackson Women's Health Organization*, 597 U.S. (2022), https://supreme
.justia.com/cases/federal/us/597/19-1392/.

51. Elisa Wells, 2023 and 2024 interviews with author. See also Grace Carroll, "Abortion Pills Are Under Threat—This Nonprofit Is Pushing Back," *Fast Company*, July
6, 2023, https://www.fastcompany.com/90910514/plan-c-medication-abortion
-pills.

52. Susan Yanow, 2023 interview with author.

CHAPTER 15: "THIS LAWSUIT IS FRIVOLOUS"

1. Renee Bracey Sherman, 2023 interview with author. See also US Congress, House
of Representatives, Energy & Commerce Committee, *Roe Reversal: The Impacts of
Taking Away the Constitutional Right to an Abortion: Hearing Before the Subcom-
mittee on Oversight and Investigations*, 117th Congress, 2022 (statement of Renee
Bracey Sherman), https://www.congress.gov/117/meeting/house/114995/witnesses
/HHRG-117-IF02-Wstate-BraceyShermanMPAR-20220719.pdf.

2. US Congress, House of Representatives, Energy & Commerce Committee, *Roe
Reversal*.

3. Lauren Gambino, "What Democrats Achieved—and Didn't—in Two Years Controlling Congress," *The Guardian*, Jan. 1, 2023, https://www.theguardian.com/us-news/2023/jan/01/democrats-congress-control-achievements-joe-biden.

4. "Executive Order 14076 of July 8, 2022, Protecting Access to Reproductive Healthcare Services," *Federal Register* 87, no. 133 (July 13, 2022): 42053, https://www.govinfo.gov/content/pkg/FR-2022-07-13/pdf/2022-15138.pdf.

5. Shefali Luthra, "Biden Signs Executive Order on Abortion Access and Legal Backing," *The 19th*, July 8, 2022, https://19thnews.org/2022/07/biden-executive-order-abortion/.

6. Abigail Higgins, "Why Doesn't Biden Use the Word 'Abortion' More?" *Washington Post*, Dec. 14, 2021, https://www.washingtonpost.com/gender-identity/why-doesnt-biden-use-the-word-abortion-more/. Also see Renee Bracey Sherman's campaign, "Did Biden Say Abortion Yet?," https://didbidensayabortionyet.org/, accessed 2024.

7. Renee Bracey Sherman and Regina Mahone, *Liberating Abortion: Claiming Our History, Sharing Our Stories, and Building the Reproductive Future We Deserve* (New York, NY: Amistad, 2024).

8. US Congress, House of Representatives, Energy & Commerce Committee, *Roe Reversal*.

9. US Congress, House of Representatives, Energy & Commerce Committee, *Roe Reversal*.

10. Alex Woodward, "Witness Tells Congress How to Self-Manage Abortion With Pills in First of Its Kind Testimony," *The Independent*, July 19, 2022, https://www.the-independent.com/news/world/americas/us-politics/self-managed-abortion-congress-b2126775.html.

11. US Congress, House of Representatives, Energy & Commerce Committee, *Roe Reversal*.

12. Dylan Lysen, Laura Ziegler, and Blaise Mesa, "Voters in Kansas Decide to Keep Abortion Legal in the State, Rejecting an Amendment," NPR, Aug. 3, 2022, https://www.npr.org/sections/2022-live-primary-election-race-results/2022/08/02/1115317596/kansas-voters-abortion-legal-reject-constitutional-amendment.

13. Lysen, Ziegler, and Mesa, "Voters in Kansas Decide to Keep Abortion Legal in the State, Rejecting an Amendment"; Becca Andrews, "Inside a Kansas Clinic Where the Battle over Abortion Is Still Raging," *Mother Jones*, Sept./Oct. 2022, https://www.motherjones.com/politics/2022/08/inside-a-kansas-clinic-where-the-battle-over-abortion-is-still-raging/.

14. Lysen, Ziegler, and Mesa, "Voters in Kansas Decide to Keep Abortion Legal in the State, Rejecting an Amendment."

15. "Ballot Tracker: Outcome of Abortion-Related State Constitutional Amendment Measures in the 2024 Election," *KFF*, last updated Nov. 6, 2024, https://www.kff.org/womens-health-policy/dashboard/ballot-tracker-status-of-abortion-related-state-constitutional-amendment-measures/.

16. Mary Ziegler, "The GOP's New Tactic to Block Abortion Votes Is Startlingly Successful," *Slate*, Sept. 12, 2024, https://slate.com/news-and-politics/2024/09/gop-blocks-abortion-votes-missouri-nebraska.html.

17. Amy Littlefield, "Look Up! *Roe* Is the Floor, Not the Ceiling," *The Nation*, Sept. 12, 2023, https://www.thenation.com/article/activism/abortion-ballot-initiatives-viability/.

18. *Alliance for Hippocratic Medicine v. Food and Drug Administration*, Case 2:22-cv-00223-Z (N.D. Tex. 2023), https://adfmedialegalfiles.blob.core.windows.net/files/AllianceForHippocraticMedicineComplaint.pdf.

19. For an explainer on this case, see Suhasini Ravi and Rebecca Reingold, "FDA v. Alliance for Hippocratic Medicine: Recapping the Supreme Court's Oral Argument," *O'Neill Institute for National and Global Health Law at Georgetown University Law Center*, Apr. 10, 2024, https://oneill.law.georgetown.edu/fda-v-alliance-for-hippocratic-medicine-recapping-the-supreme-courts-oral-argument/.

20. Amy Schoenfeld Walker et al., "Are Abortion Pills Safe? Here's the Evidence." *New York Times*, originally Apr. 1, 2023, updated Mar. 25, 2024, https://www.nytimes.com/interactive/2023/04/01/health/abortion-pill-safety.html.

21. Miriam Berger and Mikhail Klimentov, "Abortion Pill at Heart of Supreme Court Rulings Is Approved in over 90 Countries," *Washington Post*, originally Apr. 19, 2023, updated Mar. 26, 2024, https://www.washingtonpost.com/world/2023/04/19/abortion-pill-mifepristone-global-approved/.

22. *Alliance for Hippocratic Medicine v. Food and Drug Administration*.

23. *Alliance for Hippocratic Medicine v. Food and Drug Administration*.

24. US Congress, House of Representatives, Committee on Government Reform, *RU-486: Demonstrating a Low Standard for Women's Health? Hearing Before the Subcommittee on Criminal Justice, Drug Policy, and Human Resources*, 109th Congress, 2006, https://www.govinfo.gov/content/pkg/CHRG-109hhrg31397/html/CHRG-109hhrg31397.htm.

25. Southern Poverty Law Center, "Alliance Defending Freedom," Southern Poverty Law Center, accessed 2024, https://www.splcenter.org/fighting-hate/extremist-files/group/alliance-defending-freedom.

26. Ian Ward, "The Group Behind Dobbs Does Not Want to Talk About What Comes Next," *Politico*, Mar. 25, 2024, https://www.politico.com/news/magazine/2024/03/25/head-of-alliance-defending-freedom-kristen-waggoner-speaks-on-mifepristone-00148565.

27. Mitchell Creinin, 2023 interviews with author.

28. Mara Gordon, "Safety Problems Lead to Early End for Study of 'Abortion Pill Reversal,'" NPR, Dec. 5, 2019, https://www.npr.org/sections/health-shots/2019/12/05/785262221/safety-problems-lead-to-early-end-for-study-of-abortion-pill-reversal.

29. Mitchell D. Creinin et al., "Mifepristone Antagonization With Progesterone to Prevent Medical Abortion: A Randomized Controlled Trial," *Obstetrics & Gynecology* 135, no. 1 (2020): 158–165, doi:10.1097/AOG.0000000000003620, https://journals.lww.com/greenjournal/abstract/2020/01000/mifepristone_antagonization_with_progesterone_to.21.aspx.

30. American College of Obstetricians and Gynecologists, "Facts Are Important: Medication Abortion 'Reversal' Is Not Supported by Science," American College of Obstetricians and Gynecologists, accessed 2024, https://www.acog.org/advocacy/facts-are-important/medication-abortion-reversal-is-not-supported-by-science.

31. Greer Donley, 2023 interview with author.

32. Caroline Kitchener and Ann E. Marimow, "The Texas Judge Who Could Take Down the Abortion Pill," *Washington Post*, Feb. 25, 2023, https://www.washingtonpost.com/politics/2023/02/25/texas-judge-abortion-pill-decision/.

33. Heather Skanes, 2024 interview with author.

34. J. Fontenot et al., *Where You Live Matters: Maternity Care Deserts and the Crisis of Access and Equity in Alabama*, March of Dimes, 2023, https://www.marchofdimes.org/peristats/assets/s3/reports/mcd/Maternity-Care-Report-Alabama.pdf.

35. Katherine Sacks, Lawson Mansell, and Brooke Shearon, *Maternal Mortality Among Vulnerable US Communities*, Milken Institute, Aug. 2023, https://milkeninstitute.org/sites/default/files/2023-07/MaternalMortalityamongVulnerableUSCommunities.pdf.

36. Sacks, Mansell, and Shearon, *Maternal Mortality Among Vulnerable US Communities*.

37. Steven Ross Johnson, "The 10 States With the Highest Poverty Rates," *US News & World Report*, May 7, 2024, https://www.usnews.com/news/best-states/slideshows/us-states-with-the-highest-poverty-rates?slide=5.

38. *KFF*, "Abortion in the United States Dashboard," updated Nov. 6, 2024, accessed Nov. 6, 2024, https://www.kff.org/womens-health-policy/dashboard/abortion-in-the-u-s-dashboard/.

39. "Abortion Prohibited Where Postfertilization Age of Unborn Child at Least 20 Weeks; Exception," *Alabama Code* § 26–23B-5 (2023), https://law.justia.com/codes/alabama/title-26/chapter-23b/section-26-23b-5/; and *Robinson v. Marshall*, Case No. 2:19-cv-00365-MHT (M.D. Ala. Jun. 24, 2022), https://law.justia.com/cases/federal/district-courts/alabama/almdce/2:2019cv00365/69868/145/.

40. "Abortion Prohibited Where Postfertilization Age of Unborn Child at Least 20 Weeks; Exception."

41. *Alabama Code* § 26–23H-6 (1975), https://casetext.com/statute/code-of-alabama /title-26-infants-and-incompetents/chapter-23h-the-alabama-human-life-protection -act/section-26-23h-6-violations#:~:text=Current%20through%20the%202024% 20Regular,is%20a%20Class%20C%20felony and H.B 314, 2019 Leg § 6 (Ala. 2019); "Sentences of Imprisonment for Felonies," *Alabama Code* § 13A-5–6 (2022), https:// law.justia.com/codes/alabama/2022/title-13a/chapter-5/article-1/section-13a-5-6/.

42. "Abortion Prohibited Where Postfertilization Age of Unborn Child at Least 20 Weeks; Exception"; *Robinson v. Marshall*, Case No. 2:19-cv-00365-MHT (M.D. Ala. Jun. 24, 2022); "Sentences of Imprisonment for Felonies."

43. "Abortion Prohibited Where Postfertilization Age of Unborn Child at Least 20 Weeks; Exception"; *Robinson v. Marshall.*

44. Kylie Cheung, "Abortion Funds Sued Alabama's Attorney General for His 'Fringe' Threats. But the Damage Was Already Done," *Jezebel*, Aug. 16, 2024, https://www .jezebel.com/abortion-funds-sued-alabamas-attorney-general-for-his-fringe-threats -but-the-damage-was-already-done.

45. Jenice Fountain, director of Yellowhammer Fund, 2024 interview with author.

46. Fountain, 2024 interview with author.

47. Heather Skanes, 2024 interview with author; Fountain, 2024 interview with author.

48. Elisa Wells, 2023 and 2024 interviews with author; Francine Coeytaux, 2023 interview with author.

49. Emily Bazelon, "Risking Everything to Offer Abortions Across State Lines," *New York Times*, Oct. 4, 2022, https://www.nytimes.com/2022/10/04/magazine/abortion -interstate-travel-post-roe.html.

50. Linda Prine, 2023 interview with author.

51. Prine, 2023 interview with author.

52. David S. Cohen, Greer Donley, and Rachel Rebouché, "The New Abortion Battleground," *Columbia Law Review* 123 (first draft released online in 2022, final publication 2023), https://scholarship.law.pitt.edu/cgi/viewcontent.cgi?article=1515 &context=fac_articles.

53. Eleanor Klibanoff, "Texas Abortion Funds Likely Safe from Prosecution, Federal Judge Rules," *Texas Tribune*, Feb. 24, 2023, https://www.texastribune.org/2023/02 /24/texas-abortion-funds-ruling/.

54. Margot Sanger-Katz, Claire Cain Miller, and Quoctrung Bui, "Who Gets Abortions in America?" *New York Times*, Dec. 14, 2021, https://www.nytimes.com/interactive /2021/12/14/upshot/who-gets-abortions-in-america.html#:~:text=Six%20in%2010 %20women%20who,for%20Disease%20Control%20and%20Prevention.

55. *Yellowhammer Fund v. Marshall*, Civil Action 2:23cv450-MHT (WO) (M.D. Ala. Aug. 21, 2023), https://cases.justia.com/federal/district-courts/alabama/almdce /2:2023cv00450/80824/48/0.pdf?ts=1715095958.

56. Deidre McPhillips, "Travel Time to Abortion Facilities Grew Significantly After Supreme Court Overturned Roe v. Wade," CNN, Nov. 1, 2022, https://www.cnn.com /2022/11/01/health/abortion-access-travel-time/index.html.

CHAPTER 16: "I FELT LIKE I WAS ABANDONED"

1. Eleanor Klibanoff, "Federal Judge in Texas Suspends FDA Approval of Abortion Pill," *Texas Tribune*, Apr. 7, 2023, https://www.texastribune.org/2023/04/07/texas -abortion-drugs-fda-ruling/.

2. *Alliance for Hippocratic Medicine v. US Food and Drug Administration*, Case 2:22-cv-00223-Z (N. Texas Apr. 7, 2023), https://storage.courtlistener.com/recap /gov.uscourts.txnd.370067/gov.uscourts.txnd.370067.137.0_8.pdf.

3. *Alliance for Hippocratic Medicine v. US Food and Drug Administration.*

4. *Alliance for Hippocratic Medicine v. US Food and Drug Administration.*

5. US Government Accountability Office, *Food and Drug Administration: Approval and Oversight of the Drug Mifeprex*, GAO-08–751 (Washington, DC, 2008), https://www.gao.gov/assets/gao-08-751.pdf.

6. Amy Howe, "Biden Administration and Drug Manufacturer Ask Court to Block Suspension of Mifepristone Approval," *SCOTUSblog*, Apr. 14, 2023, https://www.scotusblog.com/2023/04/supreme-court-biden-administration-and-drug-manufacturer-ask-court-to-block-suspension-of-mifepristone-abortion-approval/.

7. Tierney Sneed, "Takeaways from the 5th Circuit Arguments over Abortion Drug Access," CNN, May 17, 2023, https://www.cnn.com/2023/05/17/politics/abortion-drug-mifepristone-5th-circuit-hearing-takeaways/index.html.

8. *Alliance for Hippocratic Medicine v. US Food and Drug Administration v. Danco*, Case No. 23–10362 (5th Cir. 2023), https://www.ca5.uscourts.gov/opinions/pub/23/23-10362-CV1.pdf.

9. *Alliance for Hippocratic Medicine v. US Food and Drug Administration v. Danco*.

10. Suhasini Ravi and Rebecca Reingold, "FDA v. Alliance for Hippocratic Medicine: Recapping the Supreme Court's Oral Argument," *O'Neill Institute for National and Global Health Law at Georgetown University Law Center*, Apr. 10, 2024, https://oneill.law.georgetown.edu/fda-v-alliance-for-hippocratic-medicine-recapping-the-supreme-courts-oral-argument/.

11. Brief of Former FDA Officials as *Amici Curiae* in Support of Appellants, *Alliance for Hippocratic Medicine v. US Food and Drug Administration v. Danco*, Case No. 23-10362 (5th Cir. 2023), https://reproductiverights.org/wp-content/uploads/2023/05/2023-05-01-264-Brief-of-Amici-Curiae-Former-FDA-Officials-ISO-Appellants.pdf.

12. Stef W. Kight, "The Moments That Stole a Divided America's Attention in 2023," *Axios*, https://www.axios.com/2023/12/29/google-trends-taylor-swift-donald-trump.

13. Amnesty International, "Obstacles to Autonomy: Post-*Roe* Removal of Abortion Information Online," Amnesty International Ltd., July 2024, https://www.amnestyusa.org/reports/obstacles-to-autonomy-post-roe-removal-of-abortion-information-online/.

14. Amy Littlefield, "'She Had a Heartbeat Too': Waiting for One Dead Woman," *The Nation*, Mar. 14, 2023, https://www.thenation.com/article/society/texas-abortion-lawsuit/.

15. Petition for Declaratory Judgment and Application for Permanent Injunction, *Amanda Zurawski v. State of Texas*, Case No. 23–0629 (Tex. 2023), https://reproductiverights.org/wp-content/uploads/2023/03/Zurawski-v-State-of-Texas-Complaint.pdf.

16. Amanda Seitz, "More Women Who Were Denied Abortions in Texas Join Lawsuit Challenging State's Abortion Law," *Associated Press* (PBS *Newshour* reprinted), May 22, 2023, https://www.pbs.org/newshour/nation/more-women-who-were-denied-abortions-in-texas-join-lawsuit-challenging-states-abortion-law.

17. Aria Bendix, "Woman Suing Texas over Abortion Ban Vomits on the Stand in Emotional Reaction During Dramatic Hearing," *NBC News*, July 19, 2023, https://www.nbcnews.com/health/health-news/woman-suing-texas-abortion-ban-vomits-on-stand-rcna95162.

18. *State of Texas v. Amanda Zurawski*, Case No. 23–0629 (Tex. 2023), https://www.txcourts.gov/media/1458610/230629.pdf.

19. Jericka Duncan, "Brittany Watts, Ohio Woman Charged With Felony After Miscarriage at Home, Describes Shock of Her Arrest," *CBS News*, Oct. 21, 2024, https://www.cbsnews.com/news/brittany-watts-the-ohio-woman-charged-with-a-felony-after-a-miscarriage-talks-shock-of-her-arrest/.

20. Duncan, "Brittany Watts, Ohio Woman Charged With Felony After Miscarriage at Home, Describes Shock of Her Arrest."

21. Duncan, "Brittany Watts, Ohio Woman Charged With Felony After Miscarriage at Home, Describes Shock of Her Arrest."

22. *Kate Cox v. State of Texas*, D-1-GN-23–008611 (District Court of Travis Co., Tex., 2023), https://reproductiverights.org/wp-content/uploads/2023/12/Cox-v.-Texas -original-petition-FINAL-1.pdf.

23. Eleanor Klibanoff, "Texas Woman Asks Judge To Let Her Terminate Pregnancy After Lethal Fetal Diagnosis," *Texas Tribune*, Dec. 5, 2023, https://www.texastribune .org/2023/12/05/texas-abortion-lawsuit/.

24. Pradnya Joshi, "Texas Judge Allows Abortion in Cox Case as AG Paxton Threatens Legal Action," *Washington Post*, Dec. 7, 2023, https://www.washingtonpost.com /politics/2023/12/07/texas-abortion-judge-ruling/.

25. Attorney General of Texas, "Attorney General Ken Paxton Responds to Travis County TRO," Press Release, Dec. 7, 2023, https://www.texasattorneygeneral.gov /news/releases/attorney-general-ken-paxton-responds-travis-county-tro.

26. Tracy Smith, "Texas Mother Kate Cox on the Outcome of Her Legal Fight for an Abortion: 'It Was Crushing,'" *CBS News*, Jan. 14, 2024, https://www.cbsnews.com /news/kate-cox-on-her-legal-fight-for-abortion-trisomy-18/.

27. Smith, "Texas Mother Kate Cox on the Outcome of Her Legal Fight for an Abortion."

28. Stephania Taladrid, "Did An Abortion Ban Cost a Young Texas Woman Her Life?" *New Yorker*, Jan. 8, 2024, https://www.newyorker.com/magazine/2024/01/15 /abortion-high-risk-pregnancy-yeni-glick.

29. Taladrid, "Did an Abortion Ban Cost a Young Texas Woman Her Life?"

30. Lisiane Freitas Leal et al., "Maternal Mortality in Brazil, 1990 to 2019: A Systematic Analysis of the Global Burden of Disease Study 2019," *Revista da Sociedade Brasileira de Medicina Tropical* no. 55, suppl. 1 e0279. 28 (2022), doi:10.1590/0037 –8682–0279–2021, https://pmc.ncbi.nlm.nih.gov/articles/PMC9009438/pdf/1678 -9849-rsbmt-55-s01-e0279-2021.pdf; Regine A. Douthard et al., "US Maternal Mortality Within a Global Context: Historical Trends, Current State, and Future Directions," *Journal of Women's Health* 30, no. 2 (2021): 168–77, doi:10.1089 /jwh.2020.8863, https://pmc.ncbi.nlm.nih.gov/articles/PMC8020556/pdf/jwh.2020 .8863.pdf.

31. L. G. Fleszar et al., "Trends in State-Level Maternal Mortality by Racial and Ethnic Group in the United States," *JAMA* 330, no. 1 (2023): 52–61, doi:10.1001/jama .2023.9043, https://jamanetwork.com/journals/jama/fullarticle/2806661.

32. Melody Shreiber, "'One Death Is Too Many': Abortion Bans Usher in US Maternal Mortality Crisis," *The Guardian*, Sept. 25, 2024, https://www.theguardian.com /world/2024/sep/25/abortion-bans-healthcare-maternal-mortality.

33. A. Gemmill et al., "Infant Deaths After Texas' 2021 Ban on Abortion in Early Pregnancy," *JAMA Pediatrics* 178, no. 8 (2024): 784–91, doi:10.1001/jama pediatrics.2024.0885, https://jamanetwork.com/journals/jamapediatrics/article -abstract/2819785.

34. Eleanor Klibanoff, "Anti-Abortion Doctor Appointed To Texas Maternal Death Review Committee," *Texas Tribune*, May 22, 2024, https://www.texastribune.org /2024/05/22/texas-maternal-mortality-committee-ingrid-skop-abortion-doctor/.

35. Mary Tuma, "Texas Doctor Who Said Nine-Year-Olds Can Safely Give Birth Appointed to Maternal Mortality Committee," *The Guardian*, May 23, 2024, https:// www.theguardian.com/us-news/article/2024/may/23/texas-anti-abortion-activist.

36. Pew Research Center, "Public Opinion on Abortion," Pew Research Center, May 13, 2024, https://www.pewresearch.org/religion/fact-sheet/public-opinion-on-abortion/.

37. Steve Inskeep and Domenico Montanaro, "Poll: Americans Overwhelmingly Reject Criminalizing Abortion, Divided on Other Issues," NPR, Apr. 3, 2024, https://www .npr.org/2024/04/03/1242451899/poll-americans-overwhelmingly-reject-criminalizing -abortion-divided-on-other-iss.

38. Jessica Valenti, "New Poll: Americans Support Abortion Throughout Pregnancy," *Abortion, Every Day*, June 18, 2024, https://jessica.substack.com/p/new-poll -americans-support-abortion.

39. Pam Belluck, "Abortion Shield Laws: A New War Between the States," *New York Times*, Feb. 22, 2024, https://www.nytimes.com/2024/02/22/health/abortion-shield-laws-telemedicine.html; as of March 2025, Rhode Island and Maine also passed telehealth abortion shield laws, see Rosemary Westwood, "After Historic Indictment, Doctors Will Keep Mailing Abortion Pills Over State Lines," NPR, Mar. 19, 2025, https://www.npr.org/sections/shots-health-news/2025/03/19/nx-s1-5312115/margaret-carpenter-indictment-telemedicine-abortion-louisiana-mail-mifepristone-misoprostol#:~:text=Eight%20states%20%E2%80%94%20New%20York%2C%20Maine,from%20extradition%20in%20such%20cases.

40. Laura Huss, Farah Diaz-Tello, and Goleen Samari, *Self-Care, Criminalized: The Criminalization of Self-Managed Abortion from 2000 to 2020*, If/When/How: Lawyering for Reproductive Justice, 2023, https://ifwhenhow.org/wp-content/uploads/2023/10/Self-Care-Criminalized-2023-Report.pdf.

41. KFF, "Policy Tracker: Exceptions to State Abortion Bans and Early Gestational Limits," *KFF*, accessed Nov. 2024, last updated Oct. 8, 2024, https://www.kff.org/womens-health-policy/dashboard/exceptions-in-state-abortion-bans-and-early-gestational-limits/.

42. Dana M. Johnson, Abigail R. Aiken, and Terri-Ann Thompson, "Telehealth Enables Safe Medication Abortion in Shifting Health and Legal Contexts," *Nature Medicine* 30 (2024): 946–47, https://doi.org/10.1038/s41591-024-02876-0.

43. Latoya Hill et al., "What Are the Implications of the Dobbs Ruling for Racial Disparities?" *KFF*, Apr. 24, 2024, https://www.kff.org/womens-health-policy/issue-brief/what-are-the-implications-of-the-dobbs-ruling-for-racial-disparities/.

44. Hill et al., "What Are the Implications of the Dobbs Ruling for Racial Disparities?"

45. Belluck, "Abortion Shield Laws: A New War Between the States."

46. US Department of Health and Human Services, Office of the Assistant Secretary of Planning and Evaluation, "Prior HHS Poverty Guidelines and Federal Register References," accessed 2024, https://aspe.hhs.gov/topics/poverty-economic-mobility/poverty-guidelines/prior-hhs-poverty-guidelines-federal-register-references; Diana Greene Foster et al., "Socioeconomic Outcomes of Women Who Receive and Women Who Are Denied Wanted Abortions in the United States," *American Journal of Public Health* 108, no. 3 (2018): 407–13, doi:10.2105/AJPH.2017.304247, https://pmc.ncbi.nlm.nih.gov/articles/PMC5803812/pdf/AJPH.2017.304247.pdf.

47. Foster et al., "Socioeconomic Outcomes of Women Who Receive and Women Who Are Denied Wanted Abortions in the United States," 407–13.

48. Foster et al., "Socioeconomic Outcomes of Women Who Receive and Women Who Are Denied Wanted Abortions in the United States."

49. Amy Littlefield, "The Abortion-Pill Underground," *The Nation*, May 7, 2024, https://www.thenation.com/article/society/telehealth-abortion-shield-laws/.

50. Garnet Henderson, "Following National Funding Cuts, 'July Was Pure Hell' for Abortion Funds," *Rewire News Group*, Aug. 13, 2024, https://rewirenewsgroup.com/2024/08/13/following-national-funding-cuts-july-was-pure-hell-for-abortion-funds/.

51. More than a dozen sources in the American reproductive rights, health, and justice movement, 2023 and 2024 interviews with author.

52. Shira Stein, "The Unexpected Opponent to Telehealth Abortion Shield Laws: Planned Parenthood," *San Francisco Chronicle*, June 11, 2024, https://www.sfchronicle.com/politics/article/planned-parenthood-telehealth-abortion-19494709.php.

53. More than a dozen sources in the American reproductive rights, health, and justice movement, 2023 and 2024 interviews with author.

54. Abigail R. A. Aiken, Jennifer E. Starling, and Rebecca Gomperts, "Factors Associated With Use of an Online Telemedicine Service to Access Self-managed Medical Abortion in the US," *JAMA Network Open* 4, no. 5 (2021), doi:10.1001/jamanetworkopen.2021.11852, https://jamanetwork.com/journals/jamanetworkopen/fullarticle/2780272.

55. Melissa Madera et al., "Experiences Seeking, Sourcing, and Using Abortion Pills at Home in the United States Through an Online Telemedicine Service," *SSM. Qualitative Research in Health* 2 (2022): 100075, doi:10.1016/j.ssmqr.2022.100075, https://pmc.ncbi.nlm.nih.gov/articles/PMC10372773/pdf/nihms-1903375.pdf.

56. Madera et al., "Experiences Seeking, Sourcing, and Using Abortion Pills at Home in the United States Through an Online Telemedicine Service."

57. A. R. A. Aiken et al., "Requests for Self-managed Medication Abortion Provided Using Online Telemedicine in 30 US States Before and After the *Dobbs v Jackson Women's Health Organization* Decision," *JAMA* 328, no. 17 (2022):1768–70, doi:10.1001/jama.2022.18865, https://jamanetwork.com/journals/jama/fullarticle/2797883.

58. Abortion Care Network, *Communities Need Clinics: The Abortion Care Ecosystem Depends on Independent Clinics* (2023), Abortion Care Network, https://abortioncarenetwork.org/wp-content/uploads/2023/12/cnc23-v5-WEB.pdf.

59. Tess Solomon et al., "Bigger and Bigger: The Growth of Catholic Health Systems," *Community Catalyst*, 2020, https://www.communitycatalyst.org/wp-content/uploads/2022/11/2020-Cath-Hosp-Report-2020-31.pdf.

60. Rachana Pradhan and Hannah Recht, "The Powerful Constraints on Medical Care in Catholic Hospitals Across America," *KFF Health News*, Feb. 17, 2024, https://kffhealthnews.org/news/article/catholic-hospitals-affiliates-ethical-religious-directives-reproductive-care/.

61. Kavita Vinekar et al., "Abortion Training in US Obstetrics and Gynecology Residency Programs in a Post-*Dobbs* Era," *Contraception* 130, 110291 (2024), https://doi.org/10.1016/j.contraception.2023.110291.

62. Isaac Maddow-Zimet and Candace Gibson, *Despite Bans, Number of Abortions in the United States Increased in 2023*, Guttmacher Institute, 2024, https://www.guttmacher.org/2024/03/despite-bans-number-abortions-united-states-increased-2023.

63. Rachel Jones and Amy Friedrich-Karnik, *Medication Abortion Accounted for 63% of All US Abortions in 2023—an Increase from 53% in 2020*, Guttmacher Institute, 2024, https://www.guttmacher.org/2024/03/medication-abortion-accounted-63-all-us-abortions-2023-increase-53-2020.

64. Maddow-Zimet and Gibson, *Despite Bans, Number of Abortions in the United States Increased in 2023*.

65. Society of Family Planning, *#WeCount Report: April 2022 to December 2023*, Society of Family Planning, May 14, 2024, https://doi.org/10.46621/970371hxrbsk.

66. Deidre McPhillips, "Telehealth Abortions Now Account for Nearly 1 in 5 in US, With Thousands Accessed under Shield Laws Each Month, Report Says," CNN, May 14, 2024, https://www.cnn.com/2024/05/14/health/abortion-telehealth-shield-laws-wecount-report/index.html.

67. Abigail Aiken et al., "Provision of Medications for Self-Managed Abortion Before and After the *Dobbs v Jackson Women's Health Organization* Decision," *JAMA* 331, no. 18 (2024):1558–64, doi:10.1001/jama.2024.4266, https://jamanetwork.com/journals/jama/fullarticle/2816817?utm_campaign=articlePDF&utm_medium=articlePDFlink&utm_source=articlePDF&utm_content=jama.2024.4266.

68. Aiken et al., "Provision of Medications for Self-Managed Abortion Before and After the *Dobbs v Jackson Women's Health Organization* Decision."

69. Society of Family Planning, *#WeCount Report: April 2022 to December 2022*, Society of Family Planning, Apr. 11, 2023, doi:10.46621/143729dhcsyz.

70. Terri-Ann Thompson, Dana Northcraft, and Fabiola Carrión, "Addressing Structural Inequities, a Necessary Step Toward Ensuring Equitable Access to Telehealth for Medication Abortion Care During and Post COVID-19," *Frontiers in Global Women's Health*, 2022. doi: 10.3389/fgwh.2022.805767, https://www.frontiersin.org/journals/global-womens-health/articles/10.3389/fgwh.2022.805767/full.

71. Transcript of Oral Argument in *US Food and Drug Administration v. Alliance for Hippocratic Medicine*, 602 U.S. (2024), https://www.supremecourt.gov/oral_arguments/argument_transcripts/2023/23-235_g71f.pdf.

72. Transcript of Oral Argument in *US Food and Drug Administration v. Alliance for Hippocratic Medicine*.

73. Transcript of Oral Argument in *US Food and Drug Administration v. Alliance for Hippocratic Medicine*.

74. Mary Ziegler and Reva Siegel, "How Trump Could Ban Abortion Without Congress," *Politico*, Nov. 4, 2024, https://www.politico.com/news/magazine/2024/11/04/trump-abortion-congress-00186520.

75. The Heritage Foundation, "Mandate for Leadership: The Conservative Promise," *Project 2025: Presidential Transition Project*, (2023), 489, 594, https://s3.documentcloud.org/documents/24088042/project-2025s-mandate-for-leadership-the-conservative-promise.pdf.

76. *US Food and Drug Administration v. Alliance for Hippocratic Medicine.*

77. *US Food and Drug Administration v. Alliance for Hippocratic Medicine.*

78. Transcript of Oral Argument in *Moyle v. United States*, 603 U.S. (2024), https://www.supremecourt.gov/oral_arguments/argument_transcripts/2023/23-726_ggco.pdf.

79. US Department of Health and Human Services, Office of Inspector General, "The Emergency Medical Treatment and Labor Act (EMTALA)," accessed Nov. 2024, last updated Sept. 9, 2024, https://oig.hhs.gov/reports-and-publications/featured-topics/emtala/#:~:text=The%20Emergency%20Medical%20Treatment%20and%20Labor%20Act%20(EMTALA)%2C%20also,violated%20its%20obligations%20under%20EMTALA.

80. US Department of Health and Human Services, Office of Inspector General, "The Emergency Medical Treatment and Labor Act (EMTALA)."

81. *Moyle v. United States*, 603 U.S. (2024), https://www.supremecourt.gov/opinions/23pdf/23-726_6jgm.pdf.

82. *Moyle v. United States.*

83. Zeke Miller, Colleen Long, and Darlene Superville, "Biden Drops Out of 2024 Race After Disastrous Debate Inflamed Age Concerns. VP Harris Gets His Nod," *Associated Press*, July 21, 2024, https://apnews.com/article/biden-drops-out-2024-election-ddffde72838370032bdcff946cfc2ce6.

84. Seung Min Kim, "Kamala Harris Is Now Democratic Presidential Nominee, Will Face Off Against Donald Trump This Fall," *Associated Press*, Aug. 6, 2024, https://apnews.com/article/harris-democratic-presidential-nomination-eb43b6b346cc644b2d195315cb2bfb20.

85. Amanda Becker, "Republicans in House Races Are Moderating Their Words on Abortion—but Not Always Their Policies," *The 19th*, Oct. 7, 2024, https://19thnews.org/2024/10/republicans-house-races-abortion-messaging-policies/.

86. John Fritze, Tierney Sneed, and Devan Cole, "From Unanimity to 'Fear Mongering': How the Raucous Supreme Court Term Turned in Trump's Favor," CNN, July 3, 2024, https://www.cnn.com/2024/07/03/politics/supreme-court-term-trump-favor.

CHAPTER 17: KNOW THE RIGHT PEOPLE

1. David Fischer and Stephany Matat, "Florida's 6-Week Abortion Ban Takes Effect as Doctors Worry Women Will Lose Access to Health Care," *Associated Press*, May 1, 2024, https://apnews.com/article/florida-abortion-ban-9509a806453e1eab50d118aaecffa2f1.

2. Ivette Gomez et al., "Abortion Experiences, Knowledge, and Attitudes Among Women in the US: Findings from the 2024 KFF Women's Health Survey," *KFF*, Aug. 14, 2024, https://www.kff.org/womens-health-policy/issue-brief/abortion-experiences-knowledge-attitudes-among-u-s-women-2024-womens-health-survey/;

Ashley Kirzinger et al., "Abortion Knowledge and Attitudes: KFF Polling and Policy Insights," *KFF*, Jan. 22, 2020, https://www.kff.org/womens-health-policy/poll-finding/abortion-knowledge-and-attitudes-kff-polling-and-policy-insights/.

3. Laura Huss, Farah Diaz-Tello, and Goleen Samari, *Self-Care, Criminalized: The Criminalization of Self-Managed Abortion from 2000 to 2020*, If/When/How: Lawyering for Reproductive Justice, 2023, https://ifwhenhow.org/wp-content/uploads/2023/10/Self-Care-Criminalized-2023-Report.pdf.

4. Kebé, Elizabeth Ling, and Kylee Sunderlin, *A Repro Legal Helpline Report: State Violence and the Far-Reaching Impact of* Dobbs, If/When/How: Lawyering for Reproductive Justice's Repro Legal Helpline, 2024, https://ifwhenhow.org/wp-content/uploads/2024/06/Repro-Legal-Helpline-Report-June-24.pdf.

5. Kylie Cheung, "Post-Dobbs, Abortion Bans Have Given Abusers a New Power," *Jezebel*, June 3, 2024, https://www.jezebel.com/post-dobbs-abortion-bans-have-given-abusers-a-new-power?utm_source=substack&utm_medium=email.

6. Diana Greene Foster, *The Turnaway Study: Ten Years, a Thousand Women, and the Consequences of Having—or Being Denied—an Abortion* (New York, NY: Scribner, 2020).

7. Abigail R. A. Aiken, Jennifer E. Starling, and Rebecca Gomperts, "Factors Associated With Use of an Online Telemedicine Service to Access Self-Managed Medical Abortion in the US," *JAMA Network Open* 4, no. 5 (2021), doi:10.1001/jamanetworkopen.2021.11852, https://jamanetwork.com/journals/jamanetworkopen/fullarticle/2780272.

8. Sara Ainsworth, May 2024 interview with author. Also see Kebé, Ling, and Sunderlin, *A Repro Legal Helpline Report.*

9. Attorney General of Washington, "Reproductive and Gender-Affirming Care: Shielding Providers, Seekers, and Helpers from Out-of-State Legal Actions," FAQ, Apr. 2023, accessed Nov. 11, 2024, https://www.atg.wa.gov/reproductive-and-gender-affirming-care-shielding-providers-seekers-and-helpers-out-state-legal#:~:text=State%20Legal%20Actions-,Reproductive%20and%20Gender%2DAffirming%20Care%3A%20Shielding%20Providers%2C%20Seekers%2C,well%20as%20gender%2Daffirming%20care.

10. The Abortion Defense Network, "About Us," *Abortion Network Defense*, https://abortiondefensenetwork.org/learn-more/, accessed Nov. 8, 2024.

11. Garnet Henderson, "Following National Funding Cuts, 'July Was Pure Hell' for Abortion Funds," *Rewire News Group*, Aug. 13, 2024, https://rewirenewsgroup.com/2024/08/13/following-national-funding-cuts-july-was-pure-hell-for-abortion-funds/.

12. Andrew Kaczynski and Em Steck, "JD Vance Said in 2020 He 'Would Like Abortion to Be Illegal Nationally,'" CNN, July 17, 2024, https://www.cnn.com/2024/07/17/politics/kfile-jd-vance-abortion-comments/index.html.

13. Chloe Atkins, "The Rise of 'Abortion Abolitionists' Targeting Women, Doctors and Donald Trump," *NBC News*, May 26, 2024, https://www.nbcnews.com/news/us-news/rise-abortion-abolitionists-targeting-women-doctors-donald-trump-rcna147187.

14. Andrew Joseph, "Why Drug Makers Share Their Prized Compound Libraries With Competitors," *STAT*, Nov. 20, 2015, https://www.statnews.com/2015/11/20/pharma-company-compound-libraries/.

15. Daina Beth Solomon, "Hidalgo Becomes Third Mexican State to Allow Abortion," *Reuters*, June 30, 2021, https://www.reuters.com/world/americas/hidalgo-becomes-third-mexican-state-allow-abortion-2021-06-30/.

16. Siobhan Quenby et al., "Miscarriage Matters: The Epidemiological, Physical, Psychological, and Economic Costs of Early Pregnancy Loss," *The Lancet* 397, no. 10285 (2021): 1658–67, doi:10.1016/S0140–6736(21)00682–6, https://www.thelancet.com/journals/lancet/article/PIIS0140-6736(21)00682-6/abstract.

17. Daina Beth Solomon, "Hidalgo Becomes Third Mexican State to Allow Abortion," *Reuters*, June 30, 2021, https://www.reuters.com/world/americas/hidalgo-becomes-third-mexican-state-allow-abortion-2021-06-30/.

18. Madeleine Belfrage, "Revolutionary Pills? Feminist Abortion, Pharmaceuticalization, and Reproductive Governance," *International Feminist Journal of Politics* 25, no. 1 (2023): 6–29, doi:10.1080/14616742.2022.2154688, https://www.tandfonline.com /doi/abs/10.1080/14616742.2022.2154688.

19. Mariana Prandini Assis and Joanna N. Erdman, "In the Name of Public Health: Misoprostol and the New Criminalization of Abortion in Brazil," *Journal of Law and the Biosciences* 8, no. 1 (2021), doi:10.1093/jlb/lsab009, https://pmc.ncbi.nlm .nih.gov/articles/PMC8132311/pdf/lsab009.pdf.

20. Rebecca Gomperts, 2022 interview with author.

21. Katy Watson, "Jair Bolsonaro: Far-Right Candidate Wins Brazil Poll," BBC, Oct. 29, 2018, https://www.bbc.com/news/world-latin-america-46013408.

22. Philip Reeves, "Dictatorship Was a 'Very Good' Period, Says Brazil's Aspiring President," NPR, July 30, 2018, https://www.npr.org/2018/07/30/631952886/dictatorship -was-a-very-good-period-says-brazil-s-aspiring-president.

23. Jack Nicas and André Spigariol, "Bolsonaro Supporters Lay Siege to Brazil's Capital," *New York Times*, Jan. 8, 2023, https://www.nytimes.com/2023/01/08/world /americas/brazil-election-protests-bolsonaro.html.

24. Jack Nicas, "Why Bolsonaro Was Barred in Brazil but Trump Can Run in the US," *New York Times*, July 1, 2023, updated July 8, 2023, https://www.nytimes.com /2023/07/01/world/americas/trump-bolsonaro-brazil-us.html.

25. Carmen Barroso, 2024 interview with author.

26. Zia Qureshi, "Rising Inequality: A Major Issue of Our Time," *Brookings Institution*, May 16, 2023, https://www.brookings.edu/articles/rising-inequality-a-major-issue-of -our-time/.

27. United Nations, *Women and Girls—Closing the Gender Gap*, 2019, https://www .un.org/en/un75/women_girls_closing_gender_gap.

28. United Nations, *Women and Girls—Closing the Gender Gap*.

29. Hayes Brown, "Republicans Keep Control of the House of Representatives, NBC News Projects," *MSNBC News*, Nov. 13, 2024, https://www.msnbc.com/top-stories /latest/republican-majority-house-control-democrat-election-defeat-rcna174560.

30. Joan E. Greve, "Effects of Republican Senate Majority Will Reverberate Through the Courts," *The Guardian*, Nov. 6, 2024, https://www.theguardian.com/us-news /2024/nov/06/republican-senate-majority-trump-courts.

31. CNN, "Election 2024: Exit Polls," CNN, Nov. 6, 2024, https://edition.cnn.com /election/2024/exit-polls/national-results/general/president/0.

32. Shefali Luthra, "Abortion Rights Won in Seven States—but a Trump Presidency Makes Them Vulnerable," *The 19th*, Nov. 6, 2024, https://19thnews.org/2024/11 /abortion-rights-won-seven-states-vulnerable-trump-presidency/.

EPILOGUE

1. Rakesh Kochhar, "The Enduring Grip of the Gender Pay Gap," *Pew Research Center*, Mar. 1, 2023, https://www.pewresearch.org/social-trends/2023/03/01/the -enduring-grip-of-the-gender-pay-gap/#:~:text=The%20gender%20pay%20gap %20%E2%80%93%20the,80%20cents%20to%20the%20dollar.

INDEX

abortion: as "bringing on the menses," 25, 33, 45, 211; as common, 113–14; complex reasons for, 178–79; costs, 1, 7–8, 86, 97, 162, 183, 191; guilt about, 26, 179, 213; historical, in the US, 42–43; illegal/self-induced, 29, 33, 45; methods for, 3, 24–25; misconceptions about, 98; as murder, 5; and privacy rights, 195; as a public health issue, 105; as a right, 97–98; and stigma, 161, 173, 174, 195, 208; US vs. Mexican views, 100–101. *See also* medication abortion

Abortion (Lader), 58

abortion access: classist assumptions, 46; Clergy Consultation Service on Abortion (CCS), 45; community networks, 204–5; confusion about, 89, 178, 185–87; family medicine, 88–89; in France, 26; global power imbalances, 123; Guanajuato, Mexico, 93; legal requirements, 81; medicalizing, 43–44; national abortion bans, 197–98; post-*Dobbs* ban states, 72, 181–82, 190, 191, 202–5; post-*Dobbs* funding increases, 191–92; state and local activism, 147, 177–78; viewing as a single issue, 198. *See also* accompaniment networks; SB 8 (Senate Bill 8); shield law; SMA (self-managed abortion); telehealth abortion providers

abortion, criminalizing: historical trends, 2; legal strategies, 202; levels of legality, 131, 148, 177–78; male doctors, 43–44; in Mexico, 131; post-*Dobbs*, 205; and provider vulnerability, 137. *See also* SMA (self-managed abortion)

abortion clinics: as businesses, 192; independent, and second-trimester abortions, 193; medication abortions, 89–91

Abortion Defense Network, 204

Abortion on Our Own Terms, 152

The "Abortion Pill" (Baulieu), 26

The Abortion Pill (documentary), 67, 70

"abortion pill reversal treatment," 176

Abortion Rights Mobilization (ARM): Margaret Sanger's challenge to the Comstock Act as inspiration for RU-486 activism, 59–60; clinical trials, 79; founding, 59; production of mifepristone, 78; secrecy during mifepristone production, 78–79

Abramowitz, Phoebe, 195

Abuzz (telehealth medication abortion provider), 191

ACA (Affordable Care Act), 145–46

accompaniment networks (acompañantes): Di Ramona collective, 206–10; educational role, 97; importance, 148–49; La Revuelta, Neuquén, 128–29; Las Comadres, Ecuador, 123; models for, 94–99, 103, 141; praise for, 195; Socorristas, 130–31; success and importance, 97–101; in Texas, 165–66

ACOG v. FDA, 2020, 160

"An Act for the Suppression of Trade in, and Circulation of, Obscene Literature and Articles of Immoral Use." *See* Comstock Act, 1873

ADF (Alliance Defending Freedom), 176

AHM (Alliance for Hippocratic Medicine), 175, 198–200

Aid Access website/help desk, 157–59, 165, 181, 191, 193, 208

Aiken, Abigail, 197

Ailén (abortion patient), 128

Ainsworth, Sara, 202–4

Alabama: maternal mortality rates, 177; post-*Dobbs*, 177; Yellowhammer Fund, 179

Alblas, Marijke, 109–10, 117

Alito, Samuel, 167, 170